Decoding Delusions

A Clinician's Guide to Working With Delusions and Other Extreme Beliefs

Decoding
Delusions

A Clinician's Guide to Working With
Delusions and Other
Extreme Beliefs

Edited by

Kate V. Hardy, Clin.Psych.D.
Douglas Turkington, M.D., FRCPsych

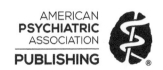

AMERICAN
PSYCHIATRIC
ASSOCIATION
PUBLISHING

Note: The authors have worked to ensure that all information in this book is accurate at the time of publication and consistent with general psychiatric and medical standards, and that information concerning drug dosages, schedules, and routes of administration is accurate at the time of publication and consistent with standards set by the U.S. Food and Drug Administration and the general medical community. As medical research and practice continue to advance, however, therapeutic standards may change. Moreover, specific situations may require a specific therapeutic response not included in this book. For these reasons and because human and mechanical errors sometimes occur, we recommend that readers follow the advice of physicians directly involved in their care or the care of a member of their family.

Books published by American Psychiatric Association Publishing represent the findings, conclusions, and views of the individual authors and do not necessarily represent the policies and opinions of American Psychiatric Association Publishing or the American Psychiatric Association.

If you wish to buy 50 or more copies of the same title, please go to www.appi.org/specialdiscounts for more information.

Copyright © 2024 American Psychiatric Association Publishing
ALL RIGHTS RESERVED
First Edition
Manufactured in the United States of America on acid-free paper
27 26 25 24 23   5 4 3 2 1

American Psychiatric Association Publishing
800 Maine Avenue SW, Suite 900
Washington, DC 20024-2812
www.appi.org

Library of Congress Cataloging-in-Publication Data
A CIP record is available from the Library of Congress.
ISBN: 9781615372959 (paperback), 9781615372966 (ebook)

British Library Cataloguing in Publication Data
A CIP record is available from the British Library.

Contents

Douglas Turkington, M.D.
Kate V. Hardy, Clin.Psych.D.

PART I

Delusions

Theoretical, Historical, and Lived Perspectives

1 **Delusional Beliefs and the Madness of Crowds: What Are Beliefs, and Why Are Some of Them**
Richard Bentall, Ph.D., FBA

2
Shaun Hunt, M.Sc., B.Sc.

3 **Considering Delusions Through**
Peter Phiri, Ph.D., RNMH, CBT (DipHE)
Farooq Naeem, Ph.D., MRCPsych
Kathryn Elliot, M.Sc.
Shanaya Rathod, D.M., MRCPsych

4
Anton P. Martinez, M.Sc.
Vyv Huddy, Ph.D.
Richard P. Bentall, Ph.D., FBA

PART III

Working With Delusions in Different Settings

Foreword

I really wish that Kate Hardy and Doug Turkington had produced this book when I was a psychiatric resident. I could have learned what they teach so effectively and used these techniques and approaches in my 30+ years working with individuals diagnosed with psychotic disorders.

One of the first things I learned, both from my family's experience with schizophrenia and then as a physician, is not to argue with people about their delusions. Regrettably, few constructive alternatives were taught. And so I, along with many of my colleagues, tried to connect with individuals experiencing delusions in a humane and respectful manner. But now we have tested methods and can learn skills and approaches that layer effective techniques and treatment approaches on this humanity and respect.

I must admit that I have tried to learn more cognitive-behavioral techniques over the years from books and lectures and never fully succeeded. I could never quite adapt them to the clinical work I was doing. But this volume speaks to me and unpacks many of the mysteries of cognitive-behavioral therapy. The authors of each chapter present a different dimension of the approach, addressing the clinical, cultural, and social contexts of illness. The volume covers what to do and how to do it. I especially value the video demonstrations that complement the text and illustrate the skills and concepts, bringing them to life.

Why does this matter? Psychosis and psychotic ideation are common, highly stigmatized, and dehumanizing. This book provides the tools for clinicians to ally with individuals experiencing thoughts that some people would characterize as extreme beliefs and others would characterize as psychosis. The method is evidence based and recovery oriented. Our competence as clinicians in cognitive-behavioral therapy for psychosis can make a difference for the people we are committed to helping.

Lisa Dixon, M.D., M.P.H.

Preface

Delusions are one of the most important but confounding symptoms of serious mental illness. Delusions are important because they frequently co-occur with hallucinations; they often have a profound effect on impairing psychosocial functioning; and they play a central role in diagnostic symptoms used to classify different psychiatric disorders, most notably schizophrenia. Delusions are confounding to nearly everyone who encounters them because by their inherent nature (or definition) they are strongly held beliefs that appear patently false to anyone who hears them but nevertheless appear impervious to change in the face of countervailing evidence. Medication can be effective at reducing and sometimes eliminating delusions altogether. For many people, however, medications are an insufficient or ineffective treatment, and other interventions are needed to reduce the suffering and functional disability associated with delusions.

Cognitive-behavioral therapy for psychosis (CBTp), or the systematic application of the principles of CBT to people with psychotic disorders, is now recognized as the most empirically supported psychotherapeutic approach to treating delusions. This book provides clinicians who are already experienced in CBTp with a comprehensive, state-of-the-art resource for improving their skills and effectiveness when working with patients with delusions.

The first six chapters, which make up Part I of the book, are devoted to defining and assessing delusions and understanding their nature, both experientially and as shaped by personal experience and culture. After providing a useful history of how delusions have been viewed over the ages and in medicine in Chapter 1, "Delusional Beliefs and the Madness of Crowds," Richard Bentall tackles the thorny issue of how to define delusions as a clinical phenomenon and what makes them different from false or outlandish beliefs that may erupt among and be widely held by many people in spite of a lack of evidence (i.e., the "madness of crowds"). Importantly, it is established that delusional beliefs cannot be distinguished from popular unsupported beliefs on the basis of their content alone; rather, one must consider the role of social factors in acquiring and potentially spreading the belief. Specifically, popular but unfounded beliefs are generally learned from other people and are spread socially, through direct interactions with people or through social or other media. Delusions, in contrast, generally do not develop through communication with other people and fail to spread from one person to the next.

In Chapter 2, "The Lived Experience of Strongly Held Beliefs," Shaun Hunt provides a helpful review of the assessment of delusions in the context of CBTp. The central role of establishing a trusting and therapeutic relationship in assessing and treating delusions is emphasized, followed by description of methods for conducting a history of the development of the delusion, understanding the phenomenology of the delusion, evaluating the function it plays in the person's life, and taking a collaborative and longitudinal approach to developing a case formulation with the patient. Hunt delves more deeply into the lived experience of having delusions and provides vital insights into connecting with and helping affected individuals. He emphasizes that the roots of delusional beliefs lie in the experiences and life history of the individual. Rather than labeling or explaining away such beliefs as symptoms of an illness, the critical task of a clinician is to help people make sense of their beliefs and the circumstances in which they arose.

In Chapter 3, "Considering Delusions Through a Cultural Lens," Peter Phiri et al. address the important role of culture in shaping the beliefs of individuals, including the specific delusions people may develop. The costs of the clinician lacking awareness of the patient's culture are discussed, including the potential for misdiagnosis, as well as mistrust and disengagement from treatment. In Chapter 4, "The Psychology of Paranoid Beliefs," Anton P. Martinez et al. examine the psychology of paranoid delusions, the most common type of delusion in people with a psychotic disorder. The role of early life adversity in the development of paranoid delusions is reviewed, as is research showing that people with such delusions tend to have more generally negative views of other people and their intentions. Ironically, the lack of trust that people with paranoia have in others results in a lack of social identity and sense of belonging, leading to feelings of loneliness. People with paranoid delusions need other people, just like everyone else, but cannot trust others enough to let them into their lives.

In Chapter 5, "Linguistic Techniques for Clinicians Working With Patients With Delusions," Nazneed Rustom and Gordon Turkington provide useful and innovative tools for helping clinicians connect with and better understand the world of their clients who experience delusions by delving deeper into language. Developing such an understanding requires attention not only to the client's thoughts, perceptions, and language, but also awareness of the clinician's own automatic thoughts about the client and treatment process. In Chapter 6, "Assessing Delusions," Dimitri Perivoliotis provides a standard outline for the assessment and treatment of simple delusions (i.e., relatively circumscribed delusions that lack complexity, bizarreness, and extensive systematization). Strategies for identifying triggering events that led to the delusion are described, as are common factors that maintain delusional beliefs and the role of safety behaviors.

Part II addresses the treatment of delusions, with all chapters containing case examples to illustrate the approaches. In Chapter 7, "Collaboration, Not Collusion," Katherine Eisen et al. begin Part II by focusing on the process of developing a collaborative and trusting relationship with the patient that serves as the foundation for all the psychotherapeutic work that follows. The use of befriending early on in the therapeutic relationship is explained, as are normalizing strongly held beliefs and showing genuine curiosity about the patient and their delusional beliefs. As noted in Chapter 2 on the lived experience of delusions, the clinician's goal is to understand the cultural context of the patient's life in which the delusions emerged without colluding or reinforcing those beliefs.

In Chapter 8, Douglas Turkington and Kate Hardy build on Chapter 7 by providing a standard outline of the treatment of paranoia. Paranoia lies on a continuum of abnormal beliefs ranging from normal beliefs to eccentric beliefs and then overvalued ideas to paranoid delusions and then primary delusions. Paranoid delusions are distinguished from primary delusions in terms of their relatively circumscribed nature and simplicity and the lack delusional mood and perception, bizarreness, and extensive systematization. After an interesting section on "Acknowledging and Investigating Our Own Strongly Held Beliefs," the authors walk readers through seven basic phases of cognitive-behavioral therapy for paranoid delusions, including 1) open-mindedness and curiosity, 2) exploring the delusion, 3) peripheral questioning, 4) reality testing and behavioral experiments, 5) generating alternative explanations, 6) anxiety reduction and linking emotions with experience, and 7) working with grief and personal beliefs. Strategies for identifying the triggering events that led to the delusion are described, as well as common factors that maintain delusional beliefs and the role of safety behaviors.

In Chapter 9, "At-Risk Mental State," Mark van der Gaag addresses the treatment of individuals at risk for psychosis, whose experience of delusions (and hallucinations) tends to be more transient. The hallmark distinction between people at risk for psychosis and those who have experienced the onset of a psychotic disorder is the greater uncertainty and doubt about the veracity of their beliefs in the at-risk group. As a result of this uncertainty, and because they have not usually experienced the momentary relief that often occurs when a delusional belief first crystallizes, at-risk individuals often have higher levels of distress than those with more frank psychotic symptoms. This higher level of distress accompanied by lower levels of delusional conviction makes individuals at risk for psychosis ideal candidates for CBTp.

In Chapter 10, "The Curious Case of Schreber," Kristin Lie Romm and Douglas Turkington provide a reinterpretation of the famous Schreber case, a classic case in the psychoanalytic literature, from a CBTp perspective. This reexamination also includes a useful discussion of how Schreber's treatment might have progressed with our current understanding of CBTp. The authors' alternative case formulation suggests how a constructive and collaborative approach to understanding and treating delusions may have helped and illustrates the humanistic nature of the CBTp approach.

In Chapter 11, "Erotomania and Sexual Delusions," Tania Lecomte et al. address the treatment of erotomania (a delusion in which a person believes that someone is in love with them) and delusions of having been sexually abused or having sexually abused others. All three types of delusions share the unique distinction in CBTp of not benefiting from the exploration of alternative explanations for the beliefs, regardless of how collaborative the process may be. The delusions experienced in erotomania are associated with feelings of exhilaration and euphoria, and patients therefore are not motivated to examine these beliefs or make them go away. Delusions of having been sexually abused or having abused others, in contrast, are based on events that supposedly happened many years ago, and attempts to find strong evidence disconfirming such delusions are doomed to failure. The authors also caution against using trauma-focused interventions that are effective in the treatment of PTSD (e.g., prolonged exposure) to treat delusions of having been sexually abused because the so-called memories are in fact distortions or transformations of other experiences in the person's life. In line with this recommendation, I have observed that when trauma-focused interventions are used to treat people with delusions of sexual abuse, rather than anxiety habituating over time with repeated and prolonged exposure to images of the events, it actually increases as further elaboration of the delusion occurs, in terms of either distressing details or entirely new events. Instead of directly focusing on delusional beliefs of this kind, the authors wisely advise spending time trying to understand the function that the delusions may play in the person's life (e.g., enhancing low self-esteem, providing a sense of purpose) and targeting the underlying needs in order to undercut the importance of holding on to the delusional beliefs.

Chapter 12, "A Bizarre and Grandiose Delusion," complements the focus of Chapter 6 on simple delusions by addressing the treatment of complex, highly systematized delusions that frequently dominate a patient's entire life. As detailed in the chapter by Douglas Turkington and Helen Spencer, the treatment of such delusions requires a rich armamentarium of

CBTp skills, patience, flexibility, and the ability to improvise to keep the therapy moving forward. The authors observe that no matter how bizarre a patient's delusions are, they always make more sense after the practitioner and patient explore the period of time before the person became psychotic and construct a timeline of events surrounding the emergence of the trauma. Numerous helpful pointers (illustrated in a detailed case example) are given for working with these challenging patients, such as the clinician initially taking the lead on completing collaboratively agreed-on homework assignments between sessions and then gradually engaging the patient in setting and following through on his or her own assignments.

In Chapter 13, "Who Are You?," Michael Garrett focuses on the nature and treatment of delusions of misidentification, the most well-known of which is the Capgras delusion (the belief that a familiar person has been replaced by a double or impostor). This group of delusions includes others, such as the Fregoli delusion (the belief that other people who appear to be different people are the same person in disguise), intermetamorphosis (the belief that a person has physically and psychically changed into another person), the delusion of subjective doubles (the belief that someone else has transformed into a physical copy of oneself), and mirrored-self misidentification (the belief that one's reflection in the mirror is someone else). The author reviews compelling evidence that delusions of misidentification are not separate disorders but rather reflect varied expressions of a singular underlying disturbance of mental representations of persons. CBTp strategies for treating delusions of misidentification are elucidated, informed, and enriched by psychoanalytic object relations theory.

In Chapter 14, "Thought Disorder or a Problem With Communication?," David Kingdon et al. focus on working with patients who have delusions and formal thought disorder (i.e., disordered language) that interferes with clear communication with others (e.g., neologisms, loose associations). Most patients with formal thought disorder also have delusions, but getting at those delusions requires attending to the individual's speech. Furthermore, formal thought disorder interferes with effective communication about other matters and can be very frustrating to patients; it is therefore important to improve the patient's speech for the person's overall social adjustment. A wide range of useful strategies for dealing with disorganized speech in the treatment of delusions are described, such as stress inoculation training.

Following Chapter 3, which addresses the influence of culture on the formation of beliefs, including delusions, in Chapter 15, "Cognitive-Behavioral Therapy for Delusions Within Japanese Culture," Akiko Kikuchi and Douglas Turkington address the importance of the clinician being familiar with the patient's culture in order to effectively treat the person's delusions.

The authors accomplish this by examining a very different culture from most cultures in North America and Europe—Japanese culture—and the implications of these differences for providing CBTp. For example, the authors describe how supportive relationships in Japanese culture are typically hierarchical, which indicates that the development of a collaborative approach in CBTp needs to occur very gradually over the course of therapy. For another example, in contrast to individualist cultures, in which the goals patients have in CBTp usually focus on desired personal changes, in collectivist cultures such as Japan, people are generally more motivated to work on changes for the betterment of the group than for themselves. This suggests a somewhat different approach from traditional goal setting in CBTp and the potential value of obtaining input from others, such as the family.

In Chapter 16, "Trauma and Delusions," Charles Heriot-Maitland addresses the treatment of delusions in people with a history of interpersonal trauma, an essential topic given the impact of early life adversities on the development of psychotic (and other) disorders. The experience of trauma results in a primary focus of attention on detecting, processing, and responding to potential threats, with delusions serving as strategies with specific functions. Trauma-informed treatment of delusions needs to be sensitive to patients' frequent perceptions of danger and vulnerability as well as their tendency to blame themselves for their victimization. Multiple clinical strategies are described for laying the groundwork needed to focus on delusions and the impact of trauma in these patients, including helping them cultivate states that signal safety and de-shaming the sense of responsibility for traumatic events through psychoeducation and collaborative examination of related beliefs.

Part III addresses the treatment of delusions across different settings, with specific chapters addressing the forensic population, the use of digital technologies, and supporting families with a loved one with delusions. In Chapter 17, "A Cognitive-Behavioral Therapy Approach to Working With Delusions in Forensic Settings," Patricia Cawthorne calls attention to the multiple problems typically faced by persons with mental illness who are involved in the criminal justice system and discusses strategies for addressing common challenges when working with these individuals, such as their lack of trust and tendency to minimize problems. In Chapter 18, "Using Digital Health Technology to Facilitate Measurement-Based Care in the Treatment of Delusions," Laura M. Tully et al. provide a useful guide to how different digital technologies can enhance the efficacy of CBTp in treating delusions. A range of different digital tools and uses are covered, such as the use of ecological momentary assessment to provide real-world tracking of symptoms, thoughts, and feelings in different situations and virtual reality environments in which people can experiment with different ways of responding in social situations.

In Chapter 19, "Cognitive-Behavioral Therapy–Informed Skills Training for Families Caring for a Loved One With Delusions," Sarah Kopelovich et al. provide important guidance on supporting the family members of patients with delusions. Families are critical supports for many people with a psychotic disorder, and they are often in a unique position to facilitate their loved one's involvement in treatment, including CBTp. However, the unique role of families in the lives of people with a major mental illness, and their potential to be allies in treatment, is all too often overlooked by mental health professionals. The authors review what families need in order to help a member get the most out of CBTp for delusions and describe approaches to addressing these needs, including psychoeducation, communication and problem-solving skills training, and the learning of CBT-informed skills.

The final chapter serves as a guide to one of the most useful resources provided by this book, a series of videos illustrating basic CBTp skills for working with patients with unusual beliefs and delusions. Douglas Turkington et al. have organized discussion of the videos into three broad categories of skills, including 1) befriending, normalizing, and questioning, 2) developing a formulation, and 3) change strategies. Of note, although most of the videos focus on the practical "how to's" of CBTp for delusions, attention is also paid to some "how *not* to's." For example, in one video, the pitfalls of colluding with a patient's delusion are illustrated, and another video shows how a lack of commitment to developing a working relationship with the patient can result in an impasse because everything the therapist says is perceived as a confrontation. These videos have much to offer both newcomers to CBTp and seasoned clinicians.

Decoding Delusions provides a comprehensive, richly textured guide to the art and science of treating patients with delusions. Although there is a wide array of technical skills to master when working with delusions, the relationship is front and center, and there is no substitute for being genuinely interested in and caring about the patient. Through collaboration and seeking to understand the unfathomable, therapists have the potential to help these distressed people make sense of their own experiences and, by doing so, to begin the process of regaining control over their lives.

Kim T. Mueser, Ph.D.

Video Guide

Callouts in the text identify the videos by name, as shown in the following example:

 Video #: Video Title

The instructional videos are streamed via the internet and can be viewed online by navigating to www.appi.org/Hardy and using the embedded video player. The videos are optimized for most current operating systems, including mobile operating systems.

Videos Discussed by Chapter

Complete descriptions of all 15 videos can be found in Chapter 20, "Decoding Delusions."

Chapter 6

Video 8: Formulation (15:44)

Chapter 7

Video 1: Befriending (3:51)
Video 2: Normalizing (7:25)
Video 3: Confrontation as an approach to avoid (5:06)
Video 4: Collusion as an approach to avoid (6:37)
Video 5: Sitting on the collaborative fence (3:56)

Chapter 8

Video 7: Socratic questioning (8:21)
Video 15: Maintaining change (8:27)
Video 10: Behavioral experiment (6:00)

Chapter 12

Chapter 13

Contributors

Richard P. Bentall, Ph.D., FBA
Professor, Clinical Psychology Unit, Department of Psychology, University of Sheffield, Sheffield, UK

H. Teresa Buckland, Ph.D., M.Ed.
Psychosis REACH Family Ambassador and Trainer in the Department of Psychiatry and Behavioral Sciences, University of Washington School of Medicine, Seattle, Washington

Patricia Cawthorne, D.N., M.Sc. (CBP), RMN
Consultant Nurse, Psychological Therapies Service, The State Hospital; Consultant Nurse, Adult Mental Health Services, Glasgow City HSCP, NHS Greater Glasgow and Clyde, Scotland, UK

Briana Cloutier
Ph.D. candidate, Department of Psychology, Université de Montréal, Montréal, Québec, Canada

Lisa Dixon, M.D., M.P.H.
Edna L. Edison Professor of Psychiatry, New York State Psychiatric Institute, Columbia University Vagelos College of Physicians and Surgeons; Director, Division of Behavioral Health Services and Policy Research and Center for Practice Innovations, New York-Presbyterian, New York, New York

Kathryn Eisen, Ph.D.
Clinical Associate Professor, Stanford University School of Medicine, Department of Psychiatry and Behavioral Sciences, Stanford, California

Kathryn Elliot, M.Sc.
Research Assistant, Research and Innovation Department, Southern Health NHS Foundation Trust, Southampton, UK

Audrey Francoeur
Ph.D. candidate, Department of Psychology, Université de Montréal, Montréal, Québec, Canada

Michael Garrett, M.D.
Professor Emeritus of Clinical Psychiatry, SUNY Downstate Medical Center, Brooklyn, New York

Christopher Komei Hakusui, B.A.
Lived Experience Junior Specialist, Department of Psychiatry, University of California, Davis, Davis, California

Kate V. Hardy, Clin.Psych.D.
Clinical Professor, Department of Psychiatry and Behavioral Sciences, Stanford University School of Medicine, Stanford, California

Charles Heriot-Maitland, Ph.D., D.Clin.Psy., M.A., B.Sc.
Clinical Psychologist and Director, Balanced Minds, Edinburgh, UK

Vyv Huddy, Ph.D.
Lecturer, Clinical Psychology Unit, Department of Psychology, University of Sheffield, Sheffield, UK

Shaun Hunt, M.Sc., B.Sc.
Lecturer, Education and Training Department, SHSC, Sheffield, UK

Akiko Kikuchi, Ph.D.
Professor, Department of Human Sciences, Musashino University, Tokyo, Japan

David Kingdon, M.D., FRCPsych
Emeritus Professor of Mental Health Care Delivery, University of Southampton, Southampton, UK

Sarah Kopelovich, Ph.D.
Associate Professor, Department of Psychiatry and Behavioral Sciences, University of Washington School of Medicine, Seattle, Washington

Melanie Lean, Clin.Psych.D.
Clinical Assistant Professor, Stanford University School of Medicine, Department of Psychiatry and Behavioral Sciences, Stanford, California

Latoyah Lebert, M.Phil.
Clinical Psychologist, Newcastle and Gateshead At Risk Mental State, CNTW NHS Foundation Trust, Cumbria, Northumberland, UK

Tania Lecomte, Ph.D.
Professor, Department of Psychology, Université de Montréal, Montréal, Québec, Canada

Anton P. Martinez, M.Sc.
Ph.D. candidate, Clinical Psychology Unit, Department of Psychology, University of Sheffield, Sheffield, UK

Maria Monroe-DeVita, Ph.D.
Associate Professor, Department of Psychiatry and Behavioral Sciences, University of Washington School of Medicine, Seattle, Washington

Kim T. Mueser, Ph.D.
Professor, Departments of Occupational Therapy and Psychological and Brain Sciences, Center for Psychiatric Rehabilitation, Boston University, Boston, Massachusetts

Karina Muro, Ph.D.
Assistant Professor, Department of Psychiatry, University of California Davis, Davis, California

Farooq Naeem, Ph.D., MRCPsych
Professor, Centre for Addiction and Mental Health, University of Toronto, Toronto, Ontario, Canada

Shannon Pagdon, B.A.
National Certified Peer Specialist, Department of Psychiatry and Behavioral Health, University of Stanford, Stanford, California; Research Coordinator, School of Social Work, University of Pittsburgh, Pittsburgh, Pennsylvania

Dimitri Perivoliotis, Ph.D.
Psychologist, VA San Diego Healthcare System; Professor, Department of Psychiatry, University of California San Diego School of Medicine, San Diego, California

Peter Phiri, Ph.D., RNMH, CBT (DipHE)
Director of Research and Innovation, Research and Innovation Department, Southern Health NHS Foundation Trust, and Visiting Fellow. School of Psychology, Faculty of Environmental and Life Sciences, University of Southampton, Southampton, UK

Shanaya Rathod, D.M., MRCPsych
Consultant Psychiatrist, Research and Innovation Department, Southern Health NHS Foundation Trust, Southampton, UK; Visiting Professor, Faculty of Science, University of Portsmouth, Portsmouth, UK

Sarah Robinson, B.Sc.
Computer Animation and VFX Department, Northumbria University, Newcastle upon Tyne, UK

Kristin Lie Romm, Ph.D., M.D.
Head of the Early Intervention in Psychosis Advisory Unit for South East Norway, Division of Mental Health and Addiction, Oslo University Hospital; Associate Professor, NORMENT, Institute of Clinical Medicine, University of Oslo, Oslo, Norway

Nazneen Rustom, Ph.D., B.A., GMBPsS
Supervised Cognitive Behavioral Therapy for Psychosis Clinician, Queen's University, School of Medicine, Department of Psychiatry, Adult Psychiatry Division, Providence Care Hospital, Kingston, Ontario, Canada

Kenneth Sandoval, Jr., M.S., M.S.W., LCSW
Program Director, Clinical Administration, California Department of State Hospitals, Patton, California

Leigh Katharine Smith, Ph.D.
Department of Psychology, University of California, Davis, Davis, California

Helen M. Spencer, B.A.
Doctoral Researcher, Cumbria, Northumberland, Tyne and Wear NHS Foundation Trust, Newcastle upon Tyne, UK

Laura M. Tully, Ph.D.
Associate Professor, Department of Psychiatry, University of California Davis, Davis, California

Douglas Turkington, M.D., FRCPsych
Professor of Psychosocial Psychiatry, Newcastle University, UK

Gordon Turkington, M.Sc., B.Sc.
Assistant Psychologist, Northumberland Children and Young Person Services, St. George's Park Hospital, Morpeth, UK

Mark van der Gaag, Ph.D.
Emeritus Professor of Clinical Psychology, Vrije Universiteit, Amsterdam,
The Netherlands

Disclosures

The following contributors have indicated that they have no financial interests or other affiliations that represent or could appear to represent a
competing interest with their contributions to this book:

H. Teresa Buckland, Ph.D., M.Ed.; Patricia Cawthorne, D.N., M.Sc.
(CBP), R.M.N.; Michael Garrett, M.D.; Kate V. Hardy, Clin.Psych.D.;
Charles Heriot-Maitland, Ph.D., D.Clin.Psy., M.A., B.Sc.; Akiko Kikuchi,
Ph.D.; Sarah Kopelovich, Ph.D.; Maria Monroe-DeVita, Ph.D., M.Ed.;
Shannon Pagdon, B.A.; Dimitri Perivoliotis, Ph.D.; Kristin Lie Romm,
Ph.D., M.D.; Nazneen Rustom; Douglas Turkington, M.D.; Mark van der
Gaag, Ph.D.

Mindful Language

Using the Term Patient

Shannon Pagdon, B.A.

Language varies immensely across communities, professional disciplines, and personal preference. Although we can try our best to be mindful and intentional with words, it is an unfortunate reality that the words we choose may not resonate with everyone. It is difficult to strike the balance between more alternative and progressive advocacy terms while still recognizing that conventional terminology is more widely used and readily recognizable. Given these complicated intersections, it is not always easy to know when speaking up is warranted. The ethics of language clue us to values that support effective communication. First, language at its core should be simple. That is, it should be easy to understand, not full of jargon or inaccessible terms. Additionally, open-ended language (in this context, terms that individuals choose to self-describe their experiences of psychosis, including unconventional beliefs) honors the individuals' autonomy in expressing their experiences in their own words (Pagdon 2022). Open-ended language invites new meanings and richer conversation, expanding the space for conversations that could be curtailed by stigmatizing labels or closed language. Essentially, ethical communication is about respect. Adhering to descriptors the individual chooses demonstrates this respect, as does allowing for people to use words differently, to communicate in their own way. These values of simplicity, openness, and respect were applied to the writing and review of this text.

Expressions contained in this text, such as *patient* or *client* spark mixed feelings, especially from service users and advocates in the mental health field (Richards 2018). Particular concerns around power dynamics in the therapeutic relationship and emphases of service users' "illness" are highlighted as difficulties with these terms (Neugerger 1999). Additionally, although many industries are shifting language they use to describe individuals who are provided services (e.g. guests, customers), the health care industry arguably continues to use outdated terms that emphasize *providing* care, not being a partner in care with the individual (Knight 2021). Given the current emphasis on person-centered care for psychosis (Allerby 2022), it is crucial to understand why some may not agree with the use of the terms patient or client. Instead, one can seek to use words that do not bear the burden of stigmatized context or invoke power dynamics. Ultimately, this is a challenging directive with mental health terminology. It is difficult to adopt new words, and it is hard for popularized language to shed connotations; both must first overcome cultural inertia and resistance. Still, it is worthwhile to seek the intersection between alternative terminology and standard language in mental health to find terms that encompass both perspectives meaningfully.

Throughout this book, readers will notice that the term *patient* has been chosen to describe individuals who are engaging with mental health services. The editors want to acknowledge that this term may not resonate with everybody. In writing and reviewing this book, simple language was valued to serve the practical ethic of being clearly discernible. The communicator bears the responsibility to be simple and comprehensible so that the text can be accessible for a global audience. This duty drove the choice of more common, if history-laden, words over alternative language.

That said, we invite you as the reader to develop your own questions and considerations around these terms. Although there are no perfect terms, some will speak to you more than others. We request that you take a moment to reflect on the language you would choose to describe these experiences, as well as why that language may resonate for you.

References

Allerby K, Goulding A, Ali L, Waern M: Increasing person-centeredness in psychosis inpatient care: staff experiences from the Person-Centered Psychosis Care (PCPC) project. BMC Health Serv Res 22(1):596, 2022 35505358

Knight S: Let's banish the term "patient" from the health care lexicon, STAT, May 13, 2021. Available at: www.statnews.com/2021/05/13/lets-banish-term-patient-from-the-health-care-lexicon. Accessed March 20, 2023.

Neuberger J: Do we need a new word for patients? Let's do away with "patients." BMJ 318(7200):1756–1757, 1999 10381717

Pagdon S, Jones N: Psychosis Outside the Box: a user-led project to amplify the diversity and richness of experiences described as psychosis. Psychiatr Serv Dec 7:appips20220488, 2022 36475822

Richards V: The importance of language in mental health care. Lancet Psychiatry 5(6):460–461, 2018 29482994

Introduction

Douglas Turkington, M.D.
Kate V. Hardy, Clin.Psych.D.

Why Do We Need a Handbook on Working With Delusions?

There can be no doubt that the management of delusions is one of the main tasks facing all mental health professionals working with individuals with psychosis. As described beautifully in Chapter 2 ("The Lived Experience of Strongly Held Beliefs") by Shaun Hunt, individuals can experience delusions as highly distressing with an enormous impact on functioning to the extent that they experience significant limitations in their lives. In addition, delusional beliefs have long captivated clinicians, with the earliest psychiatrists describing delusional beliefs and their challenges in addressing these with patients. Essential considerations for clinicians today include assessing the belief along a continuum of beliefs from nonpathological to pathological and grounding it within the individual's cultural experience and society more broadly. As Richard Bentall describes in Chapter 1 ("Delusional Beliefs and the Madness of Crowds"), this is not an easy task for the clinician, and the definition of what might be considered delusional is not a fixed entity. Thus, careful assessment of the belief is essential, as is described in Chapter 6 ("Assessing Delusions"), and it is critical that assessment be conducted within a framework of cultural humility and consideration of cultural factors (Chapter 3, "Considering Delusions Through a Cultural Lens"). Since delusions were first described in the clinical literature there have been many advances in psychosocial treatment approaches. Frequently, however, these clinical interventions are described under the broad umbrella of cognitive-behavioral therapy for psychosis (CBTp), with limited discussion of delusions specifically. In this handbook international experts on psychosis have contributed chapters that speak to different clinical approaches to working with different types of delusions within a CBTp framework, thus broadening the scope of this area and allowing readers to become familiar with a range of effective interventions.

Augmenting Medication With Other Strategies for Delusions

The cornerstone of the treatment of delusions (and psychosis generally) is psychopharmacology, and many clients will achieve effective control of the distress caused by delusions using antipsychotic medication, including clozapine. However, as Kapur (2003) clearly pointed out, this therapeutic effect only lasts for as long as the antipsychotic medication is taken, and for some individuals antipsychotics have little to no impact on the distressing experiences they may be undergoing. Clients often discontinue their medication suddenly or take it intermittently, especially when there are problems with side effects or they experience the medication as ineffective. Kapur demonstrated that other strategies are needed along with the medication to allow a fuller resolution of the delusion. CBTp is an evidence-based intervention that focuses on the individual's beliefs, including their formation and maintenance. It can be argued that for the client to gain an understanding of the delusion, and to integrate this experience into his or her life, the delusion needs to be processed psychologically and addressed directly. This book describes approaches that support the exploration of beliefs with the aim of reduced distress and meaningful recovery. Importantly, each of the clinical chapters provides clinical case examples to demonstrate the application of the techniques discussed. As practitioners who provide training in CBTp, we are frequently asked for video examples of CBTp techniques. Thus, this book includes role-play examples of key CBTp interventions for working with delusions, with further details provided in Chapter 20 ("Decoding Delusions").

What Are These Techniques?

The techniques described in this book are drawn from a variety of schools and approaches but mostly have their origin in the CBT tradition. Key techniques discussed include forming a therapeutic alliance, befriending, and normalizing experiences (Chapter 7, "Collaboration, Not Collusion"). This core principle of normalizing is also adopted throughout the chapters with the inclusion by all authors of personal reflections on experiences that have been unsettling, distressing, or confusing. To support exploration of the belief the clinician draws on the use of different questioning styles and (using guided discovery) the generation of tentative alternative explanations. Joint homework exercises can explore information relating to delusional beliefs (e.g., "Let's find out everything we can that has been published recently about telepathy, alien abduction, satellite functions, or possession by an evil spirit and then compare what we learn to your own experiences").

Throughout the book, the collaborative nature of this approach is emphasized. This collaborative nature is seen, in particular, when client and clinician are engaged in a dialogue about the delusional content and its meaning. Unfortunately, the content of the delusion was historically dismissed as irrelevant by some practitioners. However, we know that it is important to understand the function of the delusion in order to better explore why the belief may have formed and what role it may play for the individual. This can be done by exploring the timeline by considering the pre-psychotic period to look for triggers and relevant life events from childhood and adolescence (see Chapter 12, "A Bizarre and Grandiose Delusion," for an example of this). This book incorporates a number of third-wave therapies, including positive psychology, linguistic approaches, and compassion-focused techniques. The range of interventions for clinicians has expanded dramatically in recent years and continues to evolve. This book offers a summary of the primary interventions currently available.

When to Refer for Expert Psychological Treatment of Delusions

It is our position that all mental health professionals can benefit from understanding how to assess and address delusional beliefs rather than this being seen as the purview of specialist practitioners. CBTp-informed skills support the clinician to draw on key techniques within a recovery-oriented framework with the overarching aim of supporting a reduction in distress and the attainment of goals that are meaningful to the individual. However, there are instances when referral to expert clinicians with specialized training is warranted. In particular, this may include, for example, when one is working with individuals with complex delusional systems with minimal motivation for engagement in treatment or when a specialized intervention, such as eye movement desensitization and reprocessing, is warranted to address trauma.

Integrating a Dispersed Literature on Delusions

After the pioneering phenomenological work of Jaspers (1913/1963), there followed many decades when it was accepted as a self-evident truth that delusions were dichotomous psychotic symptoms with strong diagnostic validity. However, since the 1990s spectrum models of delusions have been increasingly described and investigated (Kingdon and Turkington 1994), and it is now accepted that delusions are more accurately described as existing on a spectrum of overvalued ideas, eccentric normal beliefs, overvalued yet nonpathological beliefs, and "normal" beliefs (see Chapter 1 for more details). It is also increasingly accepted that delusions can show fluctuation in conviction and linked distress and can be amenable to questioning approaches and an examination of the evidence (reality testing). This dispersed literature on the psychology of delusions has been brought together in this volume. In clinical practice, the term *delusion* is frequently applied very broadly; however, it is important to note that there are many different types of delusions seen in clinical practice, such as Capgras syndrome (a delusion of misidentification), Othello syndrome (delusional jealousy), Ekbom syndrome (a delusion of infestation), and de Clérambault syndrome (a delusion of being loved), to name but a few. It is essential for treatment planning that the form of the delusion be accurately assessed and formulated to determine the most effective intervention approach. This book provides clinically oriented chapters that focus on several common delusions (Capgras syndrome, erotomania, persecutory paranoia) as well as consider different pathways to the emergence of delusions (e.g., trauma and the presentation of those at risk for developing psychosis).

Scope of This Handbook

This book is divided into three parts, with Part I bringing readers up to date on the current state of the research literature on the etiology, characteristics, and parameters of delusions. This first section includes a chapter on recent breakthroughs in the linguistics of delusions and how this can be integrated into clinical practice. This introductory section grounds readers in how delusions are conceptualized historically and currently while also critically providing a lived experience perspective of living with delusions.

We then move into Part II, the main clinical section of the book, in which expert authors discuss formulation and intervention for different delusional presentations with corresponding clinical examples framed within a cultural context. Importantly, each author also provides a personal reflection to highlight how common it is for anyone to experience unusual thoughts and belief changes. This section includes a historical review of the Schreber case (Chapter 10, "The Curious Case of Schreber") and discusses how Schreber's bizarre delusional system of being the bride of God and yet persecuted by God might be understood today. This chapter provides a historical perspective on the understanding of delusions while also grounding it in current treatment modalities and highlights the shift in how we understand delusion formation and treatment. Part II incorporates third-wave CBTp models, including compassion-focused therapy utilized to explore the role of trauma and delusions (Chapter 16, "Trauma and Delusions"), and explores the integration of psychodynamic and cognitive-behavioral interventions (Chapter 13, "Who Are You?"). This is particularly important because these two approaches are frequently set up in opposition to each other; however, Michael Garrett deftly demonstrates the potential for integrating these two models and shows that the benefits of integrating them far outweigh the dismissal of either model by followers of CBT or psychoanalysis. Part II concludes with a discussion of CBTp in cultural settings, such as Japanese culture (Chapter 15, "Cognitive-Behavioral Therapy for Delusions Within Japanese Culture").

Treating Delusions in Specific Settings

Part III explores the management of delusions in specific settings, with unique chapters about working with delusions in forensic settings and about working with delusions remotely using Zoom and digital media. It must be said that it is increasingly the case that clients with delusions are treated remotely and that this is, perhaps surprisingly, often more acceptable than a face-to-face session and a viable means of engaging individuals in care (Kopelovich and Turkington 2021). The most common delusion is of course persecutory paranoia, and when one is experiencing this delusion even making the journey to the clinician's office can be a terrifying experience. Such clients can often feel more relaxed in their home environment interacting with the clinician via Zoom or Microsoft Teams as they begin to develop coping strategies and other possible alternative explanations that they can begin gradually to test out.

What Can Families and Friends Do?

Very often when we are delivering workshops and webinars families ask whether they can talk to their loved one about their delusions and how exactly to do this. This book provides insight into curious questioning and incorporates information for friends and families of those with delusions. There are many chapters that will be useful in terms of understanding delusions, including a chapter by an expert-by-experience (Chapter 2), the chapters on communication (Chapters 7, 14, and 16) and the link with trauma (Chapter 15), and the full chapter on CBT-informed caring for families who have a loved one with a delusion (Chapter 19, "Cognitive-Behavioral Therapy–Informed Skills Training for Families Caring for a Loved One With Delusions").

Decoding Delusions: Future Evolution

As mentioned earlier, the treatment of delusions has come a long way since delusions were first described in the clinical case literature. Digital technologies offer an exciting new frontier for intervention, with advances in this area described in Chapter 18 ("Using Digital Health Technology to Facilitate Measurement-Based Care in the Treatment of Delusions"). We await with anticipation the impact of virtual reality interventions such as gameChange (Freeman et al. 2022) as these technologies become more accessible and available to the clinician and client. In addition, the field is moving toward the recognition that CBTp as an umbrella intervention has demonstrated efficacy but that we now need to focus on the presentation of distinct symptoms and utilize strong assessment and formulation to support targeted intervention. The recent publication of the impressive results of the Feeling Safe Programme trial (Freeman et al. 2021) demonstrates the impact of modular and symptom-focused interventions, and it is exciting to see what the next decade holds in terms of the further evolution of these treatments.

References

Freeman D, Lambe S, Kabir T, et al: Automated virtual reality therapy to treat agoraphobic avoidance and distress in patients with psychosis (gameChange): a multicentre, parallel-group, single-blind, randomised, controlled trial in England with mediation and moderation analyses. Lancet Psychiatry 9(5):375–388, 2022 35395204

Freeman D, Emsley R, Diamond R, et al: Comparison of a theoretically driven cognitive therapy (the Feeling Safe Programme) with befriending for the treatment of persistent persecutory delusions: a parallel, single-blind, randomised controlled trial. Lancet Psychiatry 8(8):696–707, 2021 34246324

Jaspers K: General Psychopathology (1913). Translated by Hoenig J, Hamilton MW. Manchester, UK, Manchester University Press, 1963

Kapur S: Psychosis as a state of aberrant salience: a framework linking biology, phenomenology and pharmacology in schizophrenia. Am J Psychiatry 160(1):13–23, 2003 12505794

Kingdon DG, Turkington D: Cognitive-Behavioural Therapy of Schizophrenia. New York, Guilford, 1994

Kopelovich SL, Turkington D: Remote CBT for psychosis during the COVID-19 pandemic: challenges and opportunities. Community Ment Health J 57:30–34, 2021 33001323

PART I
Delusions
Theoretical, Historical, and Lived Perspectives

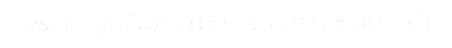

1

Delusional Beliefs and the Madness of Crowds

What Are Beliefs, and Why Are Some of Them Pathological?

Richard Bentall, Ph.D., FBA

Abnormal beliefs, otherwise described as delusions, are a common feature of severe mental illness and are often reported by patients with both nonaffective and affective psychoses (Picardi et al. 2018). In DSM-5-TR (American Psychiatric Association 2022), these kinds of beliefs are defined as

> fixed beliefs that are not amenable to change in light of conflicting evidence. Their content may include a variety of themes (e.g., persecutory, referential, somatic, religious, grandiose).... Delusions are deemed bizarre if they are clearly implausible and not understandable to same-culture peers and do not derive from ordinary life experiences. (p. 101)

This definition is a change from the third and fourth editions of DSM, which described a delusion as "a false belief based on incorrect inference about external reality that is firmly sustained despite what almost everyone else believes and despite what constitutes incontrovertible and obvious proof or evidence to the contrary" (American Psychiatric Association 1994, p. 765). This is similar to the definition contained in ICD-11:

> A belief that is demonstrably untrue or not shared by others, usually based on incorrect inference about external reality. The belief is firmly held with conviction and is not, or is only briefly, susceptible to modification by experience or evidence that contradicts it. The belief is not ordinarily accepted by other members of the person's culture or subculture (i.e., it is not an article of religious faith). (World Health Organization 2018, MB26.0)

Definitions such as these raise numerous philosophical and practical quandaries. For example, some kinds of nonpathological beliefs, such as political beliefs, are notoriously resistant to counterargument or inconsistent evidence (Lodge and Taber 2013; Westen 2008). It is also unclear what would count as "incontrovertible and obvious proof or evidence to the contrary." Moreover, the idea that delusions are false beliefs collapses in the case of rare examples such as when a pathological belief is ill-founded but true (e.g., patients with delusional jealousy often drive their spouses into the arms of others) (Enoch and Trethowan 1979), when the belief is untestable (as in the case of most religious delusions), or when it is impossible in practice to determine the truth of a patient's claims (e.g., a complaint of being victimized by intelligence services may seem unlikely, but it is not obvious how it could be definitively discounted) (Cermolacce et al. 2010).

A further problem with the requirement that delusional beliefs should be false is that false beliefs are common (e.g., most people think that they are better than average compared with other people), and, rather than being products of neural dysfunction, many of these beliefs are tolerable products of normal cognitive processes, arise from reasoning biases that favor the avoidance of costly errors (trusting someone who is untrustworthy) at the expense of less costly errors (failing to trust someone who is trustworthy), or are in other ways evolutionarily adaptive (Haselton and Nettle 2006; McKay and Dennett 2009). For these reasons, many other features of delusions have been highlighted by commentators, for example, that they are idiosyncratic, seem incredible to others, are highly preoccupying, or are usually the cause of personal distress and thereby interfere with the individual's ability to cope with everyday life (Oltmanns and Maher 1988).

One approach that can be traced to the very beginning of psychiatry has been to characterize at least the most severe delusions as "bizarre." The German psychiatrist Emil Kraepelin (1856–1926), whose foundational work on the classification of psychiatric disorders I have described elsewhere (Bentall 2003), emphasized the nonsensical nature of many delusions and argued that this feature could be used to distinguish between the patients he diagnosed as having dementia praecox (the term he coined for what modern mental health professionals call schizophrenia) and those who had paranoia (a diagnosis he used to describe patients who had any kind of delusion when no other symptoms were present; Cermolacce et al. 2010). Delusions have been said to be bizarre if they depart from "culturally determined consensual reality" (Kendler et al. 1983) or violate agreed-on understandings about what is possible (e.g., in the case of a patient who believes that his neighbor is stealing electricity through the walls of his home) (Mullen 2003). However, although clinicians can usually agree which of their patients are deluded, the distinction between bizarre and nonbizarre beliefs has proven difficult to operationalize, with the consequence that the reliability of this distinction is poor (Bell et al. 2006; Spitzer et al. 1993).

A fundamental challenge to these efforts is the propensity of ordinary people to believe weird things that seem in many ways as irrational or incomprehensible as those seen on any psychiatric ward. Indeed, it has been argued that the drawing of a line between delusions and widely accepted but arguably irrational beliefs is a fundamental Hilbert problem that must be solved to progress psychology as a science (Ross and McKay 2017). (The term *Hilbert problem* comes from the German mathematician David Hilbert (1862–1943), who in 1900 identified 23 fundamental but unsolved problems in mathematics. Hilbert's list has been influential in driving mathematical research up to the present time.) In this chapter, I explore the similarities and differences between delusions and beliefs and attitudes that are widely accepted as nonpathological (in particular religious and political beliefs) and show how confusion about this issue reflects misconceptions and naiveté about the nature of belief systems in general. Following this analysis, I make a new proposal about why delusions are different from nonpathological beliefs.

Psychotic Delusions and the Madness of Crowds

To begin, it is helpful to consider the weird beliefs of ordinary people. An attempt to catalog these kinds of beliefs was made by the Scottish journalist Charles Mackay (1814–1889), whose work *Memoirs of Extraordinary Popular Delusions and the Madness of Crowds* was first published in three volumes (Mackay 1841) with a preface that begins as follows:

> In reading the history of nations, we find that, like individuals, they have their whims and their peculiarities; their seasons of excitement and recklessness, when they care not what they do. We find that whole communities suddenly fix their minds upon one object and go mad in its pursuit; that mil-

lions of people become simultaneously impressed with one delusion, and run after it, till their attention is caught by some new folly more captivating than the first. We see one nation suddenly seized, from its highest to its lowest members, with a fierce desire for military glory; another as suddenly becomes crazed upon a religious scruple, and neither of them recovering its senses until it has shed rivers of blood and sowed a harvest of groans and tears, to be reaped by its posterity. (p. 1)

Mackay's first volume dealt with what he called "national delusions," in which he included economic bubbles (e.g., the Mississippi scheme, in which French investors in 1720 lost huge amounts of money after speculating on land for French settlements in Louisiana), prophecies such as those of Nostradamus, and "the influence of politics and religion on the hair and beard" (Mackay 1841, p. 1). The second volume, on "peculiar follies," included long accounts of the Crusades and the witch-hunting epidemic in Europe during the sixteenth and seventeenth centuries, endeavors that Mackay regarded as ultimately self-defeating. Finally, Mackay discussed "philosophical delusions," such as alchemy (a pseudoscience and the precursor of modern chemistry in which believers hoped to find a way of turning base metals into gold) and the "magnetizers" (i.e., medical practitioners who, at various times, had claimed the ability to cure diseases by manipulating magnetic fields; these approaches included Mesmerism, which was a forerunner of modern hypnotism).

History has since provided any modern cartographer of belief with numerous further examples that would expand Mackay's list enormously. For example, shortly after Mackay's book was published, in 1856, the Xhosa nation in the Eastern Cape, who were locked in a long series of wars with white settlers, embraced a prophecy by a teenage girl named Nongqawuse that if they killed their cattle and destroyed their crops, their ancestors would reward them with a mighty army that would rise from the sea and defeat the British; so many joined what became known as the "cattle-killing cult" that an estimated 40,000 died of starvation and the survivors were reduced to servitude to their sworn enemies (Peires 1989).

Another striking example of a national delusion was, arguably, the rise of Nazi ideology in the 1930s, which was fueled by myths about German history, notably the "stab-in-the-back" myth that the country's capitulation at the end of the First World War was caused by Jews and German socialists (Evans 2021). The U.S. subprime mortgage crisis, which sparked the global recession of 2007–2008, would have to be included as an example of an economic bubble (Lewis 2010). Additional examples of national delusions include numerous new pseudosciences, such as creation science, which claims to provide scientific evidence for the biblical account of the origins of the universe (Pigliucci 2018); quack medicines, such as homeopathy, which claims that drugs become more potent the more they are diluted with water; varieties of medical skepticism, such as the belief that vaccines cause autism; conspiracy theories, such as the belief that NASA faked the Moon landing in 1969 (Brotherton 2015); and exotic new-age religions. Indeed, the number and variety of "crazy" belief systems seems to change with dizzying speed, which would make the task of the compiler of the catalog even more difficult. At the time of this writing, for example, believers in the QAnon conspiracy (so named because it originated from a social media post by "Q," who claimed to be an anonymous U.S. intelligence officer) believe that the 45th president of the United States, Donald J. Trump, is engaged in a secret war against a global cabal of Satan-worshipping pedophiles and sex traffickers (Roose 2020).

The willingness of a large number of the population to believe such apparent absurdities raises the intriguing question of whether there could be a type of irrational or ill-founded belief that is so widely embraced as to be nearly universal. A candidate was proposed by Lerner (1980), who marshaled a large volume of evidence to argue that the belief in a just world is such a fundamental delusion. This idea of a just world is a commonplace feature of storytelling: from an early age, we like to see heroes rewarded and villains punished (Jose and Brewer 1984). However, this has real-world consequences, one of which is victim derogation, the tendency to believe that the unfortunate bring misfortune on themselves; hence, the poor are assumed to be feckless and lazy (Bénabou and Tirole 2006), and victims of rape are criticized for wearing short skirts or for consuming too much alcohol (Russell and Hand 2017). Among the many intriguing observations made about these kinds of beliefs are historical changes documented by Malahy et al. (2009), who noticed that many social psychologists had used the same questionnaire—the Just World Scale (Rubin and Peplau 1975)—in studies conducted with U.S. college students. Examining 28 studies that had been published between 1975 (just before Ronald Reagan entered the White House and introduced neoliberal economic policies) and 2006, they found that belief in a just world *increased* across this period, correlating positively with increases in income inequality as measured by the Gini coefficient (arguably evidence that the world is unjust).

Delusions of Psychiatric Patients

Many of the efforts to characterize the delusions of psychiatric patients have focused on their content. As the current DSM-5-TR definition cited earlier states, these beliefs tend to follow particular themes. The most studied type is the persecutory or paranoid delusion (Bentall et al. 2001; Freeman 2016), in which the individual believes "that someone, or some organisation, or some force or power, is trying to harm them in some way; to damage their reputation, to cause them bodily injury, to drive them mad or to bring about their death" (Wing et al. 1974, p. 175). The central feature of this kind of belief is an extreme sense of vulnerability and of being under attack coupled with an intense feeling of apprehension or fear (Boyd and Gumley 2007). Some definitions (e.g., the one in DSM-5-TR) also include the belief that someone close to the individual is being threatened with harm, although other commentators have cautioned that beliefs of this kind do not really belong to the paranoid category (Freeman and Garety 2000). These beliefs are particularly common in patients with a diagnosis on the schizophrenia spectrum; for example, in a large clinical trial that recruited patients very soon after they first became known to psychiatric services, 235 patients (91.8%) scored above the clinical cutoff for suspiciousness when their symptoms were assessed with the Positive and Negative Syndrome Scale (Moutoussis et al. 2007).

Delusions of reference, in which innocuous events are attributed special meaning, have been much less studied than paranoid beliefs, despite also being very commonly encountered in psychiatric practice (Startup et al. 2009). Sometimes these beliefs are included within the paranoid grouping (Green et al. 2008). However, empirical studies have shown that they fall into two separate types: delusions of observation, in which the patient believes that they are being spied on or gossiped about; and delusions of communication, in which they believe that some innocuous message or sign (e.g., a radio broadcast) is directed at the self. Only the former type is associated with beliefs about persecution (Startup and Startup 2005).

Grandiose delusions have also been studied only rarely (Knowles et al. 2011) but typically involve beliefs about special identity, special talents, a special mission in life, or extreme wealth (Leff et al. 1976). One hypothesis about these beliefs, dating back at least as far as the work of the psychoanalyst Karl Abraham (1911/1927), is that they are the product of some kind of psychological defense against depression or low self-esteem. However, a recent qualitative study of recovered grandiose patients found that these beliefs more often seem to reflect a desperate need for a purpose and meaning in life rather than a need to feel superior to others (Isham et al. 2019).

Delusions of control, sometimes called *passivity phenomena*, involve the belief that feelings, drives, and volitional acts are under the control of others. These types of delusions have sometimes been considered to have special status with respect to the diagnosis of schizophrenia because German psychiatrist Kurt Schneider (1887–1967) included them in his list of first-rank symptoms that he thought were characteristic of the disorder (Schneider 1959). Phenomenologically speaking, these symptoms seem to involve a loss of the sense of agency (Gallagher 2015) or ownership of actions and feelings (Bortolotti and Broome 2008), which has led to research to try to identify the neuropsychological origins of this kind of deficit (Frith 2012). If this account is correct, one implication is that delusions of control might be closely related to hallucinatory phenomena, such as auditory-verbal hallucinations, which occur when self-generated cognitive processes such as inner speech are misattributed to an external source (Bentall 1990), rather than to the other types of delusions considered here. (See Chapter 13, "Who Are You?")

Last, it is not uncommon for delusions to have religious content (Brewerton 1994). One study estimated that about a quarter of patients experiencing a first episode of psychosis have delusions of this kind (Siddle et al. 2002). Numerous other, much rarer delusional systems have been intensively studied because they either are associated with specific neuropsychological impairments, such as Capgras syndrome, in which the individual believes that a loved one has been replaced by an impostor (Young et al. 1990), or lead to specific medical complications, such as delusional parasitosis, which frequently leads to unnecessary interventions by dermatologists (Hylwa et al. 2011; Munro 1978), but these are not considered further here.

A striking feature of these themes is that they are universal. In a meta-analysis of 102 studies from around the world (Collin et al. 2022), paranoid delusions were consistently found to be most common, present in 64.5% of the patients studied. Ideas of reference occurred in 39.7%, grandiose delusions in 28.2%, delusions of control in 21.6%, and religious delusions in 18.3%. These estimates were almost completely unaffected by various geographic and cultural covariates, such as whether the samples were from developed industrialized nations or developing nations or whether the countries considered had high or low levels of inequality. One possible interpretation of this finding is that the themes reflect common existential themes that affect all humankind, such as the need to distinguish between trustworthy and untrustworthy others (paranoia), the need to make sense of ambiguous communications (reference), and concerns about social rank and the meaning of life (grandiose and religious delusions).

However, this is not to say that delusions are uninfluenced by the social, cultural, and political milieus in which the individual lives, although these influences become evident in only a few studies that have conducted more fine-grained analyses. For example, a study of Egyptian patients found that those who were least educated tended to have religious delusions relating to Islam, whereas those who were middle-class and educated tended to have secular and science-based delusions (El Sendiony 1976). A study from Malaysia compared patients in Penang, on the northwestern coast of the country, where the population is predominantly Chinese, with patients in Kota Bharu, in Kelantan on the eastern side, where there the population is mainly Malaysian and Muslim (Azhar et al. 1995). Once again, paranoid delusions were the most common type of delusion in both communities, followed by grandiose delusions. However, the grandiose delusions of the Kelantan patients typically concerned power or wealth, whereas those of the Penang Chinese patients were more often concerned with status. Among the Kelantan patients, delusions often focused on interpretation of the Koran; for example, patients thought that they had been specially chosen by God or were descendants of the Prophet.

A striking example of how context can color delusional content was reported during the recent COVID-19 pandemic when, in population surveys conducted in four countries, it was found that a small proportion of people had developed paranoid ideas about the virus (e.g., that others were trying to infect them); it turned out that those who developed these beliefs also scored highly on more general measures of paranoid thinking (Ellett et al. 2022).

Difficult Cases

Not surprisingly, difficult cases in which mental health experts struggle to agree on the delusional status of a belief system are not uncommon. Within clinical settings, a degree of ambiguity about this issue is often tolerated by psychiatric staff, and the problem usually generates attention only in rare and extreme cases, often those in which criminal behavior or violence is involved.

For example, in July 1984, two Mormon fundamentalists, Ron and Dan Lafferty, visited the home of their brother, Allen, in the town of American Fork, Utah. Allen was away working at the time, but they were greeted by Allen's wife, Brenda. After entering the house, the two men murdered both Brenda and her 15-month-old daughter, Erica (Krakauer 2003). Arrested after a half-hearted attempt to evade law enforcement agencies, the Laffertys claimed that the murders had been carried out on the instruction of Jesus Christ; Dan later asserted that he was the Prophet Elijah. At trial, their crime presented a conundrum for mental health professionals, who were unable to agree on whether the brothers had a shared psychotic illness or were merely in the grip of an extreme religious ideology. A similar dilemma faced mental health professionals at the trial of the Norwegian mass murderer Anders Behring Breivik, who in July 2011 bombed Norwegian government offices in Oslo, killing eight people, before shooting and killing 69 young political activists attending a summer camp on the nearby island of Utøya (Melle 2013; Parnas 2013). Breivik justified his actions on the grounds that he was a member of a secret organization, the Knights Templar, that was fighting feminism, the "Islamification" of his country, and the "cultural suicide of Europe."

Legal attempts to adjudicate these kinds of cases have usually focused on questions of culpability and the possibility that a person accused of a crime should be considered not guilty on the grounds of insanity (in this context, it is important to note that insanity is a legal and not a clinical concept). In many jurisdictions, the relevant legislation employs some version of the M'Naghten rule, named after Daniel M'Naghten, a Scottish woodcutter who on January 20, 1843, shot Edward Drummond, a civil servant whom he had mistaken for the prime minister, Robert Peel. By modern standards, M'Naghten would probably be diagnosed as psychotic because he held a complex set of highly paranoid ideas about the Tory government that was in power at the time. According to the rule that now bears his name, established by the British House of Lords, a successful not guilty plea requires the defense to establish that "the party accused was labouring under such a defect of reason from disease of the mind, as not to know the nature and quality of the act he was doing, or if he did know it, that he did not know that what he was doing was wrong" (Allnutt et al. 2007, p. 294). However, in recent times this defense has rarely been successful. Many U.S. states, including Utah, where the Laffertys were tried, removed the defense from their statute books after John Hinckley Jr. tried but failed to assassinate Ronald Reagan on March 30, 1981, in an attempt to impress actress Jodie Foster. However, in many states it is still possible for the defense to raise mental health issues in mitigation or to determine whether a defendant is capable of standing trial. Norway, where Breivik was tried, has been almost unique in simply requiring proof of psychotic illness (determined by standard psychiatric criteria, with no evidence of impaired judgment required) as grounds for a not guilty verdict.

The testimonies of expert psychiatric witnesses at the trials of both Ron Lafferty and Anders Breivik ultimately proved both contradictory and controversial. (Dan was tried separately from his brother, conducted his own defense, and rejected any suggestion that his mental health was impaired.) Juries in both cases were unconvinced by the psychologists and psychiatrists who argued that the crimes of the defendants were caused by their delusions and sided with those who argued that their beliefs were not pathological. Making the case that there was nothing pathological about Ron Lafferty's beliefs, Noel Gardner, a psychiatrist at the University of Utah Medical School, while acknowledging that the defendant's beliefs were unusual, appealed to the madness of crowds:

> Many of us believe in something referred to as trans-substantiation. That is when the priest performs the Mass, that the bread and the wine become the actual blood and body of Christ. From a scientific standpoint, that is a very strange, irrational, absurd idea. But we accept that on the basis of faith,

those of us who believe that. And because it has become so familiar and common to us, that we don't even notice, in a sense, it has an irrational quality to it. Or the idea of the virgin birth, which from a medical standpoint is highly irrational.... (Krakauer 2003, p. 301)

Commenting on the Breivik case, one observer lamented that the disputes about his mental health could have been avoided if only those who had examined him had paid less attention to the content of his beliefs and instead focused more on subtle phenomenological features that marked out true delusions (Parnas 2013).

Phenomenology and the Continuum Debate

The phenomenological approach to psychiatry traces its roots to the work of European philosophers, notably Franz Brentano (1838–1917); Edmund Husserl (1859–1938); Martin Heidegger (1889–1976); and Karl Jaspers (1883–1969), who was also a psychiatrist (see Bovet and Parnas 1993; Broome et al. 2012). Clinicians working in this tradition have argued that psychosis is a disturbance of the way the individual experiences their existence in the world, which can only be revealed by the clinician who uses empathy as a tool for understanding the unique meaningful connections that compose the patient's mental life. These connections are held to be quite different from the kinds of causal relationships that are the concern of the natural sciences (Jaspers 1913/1963). It is this disturbance of experience (arguably absent in the case of Anders Breivik but less obviously so in the case of the Lafferty brothers) that is thought to prove that delusions are qualitatively different from ordinary beliefs and attitudes.

Jaspers (1913/1963) noted that the beliefs of psychiatric patients are typically held with great conviction, are resistant to counterargument, and seem bizarre to observers, but he was aware that these criteria could also be applied to other fervently held beliefs and attitudes. He therefore argued that meeting these three criteria was not sufficient for beliefs to qualify as true delusions as opposed to what he termed "overvalued" ideas. Because true delusions do not arise meaningfully from the individual's personality and life experiences, the clinician would fail to empathize with the patient, no matter how hard he or she tries. Delusions, therefore, could only be "explained," presumably as some kind of disorder of the CNS. They are the consequence of a sudden, more or less sudden, breakdown in meaning (Jaspers 1913/1963). Taking this argument to its logical extreme, a later phenomenologically inclined researcher not only rejected the idea that delusions are wrong beliefs but argued that they are "empty speech acts, whose informational content refers to neither world or self" (Berrios 1991, p. 12).

This approach leads to the often-made distinction between the form and content of a belief, for example as articulated by Kurt Schneider:

> Diagnosis looks for the "How" (form) not the "What?" (the theme or content). When I find thought withdrawal, then this is important to me as a mode of inner experience and as a diagnostic hint, but it is not of diagnostic significance whether it is the devil, the girlfriend or a political leader who withdraws the thoughts. Wherever one focuses on such contents, diagnostics recedes; one sees then only the biographical aspects or the existence open to interpretation. (quoted in Hoenig 1982, p. 396)

This distinction has led phenomenologists to emphasize the affective and experiential aspects of delusional thinking rather than what patients say they believe (Feyaerts et al. 2021). The plausibility of this approach, of course, depends on the success with which these mental states can be characterized. One strategy has been to focus on the period that precedes the onset of the fully developed delusional system. For example, in detailed studies of more than 100 patients with psychosis—mostly soldiers with paranoia symptoms—conducted in a military hospital during the Second World War, German psychiatrist Klaus Conrad (1905–1961) claimed to identify a series of stages through which their ideas evolved (Conrad 1958/2012; see also Bovet and Parnas 1993 and Mishara 2010). First, according to Conrad, there is an initial phase of *das Trema* (derived from Greek, colloquial for "stage fright") or delusional mood, which may last for a few days or much longer, in which the patient feels a sense of tension, that there is something in the air, but is unable to say what has changed. At first this applies only to certain events and objects, but it gradually widens to encompass everything in the patient's world, creating suspiciousness, fear, and a sense of separation from others. This leads to a state of *apophany* (revelation) in which the delusion appears suddenly, as an "a-ha!" experience, often bringing about a sense of relief. Finally, in the *anastrophe* (turning back) phase, the patient feels themself to be the passive focus around which the delusional business of the world is revolving. In psychiatric research, these ideas have been influential in attempts to identify very early prodromal or basic symptoms of psychosis (e.g., Klosterkötter et al. 2001) but otherwise have been subject to very little empirical investigation.

Without a doubt, phenomenological research has been useful in making us think more broadly about psychopathological phenomena, but it has not been without limitations. One, which will not detain us here, is the problem that people have when trying to put private experiences into words to report them; the philosopher Ludwig Wittgenstein (1953) provided a compelling analysis of the limits of language in this regard. A more important limitation for the present purposes concerns the assumption of abnormality that has been made in these studies. Phenomenologists have generally conceived "normality" in terms of either coherence (whether experiences are in agreement with other experiences) or optimality (whether experiences contribute to the richness and differentiation of intentional objects in the world) rather than in statistical terms (Heinämaa and Taipale 2018). Within this framework, it is of course still necessary to consider a variety of experiences, yet phenomenological researchers have generally focused only on those of people diagnosed as having mental illness and have neglected to consider the variety of ordinary beliefs and attitudes (Connors and Halligan 2021). This has led them to underestimate the madness of crowds.

To see how serious this oversight is, we can consider religious beliefs, which often have exactly the kind of experiential component that phenomenologists think is the key to understanding delusions. Probably the best-known example of a profound change in religious belief is the conversion to Christianity of Saul of Tarsus (later known as Paul the Apostle). Born a Roman citizen to a devout Jewish family, he was the beneficiary of a broad education by the standards of his time but, as a young man, assisted in the persecution of the early Christians. At some point between 31 and 36 C.E., while traveling on the road to Damascus, he underwent a sudden and dramatic mystical experience, the nature of which has ever since been the subject of theological as well as psychological debate, made possible because it was described differently in different passages of the New Testament. According to the most widely quoted account in the Acts of the Apostles (which describes the event in the third person):

> And as he journeyed, he came near Damascus: and suddenly there shined round about him a light from heaven.
> And he fell to the earth, and heard a voice saying unto him, Saul, Saul, why persecutest thou me?
> And he said, Who art thou, Lord? And the Lord said, I am Jesus whom thou persecutest: it is hard for thee to kick against the pricks.
> And he trembling and astonished said, Lord, what wilt thou have me to do? And the Lord said unto him, Arise, and go into the city, and it shall be told thee what thou must do.
> And the men which journeyed with him stood speechless, hearing a voice, but seeing no man.
> And Saul arose from the earth; and when his eyes were opened, he saw no man: but they led him by the hand and brought him into Damascus.
> And he was three days without sight, and neither did eat nor drink. (King James Bible, Acts 9:3–9)

Occasionally, neurologists have attempted to explain away episodes of this kind as the product of epilepsy. Indeed, modern studies have found that patients with temporal lobe epilepsy often show high levels of religiosity, and one study even claimed to have detected abnormal brain waves in a patient with epilepsy who had a messianic experience while being monitored by electroencephalogram (Tedrus et al. 2015). However, it seems very unlikely that all religious experiences can be accounted for in this way. Spiritual encounters not only have been reported by key figures in all three of the Abrahamic religions but also seem to be surprisingly common experiences in ordinary people. This was demonstrated by a research program initiated by Sir Alister Hardy (1896–1985), an Oxford-based marine zoologist and one-time Antarctic explorer, who believed that human spirituality is an evolved capacity and that the spiritual strength that results from religious experiences contributes to resilience in the face of stress. Compiling more than 6,000 first-person accounts of religious experiences sent to him by members of the general public, he reported that many people (29%) included the experience of a pattern of events that convinced the individual that they were meant to happen; others involved the experience of the direct presence of God (27%), prayers being answered (25%), being looked after or guided by a presence (22%), or an awareness of the sacred in nature (16%) (Hardy 1979). Detailed interviews conducted later with a small number of people who had contacted the center that Hardy established found that these types of experiences could not be distinguished from psychotic experiences in terms of either content or form (Jackson and Fulford 1997).

The logical alternative to the idea that delusions are qualitatively different from other beliefs, typically favored by psychologists, is to propose a continuum between normal and abnormal believing. Yet, arguably, the interpretation of the evidence that appears to support this hypothesis has also been limited by simplistic assumptions about the nature of normal beliefs and attitudes. Two kinds of evidence are often cited to support the continuum.

The first type of evidence concerns the prevalence of abnormal beliefs in the general population as revealed in epidemiological studies. For example, in a study of people attending appointments with their general practitioners in southwestern France using the Peters et al. Delusions Inventory (Peters et al. 1999b), of those who had no history of psychiatric treatment, 69.3% reported that people they knew were not who they seemed to be, 46.9% reported telepathic communication, 42.2% reported experiencing seemingly innocuous events that had double meanings, and 25.5% reported that they were being persecuted in some way (Verdoux et al. 1998). In the epidemiological Netherlands Mental Health Survey and Incidence Study (NEMESIS), 3.3% of the 7,000 participants were judged to have delusions, and 8.7% were estimated to have similar ideas that were judged to be not clinically significant because they were not associated with distress (van Os et al. 2000). A later German study confirmed that the delusions of psychiatric patients and apparently similar beliefs in nonpatients are mainly distinguishable in terms of the distress associated with them rather than by either conviction or the extent to which the individual is preoccupied with the belief (Lincoln 2007).

This evidence is not decisive because it is possible that psychopathological phenomena are more prevalent than previously supposed but nonetheless qualitatively distinct from normal psychological phenomena. Hence, the second type of evidence often appealed to in support of the continuum hypothesis has been obtained by examining the distribution of beliefs in the population more closely using appropriate statistical techniques. Studies that have attempted this have typically focused on paranoid beliefs. For example, Freeman et al. (2005) administered a checklist of paranoid thoughts to an online convenience sample of more than 1,000 predominantly female university students who were asked to rate each item (e.g., "People would harm me if given an opportunity") on frequency over the past month, conviction, and distress. The three scales were highly correlated, and total scores formed a smooth exponential decay curve, with large numbers of participants endorsing nonpathological items and rarer items being endorsed only by those who had high total scores. A subsequent study by the same group used items picked out of the 2014 U.K. Adult Psychiatric Morbidity Survey of a representative sample of 7,000 adults (Bebbington and Nayani 1995). The analysis, which used sophisticated statistical techniques, identified four separate components of paranoia—interpersonal vulnerability, ideas of reference, mistrust, and fear of persecution—and again found that total scores on the items were distributed along an exponential decay curve.

One limitation of these studies is that they included no clinical samples. Elahi et al. (2017) compiled data on more than 2,000 healthy participants (mainly students and predominantly female), 157 patients with prodromal psychosis, and 360 patients with psychosis from previous studies that had used the same paranoia measure. The study used three separate taxometric methods, which have been developed to discriminate between continua and taxa (classes of individuals with unique characteristics), and the analyses were carried out on the entire sample and the nonclinical participants alone. The findings strongly supported a continuum model when the clinical participants were both included and excluded.

Earlier I criticized the phenomenologists for simplistic assumptions about the nature of normal beliefs, and the same charge can be directed against continuum theorists. The studies I have just described, which were based on questionnaires and structured interviews focused entirely on belief content, ignored the kinds of experiential aspects of believing that the phenomenologists have highlighted and that I have previously suggested are often evident in both normal and abnormal beliefs. Indeed, for the most part, psychological research has treated beliefs simply as propositions written on an *inner list* that is accessible only to the believer but that (assuming the respondent is truthful) investigators can access by asking the right questions. What seems to be missing from both the phenomenological and the psychological approaches is an adequate understanding of what believing entails.

Understanding Belief Systems

The concept of belief is ubiquitous in the human sciences and plays a central role in disciplines as diverse as history, anthropology, sociology, economics, and psychology. Indeed, to catalog its central role in how we attempt to understand the human mind and behavior would be a formidable task. At times philosophers have attempted to dispense with the concept but failed (Stich 1996), not least because the belief that there are no such things as beliefs is, of course, a belief. There is a plausible case to be made that the central role of belief is what distinguishes the social sciences from the natural sciences; this is implicit, for example, in Winch's (1958) attempts to define the unique features of the former. It is all the more surprising, then, that there has been no serious psychological analysis of what is involved in believing.

Cultural Origins of Our Understandings of Belief

A contemporary philosophical treatment of belief begins with the following observation:

> Contemporary analytic philosophers of mind generally use the term "belief" to refer to the attitude we have, roughly, whenever we take something to be the case or regard it as true. To believe something, in this sense, need not involve actively reflecting on it: Of the vast number of things ordinary adults believe, only a few can be at the fore of the mind at any single time.... Many of the things we believe, in the relevant sense, are quite mundane: that we have heads, that it's the 21st century, that a coffee mug is on the desk. Forming beliefs is thus one of the most basic and important features of the mind. (Schwitzgebel 2015)

Given the central role of this "basic and important feature of the mind" in human affairs, it is not surprising that evidence of believing is as old as recorded culture; the oldest literary works in the Western canon, *The Iliad* and *The Odyssey*, imply the existence of a wide range of beliefs (e.g., about the role of the gods in human affairs). However, according to the *Oxford English Dictionary*, the oldest uses of the word *belief* in the English language are all theological. For example, the first recorded use of the mental conviction form of *belief* appears to be a Middle English passage in Ælfric's

Homily on the Nativity of Christ, written in about 1175. This reads as *Ðesne laf we æteð þonne we mid bileafan gað to halige husle ure hælendes lichame*, which can be translated as "This bread we eat when we with faith go to the holy Eucharist of Our Lord's body." This history is not accidental: nearly all of the earliest English language texts were written by monks, and the creation of theological doctrine implies the need for a deep contemplation about the nature of belief.

Nonetheless, the scope of the word *belief* and how people have thought about the process of believing have changed with time. From the very beginning, Christianity was a highly propositional religion, perhaps as a consequence of the early Church's need to defend itself from the many dissenting cults (Ebionites, Docetists, Gnostics, and Arians, to name a few) that were eventually eliminated after Constantine the Great made Christianity the official religion of Rome in the early fourth century (Holland 2012). In the face of these challenges, orthodoxy became the child of heresy, and the early Church devoted considerable energy to the development of checklists of beliefs, known as *creeds*, that could be used to induct members, unify congregations, and distinguish between true believers and heretics (Hinson 1979). This may be the cultural origin of the inner-list idea, in which beliefs are assumed to be propositions in the mind or brain that can be read by a skillful interrogator or clinical psychologist.

Later, in the Medieval period, when Catholic orthodoxy intruded into every aspect of daily life, to believe was simply to assent to the doctrines of the Church and therefore something that was effortless and never questioned. Inevitably, this way of thinking ended with the Reformation; the emergence of competing theologies necessitated a transformation of believing into something that was difficult, often subject to error, and that might lead to a mistaken understanding of the world (Shagan 2018). These developments ultimately led to the birth of science and our modern conception of belief as an individual assessment of the likelihood of certain facts based on an assessment of probabilities, a transformation that was associated with dramatic changes in the way that ordinary people saw the world. A typical well-educated European in 1600, for example, believed that witches and werewolves existed, that a murdered body would bleed in the presence of a murderer, that a rainbow was a sign from God, and that comets portended evil—all ideas that were widely regarded as ridiculous a century later (Wootton 2015).

These historical observations point to what appears to be a paradox: the concept of belief is indispensable, yet it would be naive in the extreme to expect human psychological processes to mirror precisely the changing conceptual architecture of the English language. Indeed, English (and presumably all other languages) includes many words that are to some extent interchangeable with the word *belief* (e.g., attitude, value, opinion, conjecture, prediction). This rich language is useful in everyday life but has probably impeded any attempts to construct a unified understanding of belief. Although it seems obviously a mistake to try to construct a separate psychological theory aligned with each of these terms, that is what has happened in practice.

To make sense of what is involved in belief, then, we must identify psychological processes that correspond approximately to the ordinary language term *belief* and its near synonyms but without assuming a precise fit. This is a challenging task that is well beyond the space available in this chapter and requires synthesizing findings from a wide range of research areas that have been largely ignored by psychopathologists, such as political psychology, the psychology of religion, and the broader disciplines of sociology and anthropology. However, it is one that I hope to show, in the few pages available to me, has immense promise for informing our understanding of the distinction between pathological and nonpathological beliefs.

There Is No Inner List

Elsewhere I have defended the view that beliefs are propositional and underpinned by the human capacity for language (Bentall 2018). Observing the family dog staring hopefully at the food cupboard at dinnertime might prompt the assumption that animals can hold beliefs, and there is clearly a lot that is belief-like about their behavior. Contemporary comparative psychology (Pearce 2008) and computational models of associative learning (Dayan and Abbott 2005) treat both Pavlovian and instrumental conditioning as complex processes in which the animal adjusts its predictions about the world, adapting to changing circumstances in a way that allows it to efficiently use the resources in its environment, a set of processes that could certainly be characterized as belief-like. It is also worth noting that animals find the state of being unable to predict the world highly aversive; Pavlov showed that dogs presented with conditioned stimuli that are impossible to distinguish become highly distressed, a phenomenon he called *conditioned neurosis* (Liddell 1947), and later research using both Pavlovian and instrumental conditioning paradigms showed similar effects in a wide range of species (Mineka and Kihlstrom 1978). All this being said, no dog has ever become either a jihadist or a political scientist.

The human capacity to form sentences allows us to use grammatical rules and word combinations to construct sophisticated descriptions of the world (e.g., the blueprint of a nuclear submarine), rules to follow (e.g., the recipe for sourdough bread), novel statements about complex contingencies (e.g., "If there is no food in the valley during winter, the next best place to look for grub is in the forest at the far side of the mountain"), and abstract concepts (e.g., $E=mc^2$) that are denied to other species. Moreover, because human beings internalize language at an early age and use it as a vehicle of thought (Fernyhough 2016; Vygotsky 1962), there is a consequent enhancement of cognitive capacity even when we decline to share our thoughts with other people. The invention of literacy was likely associated with a further expansion of human cognitive skills (Ong 1982) and enabled beliefs to be recorded and then passed on from generation to generation. It is impossible to overestimate the significance of this ability; without it there would be no culture or science.

It is important to recognize that by claiming that beliefs are propositional and language based, I am not claiming that beliefs involve *only* propositional processes. There are sound philosophical reasons for supposing that our knowledge of the world ultimately rests on a bedrock of processes that are nonpropositional (Wittgenstein 1969; see also Gipps and Rhodes 2011; Rhodes and Gipps 2008), and there is indeed experimental evidence that associative processes play an important role in many aspects of language (e.g., Colunga and Smith 2005).

Nor does claiming that beliefs are propositional necessitate an inner-list model. Stich (1996), in his attempt to dispense with the concept of belief, argued that there was nothing known to neuroscience that corresponded to the idea of a stored catalog of propositions and, moreover, that connectionist models of neural architecture could demonstrate belief-like behavior in the absence of any stored representations of this kind. This argument, as Stich later conceded, did not achieve its original goal of eliminating the need for the concept of belief, but it does undermine the inner-list notion. Moreover, the list metaphor fails for many other reasons. For example, it has difficulty accounting for novel beliefs, such as my conviction that there are no teacups on the far side of the Moon, and also inadequately captures the interdependency between beliefs (my belief about the absence of teacups on the Moon is underwritten by beliefs about the nature of the Moon and teacups). More important from a clinical perspective, it fails to reflect the dynamic, shifting ways in which beliefs are constructed and adjusted, either in the course of argument with other human beings (Edwards and Potter 1992) or when we deliberate with ourselves.

This dynamic negotiation of belief is evident when psychiatric patients discuss their beliefs with other people (Georgaca 2000) and during the evolution of delusional systems. For example, Peter Chadwick (2008), a British psychologist who became psychotic after suspecting that his neighbors knew about his bisexuality and transvestism, described how he spent many months constructing the all-preoccupying narrative that eventually became his delusional system:

But all [of these events earlier in his life] were eventually collected up, knitted together and turned into a delusional web of thoughts and feelings that in the end drove me to multiple suicide attempts that very nearly succeeded in killing me. In madness, no moment of one's existence seems to be wasted; it is as if one's whole life, and the depths of one's very being in selective perspective, have been made magically clear in their awful and portentous significance. (p. 5)

To borrow a metaphor from the philosopher Dan Dennett (1991): When we administer a questionnaire or ask someone what they believe, we are not asking our interlocutor to read out from an inner list; instead, we are prompting the person to author the latest in an endless series of multiple drafts of what they believe. This draft will, in due course, be followed by many further drafts in the future.

Certainty

As noted in the subsection "Delusions of Psychiatric Patients," it has often been said that delusions are unusual in being held with extraordinary conviction. Many studies, either using interview methods (e.g., So et al. 2012) or using experimental methods to observe how patients change their minds in the face of conflicting information (e.g., Woodward et al. 2008), have shown that belief inflexibility is associated with the certainty with which patients hold their delusional beliefs (Zhu et al. 2018). At the same time, other theorists have attempted to analyze belief inflexibility in terms of problems of updating prior beliefs (McKay 2012) or as a neurobiological error in the mechanisms responsible for processing discrepancies (errors) between expected events and those that actually occur (Corlett 2018).

A general problem with these approaches is that they have given insufficient attention to the resistance to attitude change evidenced by nonpathological but personally meaningful beliefs, such as political attitudes (Lodge and Taber 2013; Westen 2008). In a study by Colbert et al. (2010), people with delusions, people who had recovered from delusions, and healthy control subjects were asked whether they were willing to consider whether their beliefs (delusional in the case of patients, idiosyncratic but meaningful in the case of the control subjects) were mistaken. Personally meaningful beliefs were held with equal conviction, and equally inflexibly, in all three groups.

These observations highlight a feature of beliefs that is implicit in the philosophical account cited in the subsection "Cultural Origins of Our Understandings of Belief" (Schwitzgebel 2015): beliefs come, as it were, in two parts—a proposition (statement about the world) and a subjective estimate of the certainty that the proposition is true. This estimate is usually not explicitly articulated, but English (and I imagine every other human language) furnishes us with a rich variety of means to express our certainty implicitly ("I guess that...," "I think that...," "I believe that...," "I expect that...," and so on). Experimental studies show that in ordinary life, people's subjective confidence usually correlates fairly well with the accuracy of what they believe (Koriat 2012).

Intriguingly, the subjective feeling of knowing something can sometimes become completely divorced from actual knowing. A common experience of this kind is the tip-of-the-tongue phenomenon, which was elegantly described at the end of the nineteenth century by the philosopher-psychologist William James (1893):

> Suppose we try to recall a forgotten name. The state of our consciousness is peculiar. There is a gap therein; but no mere gap. It is a gap that is intensely active. A sort of wraith of the name is in it, beckoning us in a given direction, making us at moments tingle with the sense of our closeness and then letting it sink back without the longed-for term. If wrong names are proposed to us, this singularly definite gap acts immediately so as to negate them. (p. 251)

A noteworthy feature of this phenomenon is that it involves a state of awareness of knowing something that the individual does not yet know (Koriat 2000). It is therefore not far-fetched to suggest that this kind of experience might be in some way related to the *Trema* experience of something being in the offing, which Klaus Conrad (1958/2012) saw as a prelude to delusions.

Whether or not this parallel is correct, research evidence suggests that at least some patients with psychosis and people with a disposition to psychosis are impaired in their ability to estimate the certainty of their beliefs (Balzan 2016). For example, Moritz et al. (2015) asked a large population sample to rate their confidence in their answers in a game modeled after the television show "Who Wants to Be a Millionaire?" and found that a poor correlation between confidence and accuracy was associated with paranoid thinking. These observations suggest that it might be fruitful for psychopathologists to consider the processes by which human beings make these kinds of judgments and study them in clinical samples.

Cognitive psychologists studying human judgment (Koriat 2012) and consumer psychologists interested in attitudes toward commercial products (Tormala and Rucker 2018) have conducted a great deal of research on this topic. In general, the various theoretical models that they have proposed view certainty judgment as a metacognitive skill that is driven either by the direct experience of knowing or by inference from contextual factors.

The distress shown by animals when they are exposed to unpredictable environments (Liddell 1947; Mineka and Kihlstrom 1978) suggests that a direct sensitivity to uncertainty may be a fundamental feature of the non-propositional learning systems shared by all vertebrate species. Moreover, some human studies have demonstrated that certainty can be read directly from our cognitive processes. For example, easily recalled knowledge is typically judged as more certain than difficult-to-recall knowledge (Alter and Oppenheimer 2009); hence, fast response times when recalling information are generally a strong predictor of confidence in the accuracy of memories (Zakay and Tuvia 1998). People are also more likely to feel a high level of certainty about a belief if the relevant information that is available to them is highly consistent (Smith et al. 2007) or if their beliefs are based on direct personal experience rather than information they have obtained secondhand from someone else (Wu and Shaffer 1987).

However, certainty judgments are sometimes inferred from self-knowledge, which leads to unjustifiably high perceptions of certainty when self-knowledge is inaccurate. For example, certainty increases when people believe that they have spent time and effort reflecting and elaborating on their beliefs, even when they have been misled into overestimating the time they have spent on this process (Barden and Petty 2008). Similarly, simply coaxing people to think that they have personally arrived at a theory that is in fact given to them is sufficient to increase their appraisal that the theory is true (Gregg et al. 2017). A complication is that individuals with the least knowledge in a particular domain (whose beliefs are least accurate) are generally poorest at judging their own knowledge, a phenomenon that is often referred to as the *Dunning-Kruger effect* after the psychologists who first studied it (Dunning et al. 1995; Ehrlinger et al. 2008).

These kinds of studies, for the most part conducted on ordinary people, provide important clues about why some beliefs—not only delusions—are held with extraordinary conviction. However, the way that beliefs are organized likely also plays a role.

Belief Systems

In a monograph on anti-Semitism penned shortly after the Second World War, the philosopher Jean-Paul Sartre (1948) noted that Enlightenment scholars had tended to treat beliefs as atomized, rational propositions that could each be evaluated independently. Anti-Semitism, Sartre argued, dispelled this assumption because hostility toward Jews seemed to be predictably related to other beliefs and attitudes, such as authoritarianism. This observation points to one of the most important features of human beliefs, which is that far from being randomly related to one another, they are often organized into *master interpretive systems* by which individuals interpret the world and their place within it (Bentall 2018). Examples of these master interpretive systems include religious beliefs (McCauley and Graham 2020; Norenzayan and Gervais 2013), political ideologies (Huddy et al. 2013), conspiracy theories (Brotherton 2015; Douglas et al. 2017), and beliefs about the supernatural (Dean et al. 2021).

Interestingly, these systems for the most part are correlated with one another, which suggests that there might be some common factors that lead people to embrace them. It is perhaps unsurprising that religiosity is associated with belief in the supernatural (Lindeman and Svedholm-Häkkinen 2016; Thalbourne 1995), but positive correlations have also been reported between religiosity and conservatism (Schlenker et al. 2012) and between conservatism and conspiracy theories (Galliford and Furnham 2017). Studies have shown that belief in conspiracy theories, in turn, is positively correlated with religiosity (Mancosu et al. 2017; Newheiser et al. 2011) and belief in the paranormal (Darwin et al. 2011; Newheiser et al. 2011; Swami et al. 2011). Importantly, these kinds of associations transcend the division between clinical phenomena and the madness of crowds. For example, and again not surprisingly, paranoia correlates with the tendency to believe in conspiracy theories (Imhoff and Lamberty 2018), but it is also associated with paranormal beliefs (Darwin et al. 2011). Similarly, both delusionality (Peters et al. 1999a) and paranoia (Ayeni et al. 2011) have been observed to be positively associated with religiosity. Although it is not possible to do justice here to the vast research that has been conducted on each of these types of belief systems, these literatures have some very important implications for understanding delusions that can be summarized briefly. In what follows, I focus mainly on political beliefs and conspiracy theories.

An important question addressed by political psychologists concerns why beliefs form distinctive patterns or structures of the kind intuited by Sartre. For example, historically, political actors have generally fallen into two groups: those who seek stability and order versus those who seek progress and rapid reform. This difference can be traced back as far as ancient Greece (Hibbing et al. 2014) but is today most commonly referred to as the *right-left dimension*, reflecting the seating arrangements of French Estates General during the French Revolution, where those who opposed the Ancien Régime and the Bourbon monarchy sat on the left. This distinction is evident in modern political attitudes and voting behavior (Jost et al. 2009), although other ways of describing variations in political belief have also been proposed; for example, a considerable volume of research has focused on authoritarian traits, which are usually thought to align with the right end of the political spectrum (Adorno et al. 1950; Stenner 2005).

Underneath this apparently simple structure, however, lies considerable complexity. In a landmark study, the American political scientist Kenneth Converse (1964/2006) noted that associations between specific beliefs can be sustained by logical associations (e.g., the belief that government should be as small as possible implies support for low tax rates and miserly benefits for the unemployed). Political belief systems can therefore be thought of as networks of interconnected attitudes that influence one another, and the same is presumably true for other kinds of belief systems. However, when Converse analyzed both quantitative and qualitative data collected from American voters in the 1950s and early 1960s, he found that these kinds of logical relationships held only at the extreme left ("liberal" in U.S. parlance) and right ("conservative") ends of the spectrum, where ideologically committed voters had often spent many years actively refining their belief systems and developing sophisticated arguments to handle apparent contradictions. Outside these extremes, voters often cast their ballots on more flimsy grounds, such as because of niche policy promises (a new law to prevent cruelty to animals) or even a vague feeling that a particular politician is trustworthy. Consistent with Converse's findings, more recent research has shown that the correlation between attitudes toward economic conservatism (free market economics) and social conservatism (family values) is greater at either end of the political spectrum than in the center (Feldman and Johnston 2014).

Note that the interconnectivity of beliefs within a system helps to explain why these systems are highly resistant to counterargument or refuting evidence. Many psychiatric patients, like political ideologists, have often spent many years finessing their theories and eliminating any contradictions within them; the firsthand account given by Peter Chadwick quoted in the subsection "There Is No Inner List" seems to illustrate this process. As a consequence, patients' beliefs are not atomized but woven into elaborate systems analogous to those formed by committed ideologists. However, a highly interconnected network of beliefs of this kind is likely to be resistant to perturbation because each individual belief within the system is sustained by the beliefs connected to it—a change to one belief is prevented by the rigidity of all the beliefs that are associated with it.

Although these kinds of logical associations are clearly important in explaining the resilience of belief systems to challenge, they are not the only factor at work, and to see why this must be the case, it is useful to consider conspiracy theories. These theories make a particularly interesting comparison with delusions, not least because, as noted earlier, they sometimes appear to be as "mad" as any beliefs observed in the psychiatric clinic. Conspiracy theories have often been embraced by extreme political projects on both the left and right of the political spectrum; for example, they played an important role in the Nazi project to turn Germany into an authoritarian state (Evans 2021), and they have long been part of political discourse in the United States (Hofstadter 1964). Unhelpfully, they are often confused with paranoia; for example, in a seminal essay, American historian Richard Hofstadter (1964) made this mistake by talking about the "paranoid style" in American politics. As we have seen, the two kinds of beliefs are indeed often correlated (Imhoff and Lamberty 2018), but factor analytic studies have shown that they are psychologically distinct, with different psychological predictors (Alsuhibani et al. 2022). For example, whereas paranoia is associated with low self-esteem, belief in conspiracies is associated with high self-esteem and narcissism (Alsuhibani et al. 2022; Cichocka et al. 2016). Consistent with this latter finding, people who score highly on measures of conspiracy thinking are more likely to endorse conspiracy theories if they think that they are endorsed only by a minority of other people (Imhoff and Lamberty 2017).

Someone who believes in one type of conspiracy is very likely to believe in others (Brotherton et al. 2013; Bruder et al. 2013). However, this cannot be explained by logical processes. For example, there is no logical connection between the belief that the American government has imprisoned extraterrestrials in Area 51 and the belief that Donald Trump is waging a secret war against pedophiles. Indeed, people are capable of believing in conspiracies that appear, at least on the surface, logically contradictory, for example, that Princess Diana faked her own death and that she was assassinated by the British Secret Service (Alsuhibani et al. 2022; Wood et al. 2012).

So if the glue holding together the network of conspiracy beliefs is not a set of logical links between the individual beliefs, what could it be? A tempting answer is that it is some kind of hidden, superordinate belief that is linked to all of the individual propositions in the network. In the case of conspiracy theories, this superordinate belief is presumably something about the duplicitousness of governments and institutions. This hypothesis is supported by results from a recent study of conspiracy theories and paranoia in three European countries (the United Kingdom, Ireland, and Spain); in all three, conspiracy theories were uniquely associated with mistrust in political institutions, whereas paranoia was uniquely associated with a tendency to judge unfamiliar faces as untrustworthy (Martinez et al. 2022).

This general idea that there are fundamental beliefs underlying surface beliefs crops up in many places in the psychological literature. One version of this idea can be found in Beck's (1987) theory of depression, which includes as a component a negative cognitive triad of beliefs about the self, the world, and the future that, when subjected to factor analysis, seems to yield a single dimension of negative beliefs about almost everything (McIntosh and Fischer 2000). Another version can be found in the work of the social psychologist Jonathan Haidt (2013), who has argued that political ideologies can be explained in terms of variations in five moral foundations: the importance people place on caring for others, commitment to fairness, loyalty to one's group, respect for rank and status, and concerns about sanctity (purity). Lerner's (1980) proposal that human beings cling to the fundamental belief that the world is just is yet another example of this kind of theorizing. Researchers studying skeptical attitudes toward science have also pointed to the importance of understanding *root beliefs* in order to explain *surface beliefs*, such as conspiracy theories and the idea that climate change being caused by human consumption of fossil fuels is a hoax (Hornsey and Fielding 2017). Most recently, Clifton et al. (2019) built on these models in an ambitious attempt to identify a hierarchy of *primal beliefs*. According to this theory, various fundamental beliefs about the world are organized into three main kinds: beliefs that the world is safe versus dangerous, that it is enticing versus dull, and that it is alive versus mechanistic.

The problem with evoking more fundamental beliefs in the attempt to explain surface ones is that eventually we run out of beliefs. A cognitive-behavioral therapist might say that the downward arrow technique can go only so far. As Wittgenstein (1969) pointed out, there ultimately has to be a bedrock of knowledge that requires no justification on which we can anchor our propositions about the world. Indeed, although fundamental beliefs look like propositions, this is arguably only an illusion created by the fact that we have to use language to express them; the idea that we should respect rank and status or that the world is dull and unexciting cannot be evaluated for truth-value in the same way that, say, we can evaluate the belief that the Earth revolves around the Sun. Indeed, in many cases it is not hard to see how proposed fundamental beliefs map onto more basic, nonpropositional psychological processes, some of which are shared with other species. For example, the big three primal beliefs described by Clifton et al. (2019) described in the previous paragraph seem to reflect sensitivity to threat, sensitivity to reward, and specifically human cognitive processes that have evolved to allow us to understand the behavior of other human beings. Similarly, Haidt et al.'s (1997) sanctity dimension in their moral foundations appears to be related to feelings of disgust, which is why disgust sensitivity is related to political conservatism and hostility to migrants (Aarøe et al. 2017).

Belief, Culture, and the Uniqueness of Delusions

Revisiting the Laffertys

There is one final characteristic of beliefs that we must consider before returning to the question of whether and how delusions are different from the madness of crowds. To understand this property, it is helpful to consider again the beliefs of Ron and Dan Lafferty, which provoked such disagreement among the mental health professionals who testified at Ron's trial. Recall that the two brothers held that they had murdered their sister-in-law and her infant daughter on the instruction of Jesus Christ and that Dan believed, and to this day still believes, that he is the Prophet Elijah. It is worth adding that, unlike Anders Breivik (who later said that he had been deliberately exaggerating his paranoid beliefs to mislead psychiatrists), the Laffertys were reticent about sharing their beliefs with investigators and never recanted. The complete backstory to the murders was uncovered only some years later by investigative journalist Jon Krakauer (2003) in his remarkable book *Under the Banner of Heaven*.

Polygamy has long been a source of conflict among the Church of Jesus Christ of Latter-Day Saints (LDS Church; the institutional authority of the Mormon religion), the U.S. government, and some of the Church's followers. The practice was introduced by the religion's founder, Joseph Smith, in Illinois in the 1830s and was officially advocated by the LDS Church from 1852 onward, by which time the membership had moved and become a dominant force in the territory of Utah. Although an 1862 law passed by the U.S. Congress prohibited plural marriage, many Mormons were undeterred, believing that they were protected by the First Amendment of the U.S. Constitution. This position became untenable in 1879, when the U.S. Supreme Court ruled that the amendment protected religious belief but not all religiously inspired practices. In 1890, the LDS Church officially rejected polygamy, which allowed Utah to be recognized as a U.S. state. However, a substantial minority of Mormons interpreted this rejection as a betrayal of one of their core values, and some fundamentalists continue to practice plural marriage today. In a small number of communities in the borderlands where Nevada, Arizona, and Utah meet, this practice has led to widespread sexual abuse of young (often underage) women, who have been passed from one Mormon elder to another. In 2006, Mormon fundamentalist leader Warren Jeffs was placed on the Federal Bureau of Investigation's Ten Most Wanted Fugitives list, and he is currently serving a long jail sentence for multiple sexual offenses against children.

The Laffertys came from a strict Mormon family ruled by an authoritarian and violent father. In adulthood they drifted toward fundamentalism, and they mixed with various fundamentalist cults in the months preceding their murder of Brenda and Erica, including a group who called themselves The Prophets, who believed that they could teach people how to receive messages directly from Jesus Christ. It was during this period that Ron's wife divorced him after he demanded a plural marriage. He was also excommunicated by the mainstream LDS Church. Ron and Dan blamed these events on their brother's wife, Brenda, who was vocally opposed to plural marriage. It was in these circumstances that Ron believed he had been told by Jesus to "remove" Brenda and Erica. Hence, the Lafferty brothers' behavior and beliefs can be understood once the cultural context is known. To appreciate the implications of this observation for delusions, we need to unpack what it means when we say that a belief can be understood in its cultural context.

Belief Propagation

An important feature of beliefs is that they are transmittable. Indeed, this is one of the main evolutionary advantages conferred by language: propositions expressed in words can be passed from one person to another, either through direct speech or via intermediate media (e.g., television programs, articles, or chapters such as this one), allowing knowledge to be shared and accumulated across time. A culture emerges when a large number of people, typically but not always located in the same geographic area, share a set of representations that can be normative (e.g., "With fish, drink white wine"), complex (e.g., common law or Einstein's theory of relativity), nonverbal (e.g., national flags), or multimedia (e.g., the saying of Mass). Of course, these representations include beliefs, and therefore, to a large extent, to be interested in culture is to be interested in the epidemiology of beliefs (Sperber 1996).

The processes involved in belief dissemination are complex, and there is space to make only a few brief observations about them here. A popular metaphor famously proposed by Richard Dawkins (1976) involves comparing beliefs to genes, with a focus on selection processes that determine whether a meme survives transmission from one person to another. It is ironic, therefore, that this model, despite receiving considerable attention for a while (Blackmore 1999) and even provoking the creation of a new journal (the *Journal of Memetics*), has not survived the process of academic natural selection (the journal closed in 2005 after just 8 years). Among the theory's limitations is that it failed to generate testable hypotheses about the conditions under which selection would occur or the cognitive capacities required for someone to acquire a belief and pass it on. It also fell short in explaining both the variation in human ideas and the creativity with which these ideas are expressed (Atran 2001). On the last point, it is important to recognize that human communication does not involve the exact replication of beliefs; instead, the outcome is usually some degree of resemblance between the beliefs of the speaker and those of the listener (Sperber 1996).

An older and in many ways more fruitful metaphor (although still a metaphor) that will resonate with readers in the current times involves comparing belief propagation to disease transmission. This idea goes back to the work of the Nobel Prize–winning and personally troubled discoverer of the mechanism responsible for the transmission of malaria, Ronald Ross (1857–1932), who developed mathematical models that he thought explained both the transmission of infections and the transmission of ideas (Kucharski 2020). The main virtue of this metaphor is that it allows us to break down belief propagation into several distinct subprocesses that form stages in the transmission process: the initial creation of beliefs, the vector (medium of transmission), belief characteristics that make the beliefs a good fit with the receiving person, and, finally, whether the receiving person has an adequate immune response to them. I briefly discuss each of these stages before pointing to the implications of this model for the understanding of delusions.

First, let us consider the origins of beliefs. Often, beliefs are lost in time and hard to pinpoint because, of course, many of them are elaborated, are combined with others, and morph as they go from the mind of one human being to another. However, in the case of master interpretive systems, it is sometimes possible to identify "patient zero"—Jesus, the Prophet Muhammad, Karl Marx, and Adolf Hitler come to mind, although these individuals all had their personal cultural backgrounds and never acted alone. As the philosopher Quassim Cassam (2019) pointed out, conspiracy theories are often created by conspiracy entrepreneurs who actively proselytize them, such as right-wing shock jocks in the United States (e.g., Alex Jones) or the anonymous "Q" behind the QAnon conspiracy theory. Conspiracy theories, unlike paranoia, therefore very often have a specific and easily identified political goal. It is not hard to imagine who benefits from the idea that the 2012 Sandy Hook Elementary School shooting was faked or from the idea that the 2020 U.S. presidential election was rigged.

Vectors are clearly important in the transmission of beliefs, and people who can master the most efficient vectors of their time are likely to be rewarded by seeing their beliefs proliferated far and wide. One part of Martin Luther's genius, after he nailed his 95 Theses onto the door of the chapel of Wittenberg Cathedral in 1517, was that he was able to exploit the latest transmission technology—the printing press—so that his ideas could be rapidly conveyed in pamphlets across Europe, eventually triggering the Protestant Reformation (Pettegree 2015). The Nazis were particularly adept at using radio propaganda in prewar Germany and continued to use it to consolidate their support and spread their anti-Semitic ideas once they had gained power (Adena et al. 2015). Today, of course, for better or worse, we have the internet; after Twitter conducted a purge of millions of suspected bot (automatic propaganda) accounts in 2018, a survey of elected representatives in European national parliaments found that far-right politicians experienced the greatest loss of Twitter followers (Silva and Proksch 2021), so it was pretty obvious which end of the political spectrum was making the most use of social media bots, perhaps the most efficient vector of all time.

An efficient vector can sometimes facilitate the accidental transmission of an idea, leading to what looks like an episode of mass delusion. For example, in April 1954, in Seattle, Washington, there was considerable public concern about small pits that citizens had begun to notice in the windshields of their cars. Because this occurred shortly after a series of U.S. nuclear tests in the Pacific, residents worried that these pits could have been caused by nuclear fallout, a hypothesis that was widely discussed in local newspapers, causing considerable alarm. Eventually, concern at the state and national levels (the U.S. president, Dwight D. Eisenhower, was consulted) led to a scientific inquiry that revealed there was nothing unusual about the small windshield blemishes, which usually went unnoticed. A subsequent survey revealed that most Seattle residents had first heard of the blemishes through local newspaper reports (Medalia and Larsen 1958). Presumably, once informed of the mysterious and possibly fallout-related windshield pits, the good people of Seattle inspected their cars and discovered blemishes that had always been there.

The question of fit between belief systems and the receiving person mainly concerns the extent to which the beliefs address the receiver's existential concerns. It will not have escaped most readers' notice that master interpretive systems, and the fundamental beliefs and nonpropositional processes that underlie them, all carry significance for our ability to cope with the great challenges of life, such as how to live a life that is rewarding, free of danger, and meaningful and how to maintain our status in a society of our peers while protecting ourselves and those we love from threats from outside our group. That this is so should not be a surprise; our passage through life is inherently subject to risks and hazards, and, unlike animals, we are blessed (if indeed it is a blessing) with the ability to describe and contemplate these challenges, including the fact that our lifetimes are finite (Becker 1973). Hence, existential concerns have been either explicitly or implicitly highlighted in theoretical accounts of religious beliefs (Willer 2009), political ideologies (Solomon et al. 2015), and conspiracy theories (Douglas et al. 2017) and, as we saw earlier in the subsection "Delusions of Psychiatric Patients," seem to explain the most common delusional themes observed in psychiatric patients.

The rapid proliferation of master interpretive systems will therefore depend on the extent to which contextual factors activate these concerns; as the well-known aphorism goes, "There are no atheists in foxholes" (Jong et al. 2012). Nongqawuse's 1856 prophecy that killing their cattle would help the Xhosa defeat the British in the Eastern Cape was no doubt made especially salient by the fact that the nation had already experienced a series of defeats by the white settlers and was also under threat from a lungworm epidemic that was crippling their herds (Peires 1989). Studies have shown that anxiety-provoking situations (Grzesiak-Feldman 2013) or the experience that life is uncontrollable (van Prooijen and Acker 2015) leads to a greater willingness to believe in conspiracy theories, so it is perhaps not surprising that the stab-in-the-back myth was facilitated by the sense of humiliation felt by the German people following their defeat by the Allied powers in the First World War and the economic difficulties that ensued (Evans 2021). More recently, it has been shown that people with authoritarian tendencies feel moved to vote for populist leaders, such as Trump in the United States and Marine Le Pen in France, or for populist policies, such as Brexit, only if they feel that their values are threatened (Stenner and Haidt 2018).

One type of existential threat that seems particularly powerful and yet difficult to avoid is awareness of our mortality. It is perhaps unsurprising that death anxiety is associated with religiosity, although the relationship may be complex and nonlinear (Jong et al. 2018), possibly accounted for by religion having a soothing effect in strong believers (Jong et al. 2013). Death anxiety has also been reported to be associated with paranormal and conservative beliefs (Tobacyk 2007; Wong 2012) and, interestingly, the severity of mental illness in psychiatric patients (Menzies et al. 2019). A considerable volume of work by social psychologists under the rubric of terror management theory has explored the effects of deliberately manipulating thoughts about death in laboratory experiments (Solomon et al. 2015); the general finding is that asking people to think about what it will be like to die leads not only to increased support for preexisting political ideologies but also to a shift toward the right end of the political spectrum (Burke et al. 2013) (although readers should be aware of some concerns about the replicability of these findings; Klein et al. 2022).

Of course, belief entrepreneurs often know how to exploit existential anxieties. Authoritarians, in particular, know that highlighting threats to normative values (e.g., the possibility of being "swamped" by migrants from other cultures) helps them to win votes. It is therefore no accident that populists at different times in history (e.g., Hitler in Germany, Slobodan Milošević in Serbia, and Trump in the United States) have often made the same promises to voters: to make their country great again, to regain control (often by revoking international treaties), and to keep out the culturally and ethnically different (Ben-Giat 2020). Depressingly, this seems to be a very effective formula.

Finally, someone who is exposed to a belief does not necessarily have to adopt it. The term *slow thinking* (sometimes called *analytic reasoning*) was introduced by Daniel Kahneman (2012) to describe the kind of thoughtful deliberation that allows people to decide whether something they have been told is reasonable. This style of thinking is easy to measure using simple puzzles (Frederick 2005), and individuals vary considerably in their propensity to indulge in this kind of reasoning. Some people, it seems, will believe a message as long as it is consistent with their existing worldview, whereas others think very carefully before accepting it.

It is intuitively obvious that good analytic reasoning should immunize people against bizarre theories. Most conspiracy theories do not survive the common sense test. For example, 46,000 people worked for NASA during the Moon landings, so if those landings were faked, all of those people would have to have been telling the same lie for a very long time; arguably, it would have been easier to go to the Moon (Aaranovitch 2009). A large number of studies have attempted to test the idea that good analytic reasoning is protective against belief in conspiracy theories by measuring slow thinking in relation to a wide range of belief systems. Poor analytic reasoning is associated with religiosity and belief in the paranormal (Pennycook et al. 2012, 2016), conspiracy theories (Swami et al. 2014), and an inability to spot fake news (Bronstein et al. 2019) or "pseudo-profound bullshit" (Pennycook et al. 2015). It has also recently been suggested that impaired analytic reasoning might be important in psychosis and delusions (Ward and Garety 2019), but the empirical studies carried out to date have produced mixed results. For example, Freeman et al. (2012, 2014) found that self-reported "intuitive thinking" was associated with paranoia in nonclinical samples but not in psychiatric patients. More recently, in a study that controlled for the covariation between paranoia and conspiracy theories in a large population sample, Alsuhibani et al. (2022) found that poor analytic reasoning was much more closely associated with the latter. This finding might seem surprising given the widespread assumption that the abnormal beliefs of psychiatric patients must reflect an impairment in thinking. However, perhaps it will seem less so when I explain the most important implication of this account of belief propagation for understanding delusions. This implication can be stated very simply: *Delusions do not propagate.*

Conclusion

In this chapter I have examined various attempts to distinguish between pathological and normal beliefs, noting that many proposals that have been made by psychopathologists in the past have failed to draw a clear line between the bizarre beliefs observed in the psychiatric wards and the madness of crowds. A common failure in all of these endeavors has been to underestimate the complexity of normal beliefs. For example, phenomenological researchers have assumed that the subtle characteristics they have identified in association with delusional thinking are absent in normal belief systems, but this is not the case. Many psychological researchers, by contrast, have simply focused on the content of beliefs without considering the dynamic ways that they are formed and linked to one another. An important implication of the wide range of research that I have considered here is that there is much that is inherently *social* about believing. Beliefs usually do not happen in isolation but are formed in the course of our relationships with other people.

This has led me to highlight one way in which delusions seem to differ from other types of belief systems: they do not propagate. The standard psychiatric way of describing this characteristic is to say that they are idiosyncratic, but what makes them idiosyncratic is that they are generally not formed in discussion with other people and do not get passed from one person to another. Deluded patients on psychiatric wards do not acquire their beliefs from conversations with other people, and they do not form societies to finesse their delusional doctrines or develop schemes to ensure that other people see the world as they do. There are no paranoia entrepreneurs. Why this is the case is, frankly, not known, but it is not difficult to speculate about possible explanations. Broadly, the factors that might be responsible fall into two types: features of the social world in which the deluded patient lives and abnormalities in the psychological mechanisms that sustain negotiation and belief sharing with other people.

With regard to the social world of the patient, one factor known to affect individuals' judgments about the certainty of their beliefs is consensus—among most ordinary people, a belief is judged to be more likely to be true if it is shared by others (Clarkson et al. 2013). Social isolation might therefore make it difficult for individuals to estimate the degree of consensus around their beliefs and, conceivably, lead to the acceptance of bizarre beliefs that might otherwise, before they became too rigidly developed, be rejected after discussion with others. There is considerable evidence that people with psychosis or with psychotic traits tend to be lonely and to have impoverished social networks, with some evidence that social isolation often precedes the onset of psychosis (Gayer-Anderson and Morgan 2013). Consistent with the idea that lack of social contact may facilitate the onset of delusions, epidemiological studies have found that people who are more isolated (e.g., because they lack friendships or people to communicate with) are much more likely to report positive symptoms, especially paranoid beliefs (Butter et al. 2017), and that lack of identification (the sense of belonging to groups) is also a risk factor for these kinds of beliefs (McIntyre et al. 2018). However, against the social isolation hypothesis, once patients are ill, the severity of positive symptoms does not seem to be related to social network characteristics (Degnan et al. 2018). Moreover, it is difficult to imagine that most deluded patients are unaware that their beliefs are not shared by others. A further complication when understanding the relationship between isolation and delusions is that any apparent association might be the consequence of reverse causation—people who express beliefs that seem crazy might find that their friends start to shun them.

The other possibility is that delusions are facilitated and maintained by impairments in the psychological processes that are responsible for belief sharing. Anthropologists (Boyer et al. 2015) and evolutionary psychologists (Sutcliffe et al. 2012) have argued that human beings have evolved complex psychological mechanisms that enable us to establish coalitions with others. Bell et al. (2021) recently argued that abnormalities in these kinds of mechanisms might explain why delusions are typically social in content. As they pointed out, the majority of psychological research directed toward understanding delusions has assumed that they arise from a failure of reason. Researchers have therefore tried to identify cognitive and emotional abnormalities that could explain this failure. An important implication of the evidence reviewed here is that when these mechanisms are examined, delusions do not seem to be very different from other kinds of organized belief systems. Perhaps instead of assuming that delusions are a consequence of cognitive failures, we should consider whether they arise from some kind of disruption of the processes involved in sustaining social relations.

Questions for Discussion

1. Are all religious beliefs, some religious beliefs, or no religious beliefs delusional?

2. In everyday life, how do we know how certain we are about something we believe? Is certainty a feeling?

3. Can you devise a set of criteria that would allow you to reliably distinguish between paranoid delusions and conspiracy theories?

4. If you wanted to change someone's political beliefs, how would you go about it? Would your approach be different from that taken when conducting therapy with a patient who has paranoid delusions?

5. Why are delusional beliefs not passed from one person to another? Can you conceive of a situation in which they might be?

KEY POINTS

- It has proven difficult to discover criteria that distinguish between the delusions of psychiatric patients and nonpathological but bizarre beliefs (the madness of crowds). Although *belief* is a central and indispensable concept in the social sciences, there is no coherent theory of human beliefs that could assist us in developing the required criteria.

- Human beliefs consist of language-based propositions that are sometimes organized into complex systems (e.g., religious and political ideologies, conspiracy theories), in which case they tend to be rigid and resistant to contradiction.

- Beliefs are transmittable between individuals, and the process by which transmission occurs can be broken down into components analogous to those involved in the transmission of a virus. One way in which delusions are unique is that they are not shared with others.

References

Aaranovitch D: Voodoo Histories: The Role of the Conspiracy Theory in Shaping Modern History. New York, Penguin Group, 2009

Aarøe A, Petersen MB, Arceneaux K: The behavioral immune system shapes political intuitions: why and how individual differences in disgust sensitivity underlie opposition to immigration. Am Polit Sci Rev 111:277–294, 2017

Abraham K: Notes on the psychoanalytic investigation and treatment of manic depressive insanity (1911), in Selected Papers of Karl Abraham, M.D. Translated by Bryan D, Strachey A. Edited by Jones E. London, Hogarth, 1927, pp 137–156

Adena M, Enikolopov R, Petrova M, et al: Radio and the rise of the Nazis in prewar Germany. Q J Econ 130(4):1885–1939, 2015

Adorno TW, Frenkel-Brunswik E, Levinson DJ, Sanford RN: The Authoritarian Personality. New York, Harper & Row, 1950

Allnutt S, Samuels A, O'Driscoll C: The insanity defence: from wild beasts to M'Naghten. Australas Psychiatry 15(4):292–298, 2007 17612881

Alsuhibani A, Shevlin M, Freeman D, et al: Why conspiracy theorists are not always paranoid: conspiracy theories and paranoia form separate factors with distinct psychological predictors. PLoS One 17(4):e0259053, 2022 35389988

Alter AL, Oppenheimer DM: Uniting the tribes of fluency to form a metacognitive nation. Pers Soc Psychol Rev 13(3):219–235, 2009 19638628

American Psychiatric Association: Diagnostic and Statistical Manual of Mental Disorders, 4th Edition. Washington, DC, American Psychiatric Association, 1994

American Psychiatric Association: Diagnostic and Statistical Manual of Mental Disorders, 5th Edition, Text Revision. Washington, DC, American Psychiatric Association, 2022

Atran S: The trouble with memes: inference versus imitation in cultural creation. Hum Nat 12(4):351–381, 2001 26192412

Ayeni OB, Ayenibiowo KO, Ayeni EA: Religiosity as correlates of some selected psychological disorders among psychiatric outpatients in Lagos State. IFE PsychologIA 19:114–128, 2011

Azhar MZ, Varma SL, Hakim HR: Phenomenological differences of delusions between schizophrenic patients of two cultures of Malaysia. Singapore Med J 36(3):273–275, 1995 8553090

Balzan RP: Overconfidence in psychosis: the foundation of delusional conviction? Cogent Psychol 3(1):1135855, 2016

Barden J, Petty RE: The mere perception of elaboration creates attitude certainty: exploring the thoughtfulness heuristic. J Pers Soc Psychol 95(3):489–509, 2008 18729690

Bebbington P, Nayani T: The Psychosis Screening Questionnaire. Int J Methods Psychiatr Res 5:11–19, 1995

Beck AT: Cognitive models of depression. J Cogn Psychother 1:5–37, 1987

Becker E: The Denial of Death. New York, Free Press, 1973

Bell V, Halligan PW, Ellis HD: Diagnosing delusions: a review of inter-rater reliability. Schizophr Res 86(1–3):76–79, 2006 16857345

Bell V, Raihani N, Wilkinson S: Clin Psychol Sci 9(1):24–37, 2021 33552704

Bénabou R, Tirole J: Belief in a just world and redistributive politics. Q J Econ 121:669–746, 2006

Ben-Giat R: Strongmen: How They Rise, Why They Succeed, How They Fall. London, Profile Books, 2020

Bentall RP: The illusion of reality: a review and integration of psychological research on hallucinations. Psychol Bull 107(1):82–95, 1990 2404293

Bentall RP: Madness Explained: Psychosis and Human Nature. New York, Penguin, 2003

Bentall RP: Delusions and other beliefs, in Delusions in Context. Edited by Bortolotti L. London, Palgrave Macmillan, 2018, pp 67–96

Bentall RP, Corcoran R, Howard R, et al: Persecutory delusions: a review and theoretical integration. Clin Psychol Rev 21(8):1143–1192, 2001 11702511

Berrios G: Delusions as "wrong beliefs": a conceptual history. Br J Psychiatry Suppl (14):6–13, 1991 1840782

Blackmore S: The Meme Machine. New York, Oxford University Press, 1999

Bortolotti L, Broome M: A role for ownership and authorship in the analysis of thought insertion. Phenomenol Cogn Sci 8:205–224, 2008

Bovet P, Parnas J: Schizophrenic delusions: a phenomenological approach. Schizophr Bull 19(3):579–597, 1993 8235460

Boyd T, Gumley A: An experiential perspective on persecutory paranoia: a grounded theory construction. Psychol Psychother 80(Pt 1):1–22, 2007

Boyer P, Firat R, van Leeuwen F: Safety, threat, and stress in intergroup relations: a coalitional index model. Perspect Psychol Sci 10(4):434–450, 2015 26177946

Brewerton TD: Hyperreligiosity in psychotic disorders. J Nerv Ment Dis 182(5):302–304, 1994 10678313

Bronstein MV, Pennycook G, Bear A, et al: Belief in fake news is associated with delusionality, dogmatism, religious fundamentalism, and reduced analytic thinking. J Appl Res Mem Cogn 8:108–117, 2019

Broome MR, Harland R, Owen GS, Stringaris A (eds): The Maudsley Reader in Phenomenological Psychiatry. Cambridge, UK, Cambridge University Press, 2012

Brotherton R: Suspicious Minds: Why We Believe Conspiracy Theories. London, Bloomsbury, 2015

Brotherton R, French CC, Pickering AD: Measuring belief in conspiracy theories: the Generic Conspiracist Beliefs Scale. Front Psychol 4:279, 2013 23734136

Bruder M, Haffke P, Neave N, et al: Measuring individual differences in generic beliefs in conspiracy theories across cultures: conspiracy mentality questionnaire. Front Psychol 4:225, 2013 23641227

Burke BL, Kosloff S, Landau MJ: Death goes to the polls: a meta-analysis of mortality salience effects on political attitudes. Polit Psychol 34(2):183–200, 2013

Butter S, Murphy J, Shevlin M, Houston J: Social isolation and psychosis-like experiences: a UK general population analysis. Psychosis 9:291–300, 2017

Cassam Q: Conspiracy Theories. Cambridge, UK, Polity Press, 2019

Cermolacce M, Sass L, Parnas J: What is bizarre in bizarre delusions? A critical review. Schizophr Bull 36(4):667–679, 2010 20142381

Chadwick PK: Delusional thinking from the inside: paranoia and personal growth, in Persecutory Delusions: Assessment, Theory and Treatment. Edited by Freeman D, Bentall RP, Garety P. Oxford, UK, Oxford University Press, 2008, pp 3–19

Cichocka A, Marchlewska M, de Zavala AG: Does self-love or self-hate predict conspiracy beliefs? Narcissism, self-esteem, and endorsement of conspiracy theories. Soc Psychol Personal Sci 7:157–166, 2016

Clarkson JJ, Tormala ZL, Rucker DD, Dugan RG: The malleable influence of social consensus on attitude certainty. J Exp Soc Psychol 49(6):1019–1022, 2013

Clifton JDW, Baker JD, Park CL, et al: Primal world beliefs. Psychol Assess 31(1):82–99, 2019 30299119

Colbert SM, Peters ER, Garety PA: Delusions and belief flexibility in psychosis. Psychol Psychother 83(Pt 1):45–57, 2010 19712542

Collin S, Rowse G, Martinez A, Bentall RP: The prevalence of delusional themes in clinical groups: a systematic review and meta-analyses of the global literature. submitted to Clin Psychol Rev, 2022

Colunga E, Smith LB: From the lexicon to expectations about kinds: a role for associative learning. Psychol Rev 112(2):347–382, 2005 15783290

Connors MH, Halligan PW: Phenomenology, delusions, and belief. Lancet Psychiatry 8(4):272–273, 2021 33743872

Conrad K: Beginning schizophrenia: attempt for a Gestalt-analysis of delusion (1958), in The Maudsley Reader in Phenomenological Psychiatry. Edited by Broome MR, Harland R, Owen GS, Stringaris A. Cambridge, UK, Cambridge University Press, 2012, pp 176–193

Converse P: The nature of belief systems in mass publics (1964). Critical Review 18:1–74, 2006

Corlett P: Delusions and prediction error, in Delusions in Context. Edited by Bortolotti L. London, Palgrave Macmillan, 2018, pp 35–66

Darwin H, Neave N, Holmes J: Belief in conspiracy theories: the role of paranormal belief, paranoid ideation and schizotypy. Pers Individ Dif 50:1289–1293, 2011

Dawkins R: The Selfish Gene. New York, Oxford University Press, 1976

Dayan P, Abbott LF: Theoretical Neuroscience: Computational and Mathematical Modeling of Neural Systems. Cambridge, MA, MIT Press, 2005

Dean CE, Akhtar S, Gale TM, et al: Development of the Paranormal and Supernatural Beliefs Scale using classical and modern test theory. BMC Psychol 9(1):98, 2021 34162430

Degnan A, Berry K, Sweet D, et al: Social networks and symptomatic and functional outcomes in schizophrenia: a systematic review and meta-analysis. Soc Psychiatry Psychiatr Epidemiol 53(9):873–888, 2018 29951929

Dennett DC: Consciousness Explained. London, Allen Lane, 1991

Douglas KM, Sutton RM, Cichocka A: The psychology of conspiracy theories. Curr Dir Psychol Sci 26(6):538–542, 2017 29276345

Dunning D, Leuenberger A, Sherman DA: A new look at motivated inference: are self-serving theories of success a product of motivational forces? J Pers Soc Psychol 69:58–68, 1995

Edwards D, Potter JP: Discursive Psychology. Thousand Oaks, CA, Sage, 1992

Ehrlinger J, Johnson K, Banner M, et al: Why the unskilled are unaware: further explorations of (absent) self-insight among the incompetent. Organ Behav Hum Decis Process 105(1):98–121, 2008 19568317

Elahi A, Perez Algorta G, Varese F, et al: Do paranoid delusions exist on a continuum with subclinical paranoia? A multi-method taxometric study. Schizophr Res 190:77–81, 2017 28318838

Ellett L, Schlier B, Kingston JL, et al: Pandemic paranoia in the general population: international prevalence and sociodemographic profile. Psychol Med Sep 6:1–8, 2022 36065655 Epub ahead of print

El Sendiony MF: Cultural aspects of delusions: a psychiatric study of Egypt. Aust N Z J Psychiatry 10(2):201–207, 1976 1067839

Enoch MD, Trethowan WH: Uncommon Psychiatric Syndromes, 2nd Edition. Bristol, UK, John Wright, 1979

Evans RJ: The Hitler Conspiracies: The Third Reich and the Paranoid Imagination. New York, Penguin, 2021

Feldman S, Johnston C: Understanding the determinants of political ideology: implications of structural complexity. Polit Psychol 35(4):337–358, 2014

Fernyhough C: The Voices Within. London, Profile Books, 2016

Feyaerts J, Henricksen MG, Vanheule S, et al: Delusions beyond beliefs: a critical overview of diagnostic, aetiological, and therapeutic schizophrenia research from a clinical-phenomenological perspective. Lancet Psychiatry 8(3):237–249, 2021

Frederick S: Cognitive reflection and decision making. J Econ Perspect 19:25–42, 2005

Freeman D: Persecutory delusions: a cognitive perspective on understanding and treatment. Lancet Psychiatry 3(7):685–692, 2016 27371990

Freeman D, Garety PA: Comments on the content of persecutory delusions: does the definition need clarification? Br J Clin Psychol 39(4):407–414, 2000 11107494

Freeman D, Garety PA, Bebbington PE, et al: Psychological investigation of the structure of paranoia in a non-clinical population. Br J Psychiatry 186:427–435, 2005 15863749

Freeman D, Evans N, Lister R: Gut feelings, deliberative thought, and paranoid ideation: a study of experiential and rational reasoning. Psychiatry Res 197(1–2):119–122, 2012 22406393

Freeman D, Lister R, Evans N: The use of intuitive and analytic reasoning styles by patients with persecutory delusions. J Behav Ther Exp Psychiatry 45(4):454–458, 2014 25000504

Frith C: Explaining delusions of control: the comparator model 20 years on. Conscious Cogn 21(1):52–54, 2012 21802318

Gallagher S: Relationship between agency and ownership in the case of schizophrenic thought insertion and delusions of control. Rev Philos Psychol 6:865–879, 2015

Galliford N, Furnham A: Individual difference factors and beliefs in medical and political conspiracy theories. Scand J Psychol 58(5):422–428, 2017 28782805

Gayer-Anderson C, Morgan C: Social networks, support and early psychosis: a systematic review. Epidemiol Psychiatr Sci 22(2):131–146, 2013 22831843

Georgaca E: Reality and discourse: a critical analysis of the category of "delusions." Br J Med Psychol 73(Pt 2):227–242, 2000 10874481

Gipps RGT, Rhodes JE: Delusions and the non-epistemic foundations of belief. Philos Psychiatr Psychol 18(1):89–97, 2011

Green CEL, Freeman D, Kuipers E, et al: Measuring ideas of persecution and social reference: the Green et al. Paranoid Thought Scales (GPTS). Psychol Med 38(1):101–111, 2008 17903336

Gregg AP, Mahadevan N, Sedikides C: The SPOT effect: people spontaneously prefer their own theories. Q J Exp Psychol (Hove) 70(6):996–1010, 2017 26836058

Grzesiak-Feldman M: The effect of high-anxiety situations on conspiracy thinking. Curr Psychol 32:100–118, 2013

Haidt J: The Righteous Mind: Why Good People Are Divided by Politics and Religion. New York, Penguin, 2013

Haidt J, Rozin P, McCauley C, Imada S: Body, psyche, and culture: the relationship of disgust to morality. Psychol Dev Soc J 9:107–131, 1997

Hardy A: The Spiritual Nature of Man: A Study of Contemporary Religious Experience. New York, Oxford University Press, 1979

Haselton MG, Nettle D: The paranoid optimist: an integrative evolutionary model of cognitive biases. Pers Soc Psychol Rev 10(1):47–66, 2006 16430328

Heinämaa S, Taipale J: Normality, in The Oxford Handbook of Phenomenological Psychopathology. Edited by Stanghellini G, Broome MR, Fernandez AV, et al. New York, Oxford University Press, 2018, pp 284–297

Hibbing JR, Smith KB, Alford JR: Differences in negativity bias underlie variations in political ideology. Behav Brain Sci 37(3):297–307, 2014 24970428

Hinson EG: Confessions of creeds in early Christian tradition. Review and Expositor 76:5–16, 1979

Hoenig J: Kurt Schneider and anglophone psychiatry. Compr Psychiatry 23(5):391–400, 1982 6754244

Hofstadter R: The paranoid style in American politics. Harper's Magazine, November 1964, 77–86

Holland T: In the Shadow of the Sword: The Battle for Global Empire and the End of the Ancient World. Boston, MA, Little, Brown, 2012

Hornsey MJ, Fielding KS: Attitude roots and jiu jitsu persuasion: understanding and overcoming the motivated rejection of science. Am Psychol 72(5):459–473, 2017 28726454

Huddy L, Sears DO, Levy JS (eds): The Oxford Handbook of Political Psychology, 2nd Edition. New York, Oxford University Press, 2013

Hylwa SA, Bury JE, Davis MDP, et al: Delusional infestation, including delusions of parasitosis: results of histologic examination of skin biopsy and patient-provided skin specimens. Arch Dermatol 147(9):1041–1045, 2011 21576554

Imhoff R, Lamberty PK: Too special to be duped: need for uniqueness motivates conspiracy beliefs. Eur J Soc Psychol 47:724–734, 2017

Imhoff R, Lamberty P: How paranoid are conspiracy believers? Toward a more fine-grained understanding of the connect and disconnect between paranoia and belief in conspiracy theories. Eur J Soc Psychol 48(7):909–926, 2018

Isham L, Griffith L, Boylan AM, et al: Understanding, treating, and renaming grandiose delusions: a qualitative study. Psychol Psychother 94(1):119–140, 2019 31785077

Jackson M, Fulford KWM: Spiritual experience and psychopathology. Philos Psychiatr Psychol 4(1):41–65, 1997

James W: Principles of Psychology, Vol 1. New York, Holt, 1893

Jaspers K: General Psychopathology (1913). Translated by Hoenig J, Hamilton MW. Manchester, UK, Manchester University Press, 1963

Jong J, Halberstadt J, Bluemke M: Foxhole atheism, revisited: the effects of mortality salience on explicit and implicit religious belief. J Exp Soc Psychol 48:983–989, 2012

Jong J, Bluemke M, Halberstadt J: Fear of death and supernatural beliefs: developing a new Supernatural Belief Scale to test the relationship. Eur J Pers 27:495–506, 2013

Jong J, Ross R, Philip T, et al: The religious correlates of death anxiety: a systematic review and meta-analysis. Religion Brain Behav 8:4–20, 2018

Jose PE, Brewer WF: Development of story liking: character identification, suspense, and outcome resolution. Dev Psychol 20:911–924, 1984

Jost JT, Federico CM, Napier JL: Political ideology: its structure, functions, and elective affinities. Annu Rev Psychol 60:307–337, 2009 19035826

Kahneman D: Thinking, Fast and Slow. New York, Penguin, 2012

Kendler KS, Glazer WM, Morgenstern H: Dimensions of delusional experience. Am J Psychiatry 140(4):466–469, 1983 6837787

Klein R, Cook C, Ebersole C, et al: Many Labs 4: failure to replicate mortality salience effect with and without original author involvement. Collabra: Psychology 8(1):35271, 2022

Klosterkötter J, Hellmich M, Steinmeyer EM, Schultze-Lutter F: Diagnosing schizophrenia in the initial prodromal phase. Arch Gen Psychiatry 58(2):158–164, 2001 11177117

Knowles R, McCarthy-Jones S, Rowse G: Grandiose delusions: a review and theoretical integration of cognitive and affective perspectives. Clin Psychol Rev 31(4):684–696, 2011 21482326

Koriat A: The feeling of knowing: some metatheoretical implications for consciousness and control. Conscious Cogn 9(2 Pt 1):149–171, 2000 10924234

Koriat A: The self-consistency model of subjective confidence. Psychol Rev 119(1):80–113, 2012 22022833

Krakauer J: Under the Banner of Heaven: A Story of Violent Faith. New York, Doubleday, 2003

Kucharski A: The Rules of Contagion: Why Things Spread—And Why They Stop. London, Profile Books, 2020

Leff JP, Fischer M, Bertelsen A: A cross-national epidemiological study of mania. Br J Psychiatry 129:428–442, 1976 990656

Lerner MJ: Belief in a Just World: A Fundamental Delusion. New York, Springer, 1980

Lewis M: The Big Short: Inside the Doomsday Machine. New York, WW Norton, 2010

Liddell HS: The experimental neurosis. Annu Rev Physiol 9:569–580, 1947 20288843

Lincoln TM: Relevant dimensions of delusions: continuing the continuum versus category debate. Schizophr Res 93(1–3):211–220, 2007 17398072

Lindeman M, Svedholm-Häkkinen AM: Does poor understanding of physical world predict religious and paranormal beliefs? Appl Cogn Psychol 30:736–742, 2016

Lodge M, Taber CS: The Rationalizing Voter. Cambridge, UK, Cambridge University Press, 2013

Mackay C: Memoirs of Extraordinary Popular Delusions and the Madness of Crowds: A Study in Crowd Psychology, Vols 1–3. London, Richard Bentley, 1841

Malahy LW, Rubinlicht MA, Kaiser CR: Justifying inequality: a cross-temporal investigation of U.S. income disparities and just-world beliefs from 1973 to 2006. Soc Justice Res 22:369–383, 2009

Mancosu M, Vassallo S, Vezzoni C: Believing in conspiracy theories: evidence from an exploratory analysis of Italian survey data. South Eur Soc Polit 22:327–344, 2017

Martinez A, Shevlin M, Valiente C, et al: Paranoid beliefs and conspiracy mentality are associated with different forms of mistrust: a three-nation study. Front Psychol 13:1023366 2022 36329737

McCauley RN, Graham G: Hearing Voices and Other Matters of the Mind. New York, Oxford University Press, 2020

McIntosh CN, Fischer DG: Beck's cognitive triad: one versus three factors. Can J Behav Sci 32(3):153–157, 2000

McIntyre JC, Wickham S, Barr B, Bentall RP: Social identity and psychosis: associations and psychological mechanisms. Schizophr Bull 44(3):681–690, 2018 28981888

McKay R: Delusional inference. Mind Lang 27(3):330–355, 2012

McKay RT, Dennett DC: The evolution of misbelief. Behav Brain Sci 32(6):493–510, discussion 510–561, 2009 20105353

Medalia NZ, Larsen O: Diffusion and belief in a collective delusion: the Seattle windshield pitting epidemic. Am Sociol Rev 23:180–186, 1958

Melle I: The Breivik case and what psychiatrists can learn from it. World Psychiatry 12(1):16–21, 2013 23471788

Menzies RE, Sharpe L, Dar-Nimrod I: The relationship between death anxiety and severity of mental illnesses. Br J Clin Psychol 58(4):452–467, 2019 31318066

Mineka S, Kihlstrom JF: Unpredictable and uncontrollable events: a new perspective on experimental neurosis. J Abnorm Psychol 87(2):256–271, 1978 565795

Mishara AL: Klaus Conrad (1905–1961): delusional mood, psychosis, and beginning schizophrenia. Schizophr Bull 36(1):9–13, 2010 19965934

Moritz S, Göritz AS, Gallinat J, et al: Subjective competence breeds overconfidence in errors in psychosis: a hubris account of paranoia. J Behav Ther Exp Psychiatry 48:118–124, 2015 25817242

Moutoussis M, Williams J, Dayan P, Bentall RP: Persecutory delusions and the conditioned avoidance paradigm: towards an integration of the psychology and biology of paranoia. Cogn Neuropsychiatry 12(6):495–510, 2007 17978936

Mullen R: The problem of bizarre delusions. J Nerv Ment Dis 191(8):546–548, 2003 12972859

Munro A: Monosymptomatic hypochondriacal psychosis manifesting as delusions of parasitosis: a description of four cases successfully treated with pimozide. Arch Dermatol 114(6):940–943, 1978 666333

Newheiser A-K, Farias M, Tausch N: The functional nature of conspiracy beliefs: examining the underpinnings of belief in the Da Vinci Code conspiracy. Pers Individ Dif 51:1007–1011, 2011

Norenzayan A, Gervais WM: The origins of religious disbelief. Trends Cogn Sci 17(1):20–25, 2013 23246230

Oltmanns TF, Maher BA (eds): Delusional Beliefs. Hoboken, NJ, Wiley, 1988

Ong WJ: Orality and Literacy: The Technologizing of the Word. London, Routledge, 1982

Parnas J: The Breivik case and "conditio psychiatrica." World Psychiatry 12(1):22–23, 2013 23471789

Pearce JM: Animal Learning and Cognition: An Introduction. London, Psychology Press, 2008

Peires JB: The Dead Will Arise: Nongqawuse and the Great Xhosa Cattle-Killing Movement of 1856–7. Bloomington, Indiana University Press, 1989

Pennycook G, Cheyne JA, Seli P, et al: Analytic cognitive style predicts religious and paranormal belief. Cognition 123(3):335–346, 2012 22481051

Pennycook G, Cheyne JA, Barr N, et al: On the reception and detection of pseudo-profound bullshit. Judgm Decis Mak 10:549–563, 2015

Pennycook G, Ross RM, Koehler DJ, Fugelsang JA: Atheists and agnostics are more reflective than religious believers: four empirical studies and a meta-analysis. PLoS One 11(4):e0153039, 2016 27054566

Peters E, Day S, McKenna J, Orbach G: Delusional ideation in religious and psychotic populations. Br J Clin Psychol 38(1):83–96, 1999a 10212739

Peters ER, Joseph SA, Garety PA: Measurement of delusional ideation in the normal population: introducing the PDI (Peters et al. Delusions Inventory). Schizophr Bull 25(3):553–576, 1999b 10478789

Pettegree A: Brand Luther: How an Unheralded Monk Turned His Small Town Into a Center of Publishing, Made Himself the Most Famous Man in Europe—and Started the Protestant Reformation. New York, Penguin, 2015

Picardi A, Fonzi L, Pallagrosi M, et al: Delusional themes across affective and non-affective psychoses. Front Psychiatry 9:132, 2018 29674982

Pigliucci M: Nonsense on Stilts: How to Tell Science From Bunk, 2nd Edition. Chicago, IL, University of Chicago Press, 2018

Rhodes J, Gipps RGT: Delusions, certainty and the background. Philos Psychiatr Psychol 15(4):295–310, 2008

Roose K: What is QAnon, the viral pro-Trump conspiracy theory? New York Times, October 19, 2020

Ross RM, McKay R: Why is belief in God not a delusion. Religion Brain Behav 7:316–319, 2017

Rubin Z, Peplau LA: Who believes in a just world? J Soc Issues 31:65–90, 1975

Russell KJ, Hand CJ: Rape myth acceptance, victim blame attribution and just world beliefs: a rapid evidence assessment. Aggress Violent Behav 37:153–160, 2017

Sartre J-P: Anti-Semite and Jew. New York, Schocken Books, 1948

Schlenker BR, Chambers JR, Le BM: Conservatives are happier than liberals, but why? Political ideology, personality, and life satisfaction. J Res Pers 46:127–146, 2012

Schneider K: Clinical Psychopathology. New York, Grune & Stratton, 1959

Schwitzgebel E: Belief, in The Stanford Encyclopedia of Philosophy. Stanford, CA, Stanford Center for the Study of Language and Information, 2015. Available at: https://plato.stanford.edu/archives/sum2015/entries/belief. Accessed December 12, 2021.

Shagan EH: The Birth of Modern Belief: Faith and Judgment from the Middle Ages to the Enlightenment. Princeton, NJ, Princeton University Press, 2018

Siddle R, Haddock G, Tarrier N, Faragher EB: Religious delusions in patients admitted to hospital with schizophrenia. Soc Psychiatry Psychiatr Epidemiol 37(3):130–138, 2002 11990010

Silva BC, Proksch S-E: Fake it 'til you make it: a natural experiment to identify European politicians' benefit from Twitter bots. Am Polit Sci Rev 115:316–322, 2021

Smith SM, Fabrigar LR, MacDougall BL, Wiesenthal NL: The role of amount, cognitive elaboration, and structural consistency of attitude-relevant knowledge in the formation of attitude certainty. Eur J Soc Psychol 38(2):280–295, 2007

So SH, Freeman D, Dunn G, et al: Jumping to conclusions, a lack of belief flexibility and delusional conviction in psychosis: a longitudinal investigation of the structure, frequency, and relatedness of reasoning biases. J Abnorm Psychol 121(1):129–139, 2021 21910515

Solomon S, Greenberg J, Pyszczynski T: The Worm at the Core: On the Role of Death in Life. New York, Penguin, 2015

Sperber D: Explaining Culture: A Naturalistic Approach. Oxford, UK, Blackwell, 1996

Spitzer RL, First MB, Kendler KS, Stein DJ: The reliability of three definitions of bizarre delusions. Am J Psychiatry 150(6):880–884, 1993 8494062

Startup M, Startup S: On two kinds of delusion of reference. Psychiatry Res 137(1–2):87–92, 2005 16226316

Startup M, Bucci S, Langdon R: Delusions of reference: a new theoretical model. Cogn Neuropsychiatry 14(2):110–126, 2009 19370435

Stenner K: The Authoritarian Dynamic. Cambridge, UK, Cambridge University Press, 2005

Stenner K, Haidt J: Authoritarianism is not a momentary madness, but an eternal dynamic within liberal democracies, in Can It Happen Here? Authoritarianism in America. Edited by Sunstein CR. New York, HarperCollins, 2018, pp 175–220

Stich SP: Deconstructing the Mind. New York, Oxford University Press, 1996

Sutcliffe A, Dunbar R, Binder J, Arrow H: Relationships and the social brain: integrating psychological and evolutionary perspectives. Br J Psychol 103(2):149–168, 2012 22506741

Swami V, Coles R, Stieger S, et al: Conspiracist ideation in Britain and Austria: evidence of a monological belief system and associations between individual psychological differences and real-world and fictitious conspiracy theories. Br J Psychol 102(3):443–463, 2011 21751999

Swami V, Voracek M, Stieger S, et al: Analytic thinking reduces belief in conspiracy theories. Cognition 133(3):572–585, 2014 25217762

Tedrus GMAS, Fonseca LC, Fagundes TM, da Silva GL: Religiosity aspects in patients with epilepsy. Epilepsy Behav 50:67–70, 2015 26133113

Thalbourne MA: Further studies of the measurement and correlates of belief in the paranormal. J Am Soc Psych Res 89:233–247, 1995

Tobacyk JJ: Death threat, death concerns, and paranormal belief. Death Educ 7:115–124, 2007

Tormala ZL, Rucker DD: Attitude certainty: antecedents, consequences, and new direction. Consumer Psychology Review 1:72–89, 2018

van Os J, Hanssen M, Bijl RV, Ravelli A: Strauss (1969) revisited: a psychosis continuum in the general population? Schizophr Res 45(1–2):11–20, 2000 10978868

van Prooijen J-W, Acker M: The influence of control on belief in conspiracy theories: conceptual and applied extensions. Appl Cogn Psychol 29:753–761, 2015

Verdoux H, Maurice-Tison S, Gay B, et al: A survey of delusional ideation in primary-care patients. Psychol Med 28(1):127–134, 1998 9483688

Vygotsky LS: Thought and Language. Cambridge, MA, MIT Press, 1962

Ward T, Garety PA: Fast and slow thinking in distressing delusions: a review of the literature and implications for targeted therapy. Schizophr Res 203:80–87, 2019 28927863

Westen D: The Political Brain: The Role of Emotion in Deciding the Fate of the Nation. New York, Public Affairs, 2008

Willer R: No atheists in foxholes: motivated reasoning and religious belief, in Social and Psychological Bases of Ideology and System Justification. Edited by Jost JT, Kay AC, Thorisdottir H. New York, Oxford University Press, 2009, pp 241–268

Winch P: The Idea of a Social Science and Its Relation to Philosophy. London, Routledge, 1958

Wing JK, Cooper JE, Sartorius N: The Measurement and Classification of Psychiatric Symptoms. London, Cambridge University Press, 1974

Wittgenstein L: Philosophical Investigations. Oxford, UK, Blackwell, 1953

Wittgenstein L: On Certainty. Translated by Paul D, Anscombe GEM. Edited by Anscombe GEM, von Wright GH. Oxford, UK, Blackwell, 1969

Wong SH: Does superstition help? A study of the role of superstitions and death beliefs on death anxiety amongst Chinese undergraduates in Hong Kong. Omega (Westport) 65(1):55–70, 2012 22852421

Wood MJ, Douglas KM, Sutton RM: Dead and alive: beliefs in contradictory conspiracy theories. Soc Psychol Personal Sci 3:767–773, 2012

Woodward TS, Moritz S, Menon M, Klinge R: Belief inflexibility in schizophrenia. Cogn Neuropsychiatry 13(3):267–277, 2008 18484291

Wootton D: The Invention of Science: A New History of the Scientific Revolution. New York, Allen Lane, 2015

World Health Organization: International Classification of Diseases, 11th Revision. Geneva, World Health Organization, 2018

Wu C, Shaffer DR: Susceptibility to persuasive appeals as a function of source credibility and prior experience with the attitude object. J Pers Soc Psychol 52(4):677–688, 1987

Young AW, Ellis HD, Szulecka TK, De Pauw KW: Face processing impairments and delusional misidentification. Behav Neurol 3(3):153–168, 1990 24487239

Zakay D, Tuvia R: Choice latency times as determinants of post-decisional confidence. Acta Psychol (Amst) 98:103–115, 1998

Zhu C, Sun X, So SH: Associations between belief inflexibility and dimensions of delusions: a meta-analytic review of two approaches to assessing belief flexibility. Br J Clin Psychol 57(1):59–81, 2018 28805246

2

The Lived Experience of Strongly Held Beliefs

Shaun Hunt, M.Sc., B.Sc.

Ask someone to give a definition of *paranoia* and you will generally find words such as *delusions*, *irrational*, and *unfounded* in the definition. I intend to use my own personal experience of paranoia when writing this chapter to attempt to show that, in fact, paranoid ideas have their roots in reality. When we begin to explore a person's narrative, the paranoid thoughts begin to make sense.

While living in the United Kingdom as a young man in my mid-20s, I was a talented musician on the verge of signing a recording contract with a major record label. I was playing in large venues across Europe and had radio play and interviews in the music press. I was married and had just seen the birth of my first son. From the outside my future looked bright; inside, though, a very different story was developing. It started with an element of suspicion: are people watching me and gathering information about me? Slowly but surely, little things grew into bigger things. I was making connections between people and events when there was no obvious connection. I started acting in a strange manner. I would do things like run down an alleyway and jump into an industrial bin to see if I could catch people following me. People around me (with good intentions) made things worse. They were noticing my unusual behavior and asking me, "Are you OK? You don't seem to be yourself." This only served to highlight to me that people were watching me and noticing me. My thought process on being asked these questions was, "Why are you asking? What do you want to know for? Who are you going to tell?"

I had heard voices from a young age, but these voices were generally pleasant. Around this time, though, they changed and began to encourage some of the suspicious thoughts that I was having.

I frantically tried to make sense of what was happening to me. I'd gone through several explanations in my mind, but then I finally worked it out: It was the police. They were behind everything. They were watching my every move, recruiting friends and family to gather information about my movements and hand it over to them.

The final incident was in Germany. I was just about clinging onto my sanity, mainly through the use of my music (and alcohol) to cope. I was incredibly hyperalert by this time. I was on stage playing with my band, and I noticed a man in the audience staring at me—really staring at me. Of course, you can rationalize this by thinking, "Of course he is staring at you, he has paid good money to watch you play." All rational thought had gone by this stage, though, and I got the notion that whatever it was that was going to happen with the police, it was going to happen right now in this building. So in the middle of a song, I ran off the stage, exited through the stage door, and ran and ran. Somehow, in a daze, I managed to get myself to an airport and fly home. I left thousands of pounds' worth of equipment on the stage. It was very shortly after this incident that I was admitted to a psychiatric hospital for the first time. I went on to spend the next 3 years of my life detained against my will on the ward. I was given a diagnosis of paranoid schizophrenia, and my life changed forever.

No attention was paid to my life history and my circumstances; my experiences just became meaningless symptoms of an illness. My voices became "auditory hallucinations," and my belief systems and the way that I was making sense of the world at the time became "paranoid delusions." Slowly but surely, an illness was created for me, and I was medicated on high doses of antipsychotics. The problem with this approach is that when we take a person's experiences of voices or paranoia as stand-alone things, they don't make sense. When we marry up the experiences with the person's life history (as opposed to psychiatric history), they then begin to make sense. We will never understand a person's belief systems from the outside looking in; we need to see life through that person's eyes to make sense of it.

I can look back now with the benefit of hindsight and see where some of the problems were arising. I had experienced a lot of trauma as a young child and as a teenager and had never had the opportunity to try to work through these events. When a traumatic thing happens, often we bury it as deep as we can so we don't have to deal with it, the proverbial can of worms. People often talk about not opening a can of worms, but it is my belief that this is why we have people using psychiatric services for 20, 30, 40 years. Keeping the can of worms closed certainly has not helped such people.

The thing is, a can of worms—even with a lid on—is still a can of worms, and I can recognize now that mine was beginning to rattle about that time. I did not seek or receive the help that I perhaps needed, and metaphorically speaking, I began to run away, using work and alcohol as a means of distraction. I worked a lot of antisocial hours as a sound engineer in a recording studio and played in a cover band in bars and clubs on the weekends, all on top of writing and performing for my own original band.

I can understand how, when someone presents to psychiatric care with the experiences that I was having, people may point straightaway to this being an illness. It was only when a worker began to take an interest in my past that everything began to unravel, and I told him about my childhood.

I was born in a small town and led a relatively uneventful life until I was 8 years old. It was around this time that my grandfather found out that my biological father had raped and sexually abused me on several occasions. My grandfather took me to live with him to remove me from the abuse. Shortly after I moved to live with him, it started—I began to hear voices, and I developed a strange feeling that someone was watching me. Wherever I went, whatever I was doing, someone was always watching. That feeling of being watched has never left me, even up to this day; the only thing that changes is my interpretation of it. As a young child, rather than being frightened by this, I felt quite the opposite. I felt protected, like I had a guardian angel looking out for me to keep me safe. I had never met my grandmother (she died before I was born), and I began to wonder if it was her. As there was no fear or threat involved in this feeling of being watched, it probably would not be described as paranoia, but I can certainly see that that is where it had its roots. I was very happy living with my grandfather; he was a kind, warm, and loving man. Unfortunately, when I reached age 11 my grandfather had a heart attack, and I had to return to the family home.

By this time my biological father was long gone; my mother had remarried, and the family now lived in another town. When I went to live with them, I quickly became a target for local bullies. I suffered quite severe physical harm both at school (where I was afforded no protection) and in the streets. Although the physical abuse took its toll, I think the emotional part of it was even more difficult to bear. I had no friends or allies; I could often be found walking around the edge of the playground, and no one would talk to me.

Compounding all of this was the treatment I began to receive from my stepfather. He was an incredibly violent man, but only ever to me. I have an older brother and two younger sisters, but he never laid a finger on any of them. This in itself became very confusing. Although I would have hated for anything bad to happen to my siblings, if it had been happening to them too it would have made more sense.

The feeling I had of being watched began to change. It was no longer a guardian angel; it was a feeling that someone was watching me so they could always know where I was so they would be able to harm me. I was being beaten in the streets, being beaten at school, and being beaten at home; I had no place of safety. One thing that really began to puzzle me was my mother's reaction. She did not do anything to try to stop what was happening; it was like I was not a part of the family.

Having to deal with all this at such a young age became incredibly confusing. I began to shut down emotionally, and I stopped feeling things. I'd also begun to shut down physically; when the beatings happened, I stopped feeling pain. I had begun to switch off and dissociate when people harmed me. It was as though it was not happening to me, it was happening to someone else.

I don't think children are always given the credit they deserve for being resilient and resourceful, but I eventually found a place of safety. I found a place where I would walk to where there was a lake, a river, a forest, and open countryside; it felt like I would walk 100 miles. I can honestly say that in all the time that I spent out there, I never once saw another living soul— so nobody hurt me.

The truth is, it was probably about half a mile down a country lane, but it just felt that I had moved to a whole new world where nobody hurt me. I began to spend a lot of my time in the forest. I was trying to make sense of what was happening. Why was I being singled out for this treatment? I toyed with religious ideas. I wondered if maybe I was an alien. I wondered if someone had come down from another planet and forgotten me. When they realized it, would they come back and get me?

I began to spend a lot of my time in this new place of safety, to the point that even at age 11 and 12 years I began to sleep rough out there. People often wonder, "How can a child feel safe sleeping in a forest?" But to me it was safe—out there everyone hurt me, in here nobody harmed me. I recognized the trees by individual features. It felt like I had an army behind me ready to protect me. I would catch snakes and newts and take them to the pet store in town, and the owner would buy them from me, so I now had money to buy things that I needed. At times I would spend three, four, maybe five nights sleeping in the forest.

I often used to think back and wonder, "Why did nobody notice?" There was a young child sleeping rough, always bruised and disheveled; my mother must have noticed, surely? I then began to wonder, "Why did nobody do anything?" Because they *must* have noticed. Eventually, someone did notice, and I was taken away into the care of the local authorities at age

13. I was moved into a residential facility in a new part of town, so I was now away from the bullies and my stepfather. A lot of people I have spoken to who have spent time in a children's home talk about very negative experiences of abuse and trauma, but for me it was not like that. The children's home that I was taken to had a very positive environment, both emotionally and practically. One member of the staff with whom I had a very good relationship really helped me to develop my love of music into an effective coping strategy that has stood the test of time.

When I reached age 16, it was time to leave the children's home. I moved to a new city completely on my own, with no friends or family, and just started a new life for myself. I married at 18 years old into what turned out to be a very unhappy marriage; it was the arguing around this time, coupled with the events described at the start of this chapter, that led to my first hospital admission. As I walk you through some of my experiences of being on a hospital ward in an extremely paranoid state, I just want to make one thing clear: any criticism that I have is not about people; it is about the system, how we categorize people's distress and medicalize their experiences. I can honestly say that I would not be in a position to write this chapter had I not met some of the incredible staff members whom I came across during my journey.

After I was admitted to the hospital, suspicious of everybody's motives and convinced that this was now the endgame and the police were going to harm me, my first experience was quite bizarre. I lay on my bed and noticed a man sitting on a chair, staring at me. He never spoke. I walked away and he followed me. I went to the toilet, and when I came out, he was there. I approached the nurse who had admitted me and asked her, "Can you tell this man to stop following me, please? He is frightening me." Her response was, "Oh, that is a staff nurse. You are on observations." No one had told me; my mad world had just become a whole lot madder.

As mentioned previously, my experiences were taken and were now being described as symptoms. I told people of my fears and of the things that were happening to me. This was rewritten as a story of illness and of deficit. One of my earliest observations was that moving to a hospital ward is like moving to a new country—you have to learn a whole new language. I was being spoken to in words that I had never heard before.

I was treated with antipsychotic medication, which had little effect other than to make me groggy. When one tablet did not work, I was moved to a new one and labeled *treatment resistant*. There were no talking treatments offered; it was all about diagnosis and medication.

Standing 6 foot 4 inches, I am larger than the average man, and I began to get the impression that people (staff and other patients) were wary of me. I have no history of any forms of anger or aggression; quite the opposite, I am someone who is very mindful of any anger around me, probably as a result of my violent childhood experiences. But when you are my size and you have a diagnosis of paranoid schizophrenia, people tend to expect certain behaviors from you. My overriding memory of those 3 years that I spent there was fear; I was petrified, and I just did not want to be there.

Despite the fact that I was detained under a section of the U.K. Mental Health Act, the hospital ward that I was on was very easy to escape from, and I was always absconding. I found myself in an incredibly strange paradox: I had staff members whom I was beginning to trust a little telling me that the police were not out to get me and that they were not following me, but then when I absconded, they picked the phone up and rang the police, asking them to find me and bring me back. Because this was my first hospital admission, I had no understanding of how the mental health system worked and the fact that this was the procedure they needed to follow. All this fed into my belief that I was there because of the police.

The police were very heavy-handed with me at times when they found and tried to return me, maybe because of my size, my diagnosis, and the fact that they knew my fears revolved around them. On one occasion when I had absconded, it was the early hours of the morning and I was in my apartment. The police broke down the door and came to take me back dressed in full riot equipment, with shields, visors down, and dogs. Words do not allow me to explain the sheer terror I felt at that moment. Very shortly after that incident, the police wrote a letter to the hospital. This is not part of any paranoia; I still have a copy of that letter today. Paraphrased slightly, the letter said,

> This man is a stocky, 6 foot 4 individual with schizophrenia, so will be difficult to deal with. The amount of times we are called to bring this man back is unacceptable, we request that he be moved to secure accommodation immediately.

So on police request I was moved to the local forensic ward, even though I had not committed any crime. Again, this only served to feed into my belief system that the police were out to harm me.

Shortly before the incident where I was moved to the forensic ward, I was introduced to someone who went on to help me make sense of all these things that were happening to me. It was about 18 months into the hospital admission, and my world had collapsed around me. My wife had left me, my son had been taken into foster care, my career had gone, my home had gone, and my friends had stopped visiting me. I had given up on my future, despite the fact that I was still in my 20s. I had asked a psychiatrist what this diagnosis meant for me, and I will never forget his exact words: "Every time you have an episode, it will take a little piece of you away." A nurse at the time had really gotten my trust, and I thought to myself, "Everything has disappeared; I have nothing left to lose." So I opened up to her about the sexual abuse I experienced as a child. I had never told anyone, not even my wife. When I told her, I got the impression that she did not know what to do to help me, so she found someone who did know what to do.

I was referred to see a man who was a mental health social worker but also ran a local support group set up to support specifically male survivors of sexual abuse. When he first came to see me, I did not want to speak to him because I believed that all he was going to ask me was who did what. But I was wrong. He did not want to know any of that; he wanted to know about the emotional impact the abuse had had on me. Every time he came, I absconded, because I just did not want to speak to him. This coincided with me being moved to the forensic ward, from which I could not escape. He persevered and invested a lot of time in me. He got my trust, and I began to open up to him. I told him everything about my childhood and about all the things that had happened to me.

This man worked in a very different way from what I had experienced during the hospital admission. For example, previously, I was never asked questions about the voices other than "Are they telling you to hurt yourself? Are they telling you to hurt someone else?" Other than that, they were seen as meaningless symptoms of an illness and were not discussed. Likewise, the content of my paranoia was never explored. This social worker began to ask these questions. He began to explore the roots of my fears about the police. I recall one day I had a meeting with him, and he came into the room and sat there for a few seconds in silence. He then said to me, "I am going to tell you something today, and I really want you to listen. I am going to tell you that there is absolutely nothing wrong with you." Quite taken aback, I said, "But I've been told I have schizophrenia; I have been told that I will never recover." He said, "I know what you have been told, but I am telling you there is nothing wrong with you whatsoever. This is normal, it's not illness. In the context of your life, this is normal." He then went further and said, "Given all the terrible things that you had to endure as a child, the horrible things you experienced as a young man, if you didn't hear voices, if you weren't paranoid, then there would be something wrong with you." That was the eureka moment: If this is genetic or biological, then there is not much I can do. If this is my response to undealt-with trauma, then there is something I can do.

Most of the work with the social worker began after discharge, and he helped me to see that all my responses need to be viewed through the context of my life. I will give an example of such a simplistic way of working with me. This may be difficult to believe, but it is completely true. After I had spent 2 years in the hospital, not one person had asked me why I was scared of the police. Many people had told me that the police were not going to harm me or that they were not monitoring me, but no one had asked, "Why the police?" The social worker asked, "Why are you scared of the police?" I told him that when I was a child, every time my biological father would rape or abuse me, he would say to me afterward, "If you ever tell anyone about this, the police will come and get you, take you away, and torture you. They know every single person you speak to because they are watching you all the time." Psychiatry called my adult response paranoid schizophrenia, but the social worker called it a completely normal reaction to undealt-with childhood trauma.

Having shared some of my own personal experience with you, I hope that you can see that the roots of my paranoia are not in "delusions" or a faulty brain. When we add the context and life history to a person's distressing experiences, they begin to make sense. In a purely medical sense, it could be argued that since that long hospital admission, I have not recovered. I still hear voices; I still have difficult and uncomfortable thoughts that I have to deal with. But from a personal view of recovery, I would argue that I have recovered a life.

Since my discharge from the hospital, I have been happily married to my second wife for 22 years. I went to university to study for a degree in information technology, and I went back to study for a master's degree in recovery in mental health and now work as a lecturer in the same subject. I understand now that the voices and the paranoia do not make me ill; it is the way that I respond to these experiences that makes me ill. I believe that the biggest and most damaging component of paranoia is fear. By understanding the causes and the roots of my paranoia, I have disarmed that fear and taken back control of my life.

Questions for Discussion

1. Should we always try to discuss historical trauma, the "can of worms" as written about in this chapter?

2. Can we work through and understand paranoia without the use of medication?

3. Can an individual still lead a productive and satisfying life while holding strongly held beliefs?

KEY POINTS

- Strongly held beliefs, or paranoia, have their roots in the reality of a person's lived experience and life history.

- Fear is a key component of paranoia. If we can take the fear away from an individual, then that person should be able to function while still holding the belief.

- Viewing paranoia as a symptom of an illness can prevent an individual from having the opportunity to make sense of the reality base driving the paranoia.

3

Considering Delusions Through a Cultural Lens

Peter Phiri, Ph.D., RNMH, CBT (DipHE)
Farooq Naeem, Ph.D., MRCPsych
Kathryn Elliot, M.Sc.
Shanaya Rathod, D.M., MRCPsych

Although schizophrenia and other psychotic disorders are classified as low-prevalence disorders, they constitute some of the most chronic and severe medical disorders (Insel 2010). *Active psychosis* is often characterized by distorted and impaired thinking, feelings, and behavior that result in a loss of the sense of consensus reality. In addition, it is often associated with delusional beliefs, hallucinations, and thought disorder, as well as disorganized and bizarre behavior.

The term *psychosis* refers to individual symptoms that undoubtedly vary in clinical significance, duration, severity, and diagnostic class. Several disorders encompass schizophrenia spectrum disorders at the categorical level, such as schizoaffective disorder, delusional disorder, and schizotypal personality disorder. Psychosis affects approximately 1% of the population worldwide and was ranked as the eighth leading cause of years with disability (disability-adjusted life years; Giotakos 2018). Thus, it has a significant negative impact on the quality of life of patients and their families.

Culture is commonly described as "that complex whole which includes knowledge, belief, art, law, morals, customs, and any other capabilities and habits acquired by man as a member of society" (Tylor 1871, p. 1). There are cultures that we are born into, and there are cultures we gather, including those of our university, our place of work, and so on. Over time, individuals accumulate several identities that relate to many aspects of culture, including gender, and religion. Culture joins individuals together in one group, with clear characteristics separating these individuals from individuals who do not identify with this group, thus confirming group identities. There is no dispute that culture is involved significantly in understanding what normality is and any deviance through which abnormality is defined, which is essential in both psychiatry and psychology.

Individuals are more inclined to seek help and engage with psychological therapies when their cultural views and explanatory models are acknowledged (Carter et al. 2017). The majority of psychotherapy theories have been developed in the West and thus conflict with many cultural views and beliefs of individuals from non-Western backgrounds. Therefore, over the past two decades, there has been a movement to culturally adapt psychotherapies to account for cultural variables. This growing movement of adapting interventions for individuals with delusions to be congruent with their cultural values will improve the acceptability and effectiveness of treatment.

Cultural Prevalence and Incidence of Psychosis

It was previously thought that the prevalence and incidence of schizophrenia were the same across different cultures. In psychiatry, there was a heavy bias toward discovering similarities across cultures and universals in mental disorders, with the assumption that culture has a mere pathoplastic effect on the core biological pathogenesis of these disorders. This belief has since been disregarded because much research has shown that specific societies have significantly more people who have schizophrenia than others (Bhavsar et al. 2014). It has been estimated that 4 people out of every 1,000 in England develop an active psychotic disorder annually (Kirkbride et al. 2012). Yet this prevalence can vary across different cultures around the world. For example, there is a 2% rate in Pakistan (Nawaz et al. 2020) and 0.3% in Ethiopia (Greene et al. 2021). One of the most consistent findings in epidemiology research on psychotic disorders is the elevated incidence of psychosis among migrants and ethnic minority groups over decades, within first and second generations. This overrepresentation of diagnoses of severe psychotic disorders among ethnic minority people is an area of great concern.

In an attempt to gain insight into the variability in the incidence rate of psychotic disorders, the Ethnic Minority Psychiatric Illness Rates in the

Community (EMPIRIC) study concluded that a twofold higher prevalence rate was present in individuals of Black Caribbean heritage compared with a group of white individuals (Nazroo and King 2002). Certain risk factors were highlighted, such as family history and an increased level of urbanicity that is consistently associated with a significantly higher incidence rate of diagnosed psychotic disorders. Other socioeconomic factors, such as poverty and discrimination, in combination with the negative impact of migration, can result in individuals experiencing high levels of distress, which makes them vulnerable to developing a mental health disorder. The added association of racism and stigma around mental disorders for migrants or Black, Indigenous, and other people of color further increases risk.

Consistent reports have been made of elevated incidence rates of schizophrenia in Black Caribbean people living in the United Kingdom. The multisite study Aetiology and Ethnicity of Schizophrenia and Other Psychoses (AESOP) found a ninefold increase in the risk of developing schizophrenia in Black Caribbean people compared with the white British population. This increased risk was also reported for Black Africans (5.8-fold) and South Asians (1.4-fold) (Fearon et al. 2006). These findings are at odds with incidence rates recorded in Caribbean countries. The incidence rates of schizophrenia in Barbados (Mahy et al. 1999), Trinidad (Bhugra et al. 1996), and Jamaica (Hickling and Rodgers-Johnson 1995) were all found to be similar to that of the white British population.

Several hypotheses have been put forward to attempt to account for the high incidence rate of schizophrenia in African Caribbean people living in England. One is that even though the symptoms of African Caribbean patients may meet DSM-5 (American Psychiatric Association 2013) criteria for schizophrenia, this does not mean that the symptoms have the same meaning as they do for white British patients. Thus, it can be questioned whether the high incidence rate of schizophrenia in members of the African Caribbean community can be explained by the fact that the experiences reported by individuals (e.g., voice-hearing) are those that British psychiatrists are trained to record as evidence for a diagnosis for schizophrenia. For example, in Western cultures, hallucinations are generally considered pathological; however, in non-Western cultures, hallucinatory experiences are considered holy, as evidenced in numerous religious texts.

Delusions

Introducing Delusions

Delusions are one of the most prominent symptoms used to diagnose an individual with schizophrenia. They are deemed a typical positive symptom of the disorder; however, delusions are arguably elusive phenomena within psychiatry and psychopathology (Maher and Spitzer 1993). DSM-5-TR classifies delusions as "fixed beliefs that are not amenable to change in light of conflicting evidence" (American Psychiatric Association 2022, p. 101). However, Freeman and Garety (2004) argued that conceptual definitions of delusions as being discrete and detached from everyday experience lack empirical validity. It is often a challenge to decide whether a belief is the norm, especially when the delusion experienced is reasonable in content or not peculiar (Maher and Spitzer 1993). A survey conducted by Cox and Cowling (1989) of 60,000 members of the British public reported that they commonly held beliefs that met the classification of delusions. The authors reported that 25% of the participants believed in reincarnation, 25% believed in ghosts or supernatural spirits, and 50% believed in thought transfer. Therefore, it cannot be assumed that strong beliefs, however strong they may be, are inaccurate or that they need to be changed.

Assessment of Delusions and Cultural Considerations

Determining the influence of cultural background can be very challenging, as is determining who decides whether a belief is culturally appropriate or is a delusion. Given the various ideologies and beliefs in different cultures, the criteria with which we draw concise distinctions between cultural and delusional beliefs appear to be beyond our grasp. This is striking because the only symptom of delusional ideation is the set of beliefs that an individual holds. Unfortunately, the tendency for talking therapies to isolate people from their culture means the psychotherapist will often not be able to understand whether any given belief is delusional. Also, the presentation of specific beliefs by one individual may be used as evidence for the diagnosis of a mental illness, whereas the same specific beliefs presented by another individual within a different cultural setting may not be taken as evidence of a mental illness.

Case Example: The Importance of Assessment Through a Cultural Lens

Addae was a 40-year-old woman of Ghanaian origin in an inpatient unit, to which she had been admitted with psychosis. She was not happy with the treatment and wanted to leave the hospital. She was not very keen on the idea of medication. She was a voluntary patient. Her treating psychiatrist decided to seek an opinion from a cultural point of view. Addae had moved to the United Kingdom with her family when she was 30 years old. However, her children had left home and she had recently lost her job. Her husband had had a heart attack and was recovering. Addae described the past year as the most distressing period of her life. She reported a disturbed sleep pattern and low appetite over the previous 6 months. She also described symptoms of depression and anxiety. Her main psychotic symptom was hearing the voices of her ancestors. She said that she was happy with the voices and found them to be helpful. However, one voice that informed her of bad things happening bothered her. This was the voice of her grandmother, who had been very critical of her when she was a young girl. It was because of this critical voice that Addae had made her initial contact with psychiatric services.

The psychiatrist talked to Addae's family over the phone because they were living in other cities. They confirmed that hearing the voices of ancestors is common in Ghana and did not consider it pathological. Addae warmed up as soon as she realized that the clinical team trusted her story and did not consider her psychotic ("mad" in her own words). She was provided with psychoeducation on depression and its relationship with stress. She agreed to try antidepressants and was discharged. She attended outpatient appointments and was reported to recover fully.

The common societal conception of values and beliefs appears to be particularly important for the theme of delusions and hallucinations. Delusions of grandeur, for example, hardly exist in societies where striving for a certain social status is frowned on (Stompe et al. 2006), and visual and tactile hallucinations are reported more frequently by members of social groups that take unexplainable sensory experiences as evidence of the supernatural or divine (Larøi et al. 2014). These examples illustrate that the likelihood and quality of psychotic phenomena are partly dependent on an individual's cultural environment. Moreover, the extent to which hallucinations and delusions are interpreted as appropriate or benign and socially accepted may have implications for the distress resulting from these experiences within a specific society (i.e., distress is likely to be lower when experiences are considered normative or appropriate; Luhrmann et al. 2015). Even the acceptance of psychosis and the stigma attached to it vary across cultures. For example, one study from Egypt reported that behavioral problems are more likely than other psychiatric problems to be stigmatized (Coker 2005).

Role of Culture and Trauma in Psychosis

The relationship between trauma and psychosis is complex. Psychosis may emerge as a reaction to a traumatic event (Ellason and Ross 1997). This suggestion stems from reports of high exposure to childhood sexual abuse and other severe traumas among individuals with diagnosed psychotic disorders, with the continuous influences of adverse environmental factors and negative life events that affect psychotic symptoms (Kingdon et al.

1994). The effect of trauma is a sensitive matter; events often have impacts on individuals and their families, who may believe they are to blame for their offspring developing psychosis.

It is essential that clinicians consider the impact of racial trauma on the individual and include an assessment of this in their clinical interaction. For example, the impact of the 2018 Windrush scandal highlights the complexity of trauma and how it can be present from one generation to the next. In 1948, individuals were uprooted from their homes in the Caribbean, having to leave their families and culture on the promise of better options in Britain. In 2018, individuals were falsely detained, stripped of their legal rights, and threatened with deportation by the UK government. The hope of a better life was in stark contrast to the reality of overt racism and discrimination, which have continued through the generations, leading to significant negative life events and trauma.

In 2020, international attention was paid to excessive force used by police that led to the deaths of several African Americans, including George Floyd, Ahmaud Arbery, Rayshard Brooks, and Breonna Taylor. These deaths sparked global protests and highlighted the reality of police brutality in the African American community in the United States (Jordan et al. 2021). Thus far, little research has been conducted within the Black community to assess the consequences of being exposed to lasting vicarious trauma through repeated exposure to images of Black people being harmed or killed by the police. However, recent evidence indicated the detrimental effect police killings have on the mental health of African Americans in the general population. Each police killing of an unarmed Black American to which respondents were exposed was associated with increased reports of issues with emotions, depressed symptoms, and stress (Bor et al. 2018). Further research is fundamental to comprehending the lasting psychological sequelae of trauma for Black people, which could range from maladaptive coping skills to problems with emotion regulation or abuse of harmful substances.

Case Example: Cultural Trauma and Psychosis

Shahid, a young second-generation Canadian man of Pakistani origin, was seen for a second opinion. He had been discharged after a 5-day stay in an inpatient unit because he had not been talking. He had been prescribed antidepressant medication because the attending physician believed him to be depressed. His parents had never been contacted, and they requested a second opinion. Subsequently Shahid was seen by a consultant psychiatrist/cognitive-behavioral therapist from his ethnic background. Shahid opened up when the consultant spoke to him in Urdu, a language commonly spoken in Pakistan. He related that he received messages from the Pakistani intelligence agency and that they were trying to control him. These messages told him that he should complete his education and return to his country and join the army to serve his nation. The messages were relayed through the local South Asian television channel. He had received the first of these messages 6 months before the meeting with the consultant psychiatrist.

During this time, Shahid was studying for his exams and was not sleeping well. He had no history of drug or alcohol use. Further questioning revealed historical trauma. Shahid's parents were political activists who had been tortured by a former military dictator of Pakistan for staging protests in favor of democracy, and had had to seek asylum 40 years ago. Shahid's parents related how they had been so scared that they had decided not to seek refuge in the United States, the United Kingdom, or France, which were believed to be the dictator's allies during the Afghan war of the 1980s. Following the assessment, Shahid was started on a low dose of risperidone, to which he responded well, and was referred to an early intervention in psychosis team for ongoing monitoring and care.

Recommendations for Working Through a Cultural Lens

As continued rapid mobilization of people occurs across national boundaries, it is imperative that clinicians become more mindful of cultures, subcultures, and societies. Therefore, psychotherapies must evolve and adapt to integrate the beliefs and needs of individuals from different cultures. There are two types of adaptations to treatment or the delivery of therapies: surface modifications (e.g., ethnically matching the therapist and patient, the setting in which the therapy is delivered, and the translation of the therapy) and core modifications (theoretical considerations as well as consideration of cultural values, norms, and beliefs of patients). For these adaptations to be instilled in psychotherapies, there is a clear four-step process. The cultural adaption framework includes four levels of adjustments exploring 1) philosophical orientation, 2) practical considerations, 3) theoretical considerations, and 4) technical adjustments of the therapy.

The first stage, which focuses on gathering information on different cultures and subcultures, feeds into the second stage, which is the creation of guidelines for adapting the therapy model. It is essential to comprehend the cultural views and beliefs that potentially influence the delusions being expressed. Once information has been gathered on the different cultures, the third stage focuses on adapting the therapy materials to incorporate these different cultural views and translating them into various languages to improve inclusion and engagement. Finally, the adapted therapy must be field-tested to assess whether all cultural needs have been addressed and to determine its acceptability within various cultures.

The cultural adaptation framework was developed by Rathod et al. (2015) for use when considering adaptations of psychological interventions for diverse populations and cultural backgrounds. This framework was evaluated in the first randomized controlled trial on culturally adapted cognitive-behavioral therapy for psychosis in the United Kingdom (Rathod et al. 2013) and also by Naeem et al. (2015a, 2015b). Since then, it has been used globally, including for anxiety and depression (Algahtani et al. 2019) and psychosis (Li et al. 2017).

A Biopsychosocial-Spiritual Model

People from many non–North American or non–Western European cultures use a biopsychosocial-spiritual model of psychotic illness. For example, in our qualitative study in Pakistan, patients and their carers noted masturbation (from Ayurveda), heat in the liver (from Chinese medicine), and increased phlegm in the body (from old Greek medicine) to be the causes of psychosis (Naeem et al. 2016). This same study also found that South Asians believe in religious and spiritual causes of psychosis (e.g., spirits, magic, *taweeds* [amulets]), fear of *hawai* things (e.g., ghosts), the evil eye, and God's will. Interestingly, all these patients were recruited from psychiatric clinics and were taking medication, which they accepted, possibly reflecting their belief in the biological component of the model. This model influenced their belief systems, especially those related to health, well-being, illness, and help-seeking in times of distress. Culture and religion influence beliefs about the cause-and-effect relationship. For example, the cause of an accident might be described as "the evil eye" or "God's will." People often use religious coping strategies when dealing with distress (Naeem et al. 2019). Many patients in the Global South see faith healers before they attend a psychiatric service. Their help-seeking behaviors and pathways are multifaceted.

Case Example: A Culturally Adapted Cognitive-Behavioral Therapy Intervention

Dayita was a first-generation depressed Hindu woman who believed that her young son was under the magic spell of her daughter-in-law. Her family doctor referred her for assessment of psychosis and therapy.

Dayita's son had married 18 months ago and appeared to be paying more attention to his wife, which resulted in his mother feeling upset because she assumed he was ignoring her. She began to feel depressed, believing that her son's behavior was due to a black magic spell, kala jadoo. The therapist talked to family members, which was helpful because they informed him that this was a commonly held belief in the community. The therapist did not confront Dayita and assumed a nonjudgmental approach because she was already angry with family members for not believing her.

The therapist then explored and discussed alternative explanations for the son's behaviors. Family members were encouraged to talk to Dayita about this between sessions. The therapist advised them to highlight alternative reasons for the son's behaviors to her at home rather than confront her. Dayita was also encouraged to resume her religious practice. This was very helpful, and at her next therapy session she was less distressed about the belief in the black magic spell and demonstrated a willingness to engage with the psychological input and address her presentation with depression. She did continue to believe that black magic was a possibility.

Being cognizant of Dayita's culturally derived beliefs allowed the therapist to approach her presentation sensitively, and working with family members facilitated engagement and support in reducing distress associated with the delusional belief.

The aim of cognitive-behavioral therapy is not to eliminate the delusions experienced by individuals but rather to alter what the individuals perceive about these phenomena to diminish the level of distress that occurs. Individuals with delusions tend to jump to conclusions, and in Dayita's case, she assumed that her son was ignoring her when he was not. Through therapy, she was able to reduce her distress around her delusions.

Personal Reflection: Culture Shock

One of us (F.N.), a South Asian male, started his career as a trainee psychiatrist in a Liverpool training program in England. This was his first job in the United Kingdom. He struggled with adjusting to a new culture in addition to a new system of health care. He had to cook for himself, which he was not used to doing as a firstborn South Asian male, because South Asian food was not readily available and the food in a local South Asian restaurant (e.g., chicken tikka masala, a popular dish in the United Kingdom) was not authentic. He had no friends or family and had to cope with constant rain. All these factors led to an immense amount of stress. He also found it challenging to understand the local Liverpool Scouse accent. He remembers feeling paranoid during his first few months at work when, for example, colleagues would make a joke and laugh and he wondered whether they were laughing at him. As he adjusted to these stressors and got used to the Scouse accent, his paranoid thoughts disappeared. Experiencing culture shock is common not only among people coming from another country but also among individuals who move internally within a particular country.

Questions for Discussion

1. What factors will you consider when formulating delusions and helping patients make sense of what might be causing their distress?

2. What would be your rationale for considering patients' cultural identity, cultural reference group, religious influence, and sociopolitical beliefs about their attributions of illness and explanations within their cultural context?

3. Given the impact of racism and discrimination on Black, Indigenous, and other people of color, might racism and discrimination influence threat beliefs in delusion formation?

KEY POINTS

- Delusions are one of the most prominent symptoms used to diagnose schizophrenia. However, delusions are arguably elusive phenomena when considered from a cultural viewpoint.

- Religious themes are a cardinal feature across categories and types of delusions, with a large proportion (between one-fifth and two-thirds) of delusions having a religious element.

- There are cultural variations in the formation of delusions. Also, culture influences each individual's interactions and responses to illness, treatment, and outcomes.

- A lack of cultural awareness on the part of both the patient and the clinician can lead to barriers, misunderstanding, and mistrust.

- The tendency for talking therapies to isolate individuals from their culture means that the psychotherapist may not be able to understand whether any given belief is delusional.

References

Algahtani HM, Almulhim A, AlNajjar FA, et al: Cultural adaptation of cognitive behavioural therapy (CBT) for patients with depression and anxiety in Saudi Arabia and Bahrain: a qualitative study exploring views of patients, carers, and mental health professionals. Cogn Behav Therap 12:344, 2019

American Psychiatric Association: Diagnostic and Statistical Manual of Mental Disorders, 5th Edition. Arlington, VA, American Psychiatric Association, 2013

American Psychiatric Association: Diagnostic and Statistical Manual of Mental Disorders, 5th Edition, Text Revision. Washington, DC, American Psychiatric Association, 2022

Bhavsar V, Boydell J, Murray R, Power P: Identifying aspects of neighbourhood deprivation associated with increased incidence of schizophrenia. Schizophr Res 156(1):115–121, 2014 24731617

Bhugra D, Hilwig M, Hossein B, et al: First-contact incidence rates of schizophrenia in Trinidad and one-year follow-up. Br J Psychiatry 169(5):587–592, 1996 8932887

Bor J, Venkataramani AS, Williams DR, Tsai AC: Police killings and their spillover effects on the mental health of Black Americans: a population-based, quasi-experimental study. Lancet 392(10144):302–310, 2018 29937193

Carter L, Read J, Pyle M, Morrison AP: The impact of causal explanations on outcome in people experiencing psychosis: a systematic review. Clin Psychol Psychother 24(2):332–347, 2017 26805779

Coker EM: Selfhood and social distance: toward a cultural understanding of psychiatric stigma in Egypt. Soc Sci Med 61(5):920–930, 2005 15955396

Cox D, Cowling P: Are You Normal? London, Tower Press, 1989

Ellason JW, Ross CA: Childhood trauma and psychiatric symptoms. Psychol Rep 80(2):447–450, 1997 9129365

Fearon P, Kirkbride JB, Morgan C, et al: Incidence of schizophrenia and other psychoses in ethnic minority groups: results from the MRC AESOP Study. Psychol Med 36(11):1541–1550, 2006 16938150

Freeman D, Garety PA: Paranoia: The Psychology of Persecutory Delusions. London, Psychology Press, 2004

Giotakos O: Persistence of psychosis in the population: the cost and the price for humanity [Greek]. Psychiatriki 29(4):316–326, 2018 30814041

Greene MC, Yangchen T, Lehner T, et al: The epidemiology of psychiatric disorders in Africa: a scoping review. Lancet Psychiatry 8(8):717–731, 2021 34115983

Hickling FW, Rodgers-Johnson P: The incidence of first contact schizophrenia in Jamaica. Br J Psychiatry 167(2):193–196, 1995 7582668

Insel TR: Rethinking schizophrenia. Nature 468(7321):187–193, 2010 21068826

Jordan A, Allsop AS, Collins PY: Decriminalising being Black with mental illness. Lancet Psychiatry 8(1):8–9, 2021 33341173

Kingdon D, Turkington D, John C: Cognitive behaviour therapy of schizophrenia: the amenability of delusions and hallucinations to reasoning. Br J Psychiatry 164(5):581–587, 1994 7802805

Kirkbride JB, Errazuriz A, Croudace TJ, et al: Systematic Review of the Incidence and Prevalence of Schizophrenia and Other Psychoses in England. London, Department of Health Policy Research Programme, 2012

Larøi F, Luhrmann TM, Bell V, et al: Culture and hallucinations: overview and future directions. Schizophr Bull 40(Suppl 4):S213–S220, 2014 24936082

Li W, Zhang L, Luo X, et al: A qualitative study to explore views of patients, carers and mental health professionals to inform cultural adaptation of CBT for psychosis (CBTp) in China. BMC Psychiatry 17(1):131, 2017 28390407

Luhrmann TM, Padmavati R, Tharoor H, Osei A: Hearing voices in different cultures: a social kindling hypothesis. Top Cogn Sci 7(4):646–663, 2015 26349837

Maher BA, Spitzer M: Delusions, in Symptoms of Schizophrenia (Wiley Series on Personality Processes). Edited by Costello CG. New York, Wiley, 1993, pp 92–120

Mahy GE, Mallett R, Leff J, Bhugra D: First-contact incidence rate of schizophrenia on Barbados. Br J Psychiatry 175(1):28–33, 1999 10621765

Naeem F, Gul M, Irfan M, et al: Brief culturally adapted CBT (CaCBT) for depression: a randomized controlled trial from Pakistan. J Affect Disord 177:101–107, 2015a 25766269

Naeem F, Saeed S, Irfan M, et al: Brief culturally adapted CBT for psychosis (CaCBTp): a randomized controlled trial from a low income country. Schizophr Res 164(1–3):143–148, 2015b 25757714

Naeem F, Habib N, Gul M, et al: A qualitative study to explore patients', carers' and health professionals' views to culturally adapt CBT for psychosis (CBTp) in Pakistan. Behav Cogn Psychother 44(1):43–55, 2016 25180541

Naeem F, Phiri P, Rathod S, Ayub M: Cultural adaptation of cognitive-behavioural therapy. BJPsych Adv 25(6):387–395, 2019

Nawaz R, Gul S, Amin R, et al: Overview of schizophrenia research and treatment in Pakistan. Heliyon 6(11):e05545, 2020 33294688

Nazroo J, King M: Psychosis: symptoms and estimated rates, in Ethnic Minority Psychiatric Illness Rates in the Community (EMPIRIC). Edited by Sproston K, Nazroo J. London, The Stationery Office, 2002, pp 47–62

Rathod S, Phiri P, Harris S, et al: Cognitive behaviour therapy for psychosis can be adapted for minority ethnic groups: a randomised controlled trial. Schizophr Res 143(2–3):319–326, 2013 23231878

Rathod S, Kingdon D, Pinninti N, et al: Cultural Adaptation of CBT for Serious Mental Illness: A Guide for Training and Practice. Chichester, UK, Wiley-Blackwell, 2015

Stompe T, Karakula H, Rudaleviciene P, et al: The pathoplastic effect of culture on psychotic symptoms in schizophrenia. World Cult Psychiatry Res Rev 1(3–4):157–163, 2006

Tylor EB: Primitive Culture: Researches Into the Development of Mythology, Philosophy, Religion, Art, and Custom, Vol 2. London, John Murray, 1871

4

The Psychology of Paranoid Beliefs

Anton P. Martinez, M.Sc.
Vyv Huddy, Ph.D.
Richard P. Bentall, Ph.D., FBA

Paranoid (sometimes called persecutory) delusions, one of the most common symptoms of severe mental illness (Bebbington and Freeman 2017; Bentall et al. 2001), are present in more than 90% of first-episode schizophrenia patients (Moutoussis et al. 2007). However, because of the importance of suspiciousness and mistrust in ordinary social relationships, these kinds of beliefs have been studied not only by clinical researchers but also by social and behavioral scientists. In this chapter, we explore conceptualizations of paranoia from the initial years of psychiatry through to the theoretical advances resulting from psychological research during the past 30 years. By summarizing the available evidence from clinical, experimental, and epidemiological studies, we intend to provide an up-to-date review of theories about the origins and mechanisms of paranoid beliefs that will be useful to both clinicians and researchers.

A Conceptual History

Paranoia is a word often used in ordinary life to refer to persons who feel excessively suspicious, distrustful, or persecuted for no apparent reason. However, this everyday usage is quite recent and was not much evident before World War II (the earliest use of this kind recorded in the *Oxford En-*

glish Dictionary is from Samuel Beckett's (1938) novel *Murphy*, which describes "Paranoids, feverishly covering sheets of paper with complaints against their treatment or verbatim reports of their inner voices," although the context is a description of patients with psychosis in a psychiatric ward).

The term is derived from the Greek words *para* ("beyond," "beside") and *nous* ("mind," "intellect"), creating the word *paranoia*, which was used in Greek literature to describe people who were "out of their minds." However, it was not until the eighteenth century that it was transformed into a formal clinical concept (Dowbiggin 2000). French and German psychiatrists, for example, J.E.D. Esquirol (1772–1840), J.C.A. Heinroth (1773–1843), and Karl Kahlbaum (1828–1899), used the word to describe a limited form of insanity in which abnormal beliefs affected only circumscribed areas of functioning, leaving intact other domains of reasoning and judgment (Dowbiggin 2000; Lewis 1970).

At the beginning of the twentieth century, German psychiatrist Emil Kraepelin (1856–1926), considered one of the most influential pioneers of modern psychiatry (Bentall 2003), developed the concept dementia praecox (the precursor to the modern concept of schizophrenia), which he described as a chronic mental disease marked by a deterioration of the psychic functions (e.g., volition, affect, intellect) that led to the degradation of personality (Dowbiggin 2000; Kendler 1988; Lewis 1970). Although Kraepelin recognized that dementia praecox could manifest in a paranoid form (paranoide formen dementia praecox), he came to regard paranoia as a separate nosological construct, which he conceptualized as an abnormal form of personality development characterized by a stable and uniformly connected system of coherent, nonbizarre delusions without marked mental deterioration (Kendler 2018). The two conditions were distinguished on the basis of both etiology and course: whereas Kraepelin considered dementia praecox to be a "natural disease" that led to profound mental disturbances, paranoia was conceptualized as a disorder that arose from the interaction of personality development and life experiences.

This view of paranoia as a reactive or psychogenic psychosis bore some similarities to the psychoanalytic approach developed by Sigmund Freud (1911/1950). Freud's theory was developed in his analysis of the case of the German high court judge Daniel Schreber, whom he never met (the analysis was based on Schreber's autobiography [Schreber 1903/1955]), and attributed the judge's highly disorganized and religiously themed delusions to unconscious conflicts caused by his repressed homosexual desires (see Chapter 10, "The Curious Case of Schreber").

These views influenced North American psychiatrists, who, by the middle of the twentieth century, had become highly influential in international psychiatry (Strand 2011). During this period, nosological issues became less salient because of the influence of Swiss-American psychiatrist Adolf Meyer (1866–1950), who advocated a holistic, formulation-based approach to psychiatric care (Bentall 2009). Nonetheless, after the Second World War, there was increasing pressure to develop a uniform diagnostic system for administrative, governmental, and educational purposes, which led U.S. psychiatrists to create standardized diagnostic manuals, which culminated in the publication of the *Diagnostic and Statistical Manual: Mental Disorders* (DSM-I; American Psychiatric Association 1952). This manual was heavily influenced by Meyer's approach and by psychoanalysis and embraced a very broad formulation of schizophrenia that was seen as having a paranoid subtype (Dowbiggin 2000).

The poor reliability of psychiatric diagnoses during this period (identified in a seminal paper by Spitzer and Fleiss (1974) and the wish of some psychiatrists to enhance their credibility as medical practitioners led, ultimately, to the neo-Kraepelinian movement, which aimed to return psychiatry to the principles developed by Kraepelin in the late nineteenth century (Blashfield 1984). The neo-Kraepelinians conceived psychiatric disorders as biological conditions that they believed would ultimately be explained in terms of genetic and neurochemical processes (Guze 1989) and quickly focused on the need to operationalize psychiatric diagnoses as a means of accelerating advances in research in these areas. Perhaps the most important achievement of the neo-Kraepelinians was the publication of DSM-III (American Psychiatric Association 1980), which for the first time provided precise operational criteria for each diagnostic condition (Bentall 2003).

In DSM-III, paranoia was included as a diagnosis with the stipulation that a diagnosis of schizophrenia must be excluded, a criterion that has been maintained in all subsequent editions until the present day. Only persecutory delusions were considered in the definition provided, but some U.S. psychiatrists of the period, for example, George Winokur (1977) and Kenneth Kendler (1980), were actively researching patients with delusional conditions and argued that the diagnostic criteria should be broadened. Their work was influential when DSM underwent further revisions, so that in the present DSM-5-TR (American Psychiatric Association 2022) the term *delusional disorder* is now used to describe a condition in which disorganized speech and negative symptoms are absent, hallucinations are rare, and the main symptom is nonbizarre delusions that may have themes of persecution, grandiosity, jealousy, or somatic complaints.

Challenging the Categorical Model: The Idea of Paranoia as a Continuum

The medical approach to mental disorders assumes that psychopathological syndromes are caused by an underlying common causal process—a medical condition—so that the symptoms of the disorder are explained by the latent disease (Borsboom and Cramer 2013). However, this model struggles to account for the overlap of symptoms of different disorders and the consequent high rate of comorbidity (when symptoms meet the criteria for two or more categorical diagnoses) observed in everyday clinical and research practice (Brown and Barlow 2005; Renard et al. 2017). Paranoid beliefs, for example, can be present in delusional disorder, schizophrenia, bipolar disorder, major depressive disorder, paranoid personality disorder, autism spectrum disorder, and OCD (American Psychiatric Association 2022; Bentall et al. 2009).

An alternative approach to understanding paranoia was proposed by the German psychiatrist Ernst Kretschmer (1888–1964), who claimed that paranoid beliefs develop when people with vulnerable personalities experience stressful events. Kretschmer believed that three factors were important: first, a personality characterized by hypersensitivity, exhaustibility, and psychosexual inhibitions; second, embarrassing experiences that occur when people with this kind of personality are forced to interact too intensively with others; and finally, a social environment that does not allow them any means of escape (Hoehne 1988). This concept is represented in the DSM system as paranoid personality disorder, which is considered quite distinct from delusional disorder or any of the psychiatric disorders in which delusions may be prominent. People with this kind of personality are said to harbor suspicions about being deceived and doubts about the trustworthiness of others, to bear grudges, to suspect unfounded attacks on their reputation, to doubt the fidelity of their spouses, and to infer threatening or demeaning intentions behind benign remarks. However, research that has used this construct has been limited, and debates have persisted about whether this kind of personality is related to schizophrenia or delusional disorder (Lee 2017). These debates relate to the more general question, addressed in a separate chapter in this volume (Chapter 1, "Delusional Beliefs and the Madness of Crowds"), of whether pathological beliefs are qualitatively distinct from ordinary beliefs and attitudes or exist on a continuum with them. Those who hold that paranoid delusions are distinct from subclinical paranoia usually point to subtle phenomenological features of the lived experience of paranoid patients, for example, the state of *das Trema* ("something in the offing") that immediately precedes the development of the delusional idea, the state of *apophany* (revelation) that accompanies its formation, and the state of *anastrophe* afterward (in which the patient feels passive and at the center of a delusional world) (Conrad 1958/2012; Mishara 2010).

Those who defend the continuum concept typically point to evidence that paranoid beliefs are experienced by at least 10%–15% of the general population (Freeman 2007) and to sophisticated statistical studies using either factor analysis (Bebbington et al. 2013) or taxometric methods (Elahi et al. 2017), which have led to the development of questionnaires designed to measure paranoid beliefs in both clinical samples and the general population (Freeman 2008). The continuum approach is also supported by numerous studies of social and cognitive factors, reviewed in this chapter, that have generated similar findings from patients with paranoid delusions and ordinary people who score high on paranoia scales.

Current Conceptualizations of Paranoia

In recent years, psychological researchers have developed a parsimonious conceptualization of paranoia that takes into account the heterogeneity of its manifestation as well as its characterization as a continuum rather than a category. From this viewpoint, the central aspect of paranoia is the unfounded core belief that an imminent threat against the believer is intentionally orchestrated by others (Bebbington et al. 2013; Bell and O'Driscoll 2018; Brown et al. 2019; Freeman 2016; Murphy et al. 2018; Trotta et al. 2021). This type of belief is characterized by high degrees of conviction (i.e., how strongly the belief is held), preoccupation (i.e., fixation on the belief), and distress (i.e., negativity associated with the belief) (Combs et al. 2006), but each of these dimensions varies according to the severity of the experience (Elahi et al. 2017; Freeman 2007). Depending on its severity, paranoia can manifest in different ways, from social evaluative concerns and suspiciousness to self-referential processing and persecutory ideation, culminating in delusions (Freeman 2007, 2016). The anticipation of intended harm can manifest in various ways, such as by being wary of other people's intentions (i.e., mistrust), perceiving vulnerability in the presence of others (i.e., interpersonal sensitivity), interpreting innocuous experiences as personally targeted messages (i.e., self-referential beliefs), or performing safety behaviors in order to prevent significant harm from others (i.e., anticipation of threat) (Bebbington et al. 2013; Bell and O'Driscoll 2018; Bentall et al. 2009; Freeman 2007). In short, paranoia is currently conceived as a wide spectrum that varies not only in how persecutory beliefs are experienced (e.g., rigid, distressing) but also in the way these beliefs manifest behaviorally.

An important caveat to this description concerns the extent to which people believe that they deserve to be persecuted. Trower and Chadwick (1995) proposed that paranoia occurs in two forms: "poor-me," in which individuals believe that they are the innocent victims of the malign intentions of others, and "bad-me," in which people believe that they deserve to be persecuted. In fact, bad-me paranoia is much less common in psychiatric patients than poor-me paranoia (Fornells-Ambrojo and Garety 2005), and longitudinal studies have shown that patients tend either to be stably poor-me or to fluctuate between bad-me and poor-me, with fluctuations occurring over periods of a few hours or days (Melo et al. 2006; Udachina et al. 2012). As we will see in the subsection "Paranoia as a Defense Model," this observation has been interpreted as evidence that defensive processes play an important role in paranoid beliefs.

Paranoia as a Social Phenomenon

The foregoing discussion suggests that paranoia can be conceived as a disruption of normal social relationships. Current definitions, such as those by Freeman and Garety (2000), highlight the belief that others intend to harm the individual. One psychological measure that directly assesses this kind of belief is the Ambiguous Intentions Hostility Questionnaire (AIHQ; Combs et al. 2007), which requires participants to imagine interpersonal situations and provide indications of the intentions of others. Studies using this scale have reported that people with subclinical paranoia (Combs et al. 2007) and patients with persecutory delusions (Combs et al. 2009) view other people's intentions as more hostile than do nonparanoid control groups.

However, the AIHQ does not consider potential positive or benevolent intentions of others. A study of how people with persecutory delusions responded to everyday scenarios (Huddy et al. 2014) found not only that, as expected, these patients were more likely to generate negative interpretations of other people's intentions but also that there was a concurrent *lack* of perceptions of others as holding cooperative or helpful intentions. Hence, people with paranoid beliefs may not just see others as potentially threatening but also may be less able to detect opportunities for help and support from other people.

Paranoia and Human Cooperation

Studies using game theory research methods have been used to investigate cooperative intentions in people with paranoia. These studies typically involve one participant playing an interactive game with another participant in a manner that either involves a true social interaction (Gummerum et al. 2008) or resembles one. The two players are instructed to decide independently whether to act cooperatively with each other, and the combination of their decisions governs both players' payoffs (Camerer 2003). The first strategic game used for this purpose was the prisoner's dilemma (Ellett et al. 2013), in which participants are informed that they will play one or more rounds of a game in which they have to decide to cooperate or compete with another player. In the simplest version of the game, participants choose in the knowledge that the other player will do the same. Points are then awarded depending on each player's choice: if both compete, the score is lower than if both cooperate. Ellett and colleagues (2013) found that non-clinical participants with high paranoia scores were more likely to choose to compete rather than cooperate, and they justified their choice on the basis of distrust of their opponent rather than because they sought to maximize their own benefit. Other work using a related game has found that people with a high level of paranoia are less likely to invest money with others (Fett et al. 2012; Gromann et al. 2013).

More recently, in a large online study, Raihani and Bell (2017) used a "dictator game," in which another party (the dictator) was given money and had to decide how much of it to pass on to the participant. Participants both took part in games and observed other players taking part and receiving money from the dictator. In both cases, people who scored high on a measure of paranoia were more likely to judge the dictator's decision to be unfair. This finding challenges the assumption that paranoia is mainly due to an exaggerated sense of personalized threat and suggests instead that it involves a more general tendency to hold negative beliefs about the intentions of others.

It must be acknowledged that studies that use economic games have important limitations. They frequently require participants to imagine interacting with another person or to accept the experimenter's explanation that another player is involved. However, in the study by Raihani and Bell (2017), a sizable minority of participants were not convinced that there really was another person involved. These studies also construe the utility of interactions purely in monetary terms and require discrete decisions, yielding data with a limited range, which reduces the sensitivity of the design.

Role of Trust

Almost all of our everyday interactions with other people, from small monetary transactions to voting for a political party, involve a certain degree of trust. Thus, trust is a key facet of social behavior and is probably rooted in evolutionary mechanisms, given that our ancestors would have had to rely on one another in order to survive in harsh and stressful environments (Simpson 2007). Trust is usually conceived of as the willingness to accept vulnerability to the actions of others, which involves positive expectations about the intentions of the party being trusted, the trustee (Lewicki et al. 2006). These positive expectations are held in the absence of knowledge that the other party will act accordingly (Lewicki and Brinsfield 2012), and thus the act of trusting involves placing one's personal welfare in the hands of someone else in conditions of uncertainty (Hatzakis 2009; Simpson 2007).

Trust has generally been conceptualized as a multidimensional construct that includes initial perceptual judgments based on first impressions of often unfamiliar faces (Oosterhof and Todorov 2008) and more general beliefs about the degree to which people can be trusted (i.e., interpersonal trust; Lewicki and Brinsfield 2012; Simpson 2007). Whereas the former involves fast and automatic evaluations (Todorov et al. 2009), the latter encompasses a more stable set of cognitive, affective, and behavioral dispositions about the reliability of other people's intentions (Lewicki et al. 2006). Some authors argue that trust processes become activated by uncertain situations and that in harsh environments, adopting a tendency to perceive and/or believe that others are untrustworthy allows people to minimize the risk of making the more costly error and hence avoid getting hurt by someone who was initially trusted (Haselton and Nettle 2006; Hatzakis 2009).

Mistrust tends to be considered a core feature of paranoid thinking and is regarded as a subcomponent of the paranoia spectrum (Bebbington et al. 2013; Bell and O'Driscoll 2018). However, the role of mistrust in paranoid thinking has not been studied extensively, and it is not clear if problems of trusting act as precursors of paranoid beliefs or as consequences of them.

Several studies have explored judgments about the trustworthiness of faces made by patients with schizophrenia (Baas et al. 2008; Couture et al. 2008; Strauss et al. 2012), but only a few of them have looked at this construct in specific relation to paranoia (Buck et al. 2016; Haut and MacDonald 2010; Hooker et al. 2011; Pinkham et al. 2008; Trémeau et al. 2016). Although some of these studies found positive associations between paranoia and judgments of mistrust (Buck et al. 2016; Pinkham et al. 2008), others found no association at all (Haut and MacDonald 2010; Trémeau et al. 2016). The inconsistency in these findings must be interpreted in the context of the heterogeneity of symptom presentations in the participating patients. Moreover, one study found that low levels of trust were reported by paranoid patients only after they had been primed beforehand with threatening images, which supports the notion that judgments of trustworthiness are context dependent, particularly in clinical populations (Hooker et al. 2011).

Similar research in subclinical paranoia has been less extensive. One study reported differences in ratings of trustworthiness between high- and low-paranoia participants (Kirk et al. 2013), whereas another did not (Hillmann et al. 2017). Nonetheless, in a large representative U.K. epidemiological sample, a bias toward judging unfamiliar faces as untrustworthy was found to mediate between insecure attachment styles and paranoid beliefs (Martinez et al. 2021), and in a recent study using large representative samples from three countries, this association between paranoia and judging unfamiliar faces as untrustworthy was replicated in the United Kingdom, Ireland, and Spain (Martinez et al. 2021).

The relationship between more general interpersonal trust and paranoia has been more extensively studied in nonclinical populations, with most studies reporting medium to large associations (Axelrod et al. 1997; Furnham and Crump 2015; Greenaway et al. 2019; Kong 2017; Kramer 1994; Murphy et al. 2012; Wickham et al. 2014a, 2014b). Some of these studies were conducted in the context of psychometric validation of instruments assessing subclinical paranoia (Axelrod et al. 1997; Barreto Carvalho et al. 2017; Furnham and Crump 2015) or in order to explore the mediational role of trust between social adversities (e.g., trauma, social deprivation) and paranoid beliefs (Murphy et al. 2012; Wickham et al. 2014a, 2014b). Other studies have considered trust as a potential mechanism in promoting prosocial behaviors (e.g., cooperation, coordination) and thus reducing paranoid cognitions (Greenaway et al. 2019; Kong 2017; Kramer 1994). Hence, interpersonal trust, operationalized as a personality trait or a set of cognitions that guide social behavior, seems to show a more stable association with paranoia when measured in nonclinical populations.

Genetic and Social Determinants of Paranoia

Research on the social and genetic determinants of severe mental illness during the past two decades has led to a fairly dramatic recalibration of the relative contribution of each of these causal determinants to psychosis. It was once argued that classic family, twin, and adoption studies show that schizophrenia and related conditions are so heritable (typical estimates have exceeded 80%; Sullivan et al. 2003) that there is almost no space for environmental factors to play a role (van Os and McGuffin 2003). However, this argument is based on a fundamental misunderstanding of heritability; even when it is calculated at nearly 100%, environmental factors may still be very important (for an explanation, see Bentall 2021).

Studies in molecular genetics have converged on the finding that all psychiatric disorders are highly polygenic (associated with a large number of genetic variations, each with a very small effect), although some rare genetic mutations may confer a higher risk in a small number of cases (Kendler 2015; Owen 2012). At the same time, epidemiological studies, prospective birth cohort studies, and retrospective case-control studies (in which patients' accounts of their early lives are compared with the accounts given by control participants) have revealed that severe mental illness is associated with a wide range of adverse experiences, such as poverty (Wicks et al. 2005); exposure to harsh urban environments (Vassos et al. 2012); ethnic minority status (Bosqui et al. 2014); and interpersonal trauma, especially during childhood (Varese et al. 2012).

Very little research has considered the specific role of genes in paranoid beliefs. One large study of adolescents living in the community estimated that paranoia was 50% heritable when traditional methods were used (Zavos et al. 2014), but this figure fell to only 14% when heritability was estimated using molecular data (Sieradzka et al. 2015). This discrepancy is an example of the commonly observed "missing heritability" from molecular studies that is typical when the two methods of estimating the contribution of genes are compared (Cheesman et al. 2017).

In contrast, a number of studies have examined environmental determinants, often focusing on those that have been examined in the wider psychosis literature. For example, one line of research has examined the impact of harsh and deprived urban environments. Interestingly, one of the earliest studies of the relationship between urbanicity and psychosis, by Faris and Dunham (1939), reported that patients with psychosis living in inner-city areas were especially likely to experience paranoia symptoms. In a much later study comparing residents of Juarez in Mexico with those of El Paso, just across the border in the United States, sociologists Mirowsky and Ross (1983) reported that people were more likely to report paranoid beliefs if they lived in circumstances characterized by victimization and powerlessness. Analyzing epidemiological data from the United Kingdom, Wickham et al. (2014b) found higher levels of depression and paranoia, but not hallucinations or mania, in deprived areas. A later British study used network analysis to show that paranoia symptoms appeared to be closely related to the experience of incivilities and distrust of neighbors (McElroy et al. 2019); in this study, paranoid beliefs seemed to be a bridge symptom mediating between harsh environments and symptoms of depression and anxiety, which suggests that subclinical paranoia may have a greater public health significance than is often recognized. Consistent with these findings, studies have shown that both healthy individuals (Corcoran et al. 2018) and paranoid patients (Ellett et al. 2008) feel more paranoid when they walk around deprived areas.

It has been argued that social identity, or the sense of belonging, may protect people against paranoid beliefs, and therefore an absence of identity may explain the elevated rates of psychotic symptoms observed in ethnic minorities (McIntyre et al. 2016) and other discriminated-against groups, such as people with a nonheterosexual sexual orientation (Qi et al. 2020). Consistent with this hypothesis, the sense of belonging to a neighborhood is associated with lower levels of paranoid beliefs (Elahi et al. 2018; McIntyre et al. 2018). However, the relationship between identity, minority status, and paranoia is likely complex. For example, high rates of paranoia have been observed in the United States among African American citizens if they have experienced discrimination (Combs et al. 2006), and in a survey of African Caribbeans in the United Kingdom, it was found that paranoia was explained by the interaction between identity and the experience of discrimination, so that those who identified as British were less likely to be paranoid if they had predominantly positive relationships with the white majority but were more likely to be paranoid if these relationships were perceived as negative (McIntyre et al. 2021).

Early parental relationships have also been examined with respect to paranoid beliefs. In a British epidemiological survey (Bentall et al. 2012) and a survey of people incarcerated in British prisons (Shevlin et al. 2015), paranoid beliefs were found to be specifically associated with having been raised in institutional care, which was interpreted as evidence that the disruption of early attachment relationships was a causal factor (the role of attachment in paranoia is considered further later). Consistent with this hypothesis, an analysis of a U.S. epidemiological data set found a close association between paranoid beliefs and the experience of neglect during childhood (Sitko et al. 2014), and a recent study of adolescents in the United States and United Kingdom reported that paranoid beliefs were associated with physical abuse, emotional abuse, and especially maternal indifference, whereas a high level of care was associated with a low level of paranoia (Brown et al. 2021).

Similar findings have been reported in studies of patient samples. For example, Rankin et al. (2005) found that both currently paranoid and recovered paranoid patients reported more adverse relationships with their parents compared with healthy control participants, and Wickham and Bentall (2016) found that paranoia symptoms in a group of patients with psychosis were associated with reports of childhood neglect. Overall, a clear picture emerges from both clinical and nonclinical populations: the disruption of bonds with parental figures in early life, experiences of victimization and exposure to harsh environments in later life, and weak identification with others all contribute to the development of paranoid beliefs.

Psychological Models of Paranoia

As a result of the shift in focus from construing paranoia as the symptom of an underlying illness to considering it a phenomenon in its own right and the development of the continuum model linking persecutory delusions to more widespread experiences of mistrust and suspiciousness, a number of psychological models have been developed. These models attempt to identify cognitive and emotional factors that mediate between the kinds of life experiences described earlier and both clinical and subclinical paranoid states.

Anomalous Perception Model

Perhaps the simplest psychological model was proposed in the early 1970s by the American psychologist Brendan A. Maher (1974, 1999). Maher argued that all delusions were generated as an explanation of abnormal perceptual experiences, which provided the evidence on which patients made delusional inferences. From this point of view, Maher argued that the reasoning processes involved in delusions were not impaired but rather were the same as those present in nonclinical populations. Note that these two elements of the theory are not logically connected—aberrant perceptions could be important in delusions, but reasoning could still be impaired. Note also that an aberrant perception account could be considered consistent with some of the phenomenological data (see, e.g., Conrad 1958/2012), which is usually taken as evidence that delusions are qualitatively distinct from ordinary beliefs and attitudes.

The idea that aberrant perceptions may play a critical role in the formation of delusions was partially inspired by psychological models of schizophrenia from the period, which saw deficits in filtering perceptual information as a central feature of the disorder. Maher held that aberrant perceptual experiences would inevitably lead to a state of uncertainty and anxiety, prompting a search for an explanation as a way to ameliorate these negative feelings (Bell et al. 2006). The content of the resulting delusional explanations was believed to reflect the patient's cultural background and personal experiences (Maher 1999). For example, Maher argued, on the basis of Freud's analysis of the Schreber case, that the persecutory content of the judge's beliefs was a consequence of guilt associated with his repressed homosexuality, which served as an explanation of his unusual somatic experiences (Maher 1974).

Empirical studies of both nonclinical samples (Chapman and Chapman 1988) and clinical samples (Bell et al. 2008) have not consistently supported the idea of a strong relationship between anomalous experiences (e.g., hallucinations) and delusions in general of the kind Maher's theory predicted. However, some types of rare delusional systems can be accounted for in this way. For example, in Capgras syndrome, the individual believes a loved one has been replaced by an impostor, which seems to be caused by an impairment in the ability to recognize familiar faces (Ellis et al. 1997; see Chapter 13, "Who Are You?").

In the case of paranoia, there is strong evidence that late-onset deafness sometimes plays a role. Early studies showed that progressive hearing loss in elderly people is associated with paranoid beliefs (Cooper and Curry 1976), and an association between paranoia and hearing difficulties across the life span was subsequently confirmed in several epidemiological studies (Stefanis et al. 2006; Thewissen et al. 2005). One possible explanation for this association is that people with hearing loss develop suspicions about why people are no longer communicating with them.

Several other factors that seem to contribute to paranoia can also be interpreted within an anomalous perception framework. One is the impact of cannabis consumption on paranoid thinking, which has been demonstrated experimentally (Freeman et al. 2015a). Another is the observed association between sleep disturbances (e.g., insomnia) and paranoid beliefs, which has been widely reported in clinical and nonclinical populations (Blanchard et al. 2020; Freeman et al. 2009; Kasanova et al. 2020) and supported by experimental studies in which participants have been deliberately deprived of sleep (Kahn-Greene et al. 2007; Reeve et al. 2018). However, randomized controlled trials that have been conducted in order to reduce paranoia by targeting insomnia through cognitive-behavioral treatment have led to inconsistent results, with some studies showing an effect (Freeman et al. 2017; Myers et al. 2011) but others showing no impact on paranoia symptoms despite an improvement in insomnia (Freeman et al. 2015b). Finally, the possible role of dissociative experiences should be considered within an anomalous perception framework. These experiences, which are common consequences of severe traumatic events in either adulthood or childhood (Dalenberg et al. 2012), involve a disturbance of the integration of identity (memory, personality, emotion) that can lead to feelings of detachment from the self (depersonalization) or surroundings (derealization) (American Psychiatric Association 2022). Although a robust link between dissociation and auditory hallucinations has been clearly established in the literature (Pilton et al. 2015), some researchers have argued that this kind of strange experience could lead to delusional interpretations fueled by worry and anxiety (Černis et al. 2021; Freeman et al. 2013), and a recent meta-analysis provided some support for this hypothesis (Longden et al. 2020).

Paranoia as a Defense Model

By the late 1980s, the idea that anomalous experiences could be the sole cause of delusional thinking was no longer widely accepted. Given the nature of persecutory delusions (that malevolent intentions by others were the central feature), some researchers began to consider the psychological processes by which patients judged their position in the social universe (Kaney and Bentall 1989, 1992). From this perspective, social reasoning biases, in particular the attributions (explanations) that people made about interpersonal events (Bentall et al. 2001; Kaney and Bentall 1992), seemed to be a likely candidate for this process.

Bentall and colleagues published a series of studies reporting an association between self-serving biases (the tendency to make external, especially other-blaming, attributions for negative events and internal, self-blaming attributions for positive events) and persecutory delusions (Kaney and Bentall 1989; Kinderman and Bentall 1996). Although some later studies have not found this effect, most have, and a recent meta-analysis reported that the bias was especially marked in schizophrenia patients with persecutory delusions (Müller et al. 2021).

In light of this observation, Bentall et al. (1994) hypothesized that this specific attributional style was a cognitive bias that served to protect a vulnerable self against potentially threatening information, an account that seemed to capture the clinical presentation of many paranoid patients. In this model, the bias is conceived to be a psychological defense that serves to ward off negative thoughts about the self and thereby reduce an otherwise unpleasant discrepancy between current beliefs about the *actual self* and beliefs about the *ideal self*. A later dynamic version of the model proposed by Bentall et al. (2001) was designed to accommodate evidence that self-esteem and attributions reciprocally influence each other (making an internal attribution for a negative event should lead to more negative self-esteem, and low self-esteem should make an internal attribution for a negative event more likely) and evidence that patients sometimes fluctuate between poor-me (persecution is undeserved) and bad-me (persecution is deserved) paranoia (Udachina et al. 2012). Several predictions emerge from this model. For example, paranoia should be associated with unstable self-esteem when explicit (direct) measures are used but also when discrepancies between explicit self-esteem and self-esteem are measured using indirect or implicit techniques that are less likely to trigger defenses (Murphy et al. 2018).

Many studies have been carried out in order to test these predictions, but the results have not consistently supported the defense model. For example, many researchers have noted that low self-esteem is common in paranoid patients, which seems inconsistent with the model (Garety and Freeman 1999). Indeed, a recent meta-analysis of studies with both clinical and nonclinical participants reported a consistent association between negative self-beliefs and paranoia, although a complication is that some of this effect may have been due to depression, which is a common comorbidity of persecutory delusions (Humphrey et al. 2021).

Although some studies have reported an association between implicit negative self-esteem and paranoia, other studies have reported that levels of implicit self-esteem do not differ between patients with persecutory delusions and control samples (Kesting and Lincoln 2013; Tiernan et al. 2014). A recent meta-analysis of 64 studies testing the defense theory found support for some aspects—an externalizing attributional bias (as also reported in Müller et al.'s 2021 meta-analysis) and high levels of fluctuation in self-esteem in paranoid patients but not in nonparanoid patients—but there was little evidence that the paranoid patients showed abnormal discrepancies between their scores on implicit and explicit self-esteem measures (Murphy et al. 2018).

Cognitive (Direct) Model of Paranoia

A model of paranoia that is in many ways simpler than the defense model has been developed over many years by Daniel Freeman, Philippa Garety, and colleagues. It was inspired in part by Maher's earlier anomalous perception account but also incorporates additional cognitive and emotional components (Freeman 2016; Freeman et al. 2002). The model stresses how patients' appraisals of their own experiences can be affected by emotional and cognitive biases, which leads directly to paranoid explanations. Persecutory delusions are therefore regarded as threat beliefs that arise from a search for the meaning of anomalous internal or external experiences. Once established, threat beliefs are in turn maintained by various cognitive and behavioral factors (Freeman et al. 2002; Garety and Freeman 1999), including safety behaviors, such as the avoidance of situations that might provide disconfirmatory evidence about paranoid hypotheses (Freeman et al. 2007). Hence, the model attempts to account for both the formation of paranoid beliefs as a direct reflection of the psychology of the individual rather than as a defense and how these beliefs are maintained once formed (Freeman 2007; Freeman et al. 2002).

An early attempt to characterize a cognitive bias that has subsequently been incorporated into this model was made by Hemsley and Garety (1986), who argued that the reasoning style of deluded patients deviated from Bayesian probabilistic inference, which led patients to reach a conclusion without seeking the necessary information or rendered them unable to change their minds when presented with new information that was incongruent with an established belief system (Garety et al. 1991). This type of bias has been termed a *data-gathering* or *jumping to conclusion bias*, and many studies have now been conducted to measure it, typically using the beads task. In this task, participants are shown two jars, one with predominantly red beads but some blue and the other with the ratio (typically 85:15) reversed. Participants are presented with a bead and given the choice of either deciding which jar it came from or requesting another bead (seeking more evidence); the process continues until the participant makes a decision (a number of variations of this procedure have been tried in different studies). Studies have consistently found strong associations between delusions and reaching a hasty decision compared with control subjects, such that some deluded patients make a decision after seeing only one or two beads (Garety and Freeman 2013; McLean et al. 2017; So et al. 2016). Note that this bias is believed to be specific not to paranoia but to delusions more generally. However, some studies have found that the data-gathering bias is especially strong in paranoid patients when they are assessed with probability reasoning tasks that use socially and emotionally salient stimuli rather than beads (Dudley et al. 1997; Lincoln et al. 2011; Young and Bentall 1997). More than 30 years after this task was first used, some questions about the precise psychological mechanisms involved remain. For example, some studies have shown that the bias is closely correlated with and may be indistinguishable from broader measures of executive function (Bentall et al. 2009).

A similar concept that has garnered attention more recently is the bias against disconfirmatory information (Woodward et al. 2007, 2008). This is measured with a task in which participants are shown a picture and then asked to choose which of four hypotheses most likely describes the events depicted. Additional pictures are presented, and the participants are asked to reevaluate the hypotheses. A bias against disconfirmatory information is demonstrated when information that is inconsistent with an initial hypothesis does not lead to a change in the participant's appraisal of the likelihood of the hypotheses. Again, the bias against disconfirmatory information has been consistently associated with delusions (McLean et al. 2017), although not specifically with paranoia. One significant aspect of this observation (as with most versions of the beads task) is that the content of the task is unrelated to patients' delusional beliefs, which suggests that the cognitive biases of deluded patients are general and not restricted to when these patients reason about information related to their delusions.

Role of Attachment

As noted earlier, there is consistent evidence that paranoid beliefs are associated with negative beliefs about the self (Humphrey et al. 2021) and attributional biases (Müller et al. 2021; Murphy et al. 2018). The defense model and the direct cognitive model both incorporate these biases, although the way that these biases then lead to paranoia is different in the two models: in the defense model, the individual uses attributions to reduce the distress associated with awareness of negative beliefs about the self; in the direct model, these biases cause feelings of vulnerability and help shape paranoid interpretations of anomalous experiences. Most researchers believe that these biases are likely to be mediating mechanisms that help to explain the relationship between paranoia and adverse life experiences, such as experiences of victimization and disrupted early relationships with caregivers.

Research has expanded our understanding of emotional processes in paranoia by focusing on attachment processes. Attachment styles were conceptualized by the British developmentalist John Bowlby (1969) as internalized representations of relationships with primary caregivers. These representations take the form of working models of the self and others, which in turn guide interpersonal behavior (Shaver and Mikulincer 2005). In adulthood, these styles can be secure or insecure, with the former reflecting confidence in the availability of attachment figures and the latter reflecting the contrary (Mikulincer 1995). Two underlying dimensions of attachment insecurity in adults are anxiety and avoidance. Attachment avoidance is associated with insecurity about another's intentions, preference for emotional distance, and a negative view of others; attachment anxiety reflects negative self-beliefs, fear of rejection, and excessive need for approval (Berry et al. 2007; Mikulincer 1995).

Bentall and Fernyhough (2008) proposed that an insecure attachment process might explain the relationship between early adverse experiences—in particular disrupted bonds with caregivers—and paranoid beliefs. Pickering et al. (2008) subsequently demonstrated that subclinical paranoid beliefs were associated with both anxious and avoidant styles and that this relationship was mediated by negative beliefs about the self, the anticipation of threat, and the perception of others as powerful and controlling. Later Wickham et al. (2015) showed that paranoia symptoms (but not hallucinations) in a clinical sample were also associated with both insecure styles and that this effect was mediated by low self-esteem (see also Ringer et al. 2014). These associations between insecure attachment and paranoia have since been replicated many times in both clinical and nonclinical samples (for a meta-analysis, see Murphy et al. 2020).

In a longitudinal (experience sampling) study with clinical participants, fluctuations in attachment-related cognitions were shown to predict fluctuations in paranoid beliefs, and this effect was much stronger than the association between fluctuations in self-esteem and paranoia (Sitko et al. 2016). Furthermore, a recent study with a large subclinical sample confirmed that low self-esteem was a mediator only in the case of attachment anxiety but also found that the relationship between both insecure attachment styles (anxious and avoidant) and paranoia was mediated by a tendency to judge unfamiliar faces as untrustworthy (Martinez et al. 2021). This latter finding is consistent with previous research showing that insecure attachment is related to mistrust (Fett et al. 2016; Mikulincer 1995, 1998) and suggests that mistrust may be an important factor that explains the difference between paranoia and other conditions related to insecure attachment, such as depression.

Conclusion

In this chapter we have tried to document the enormous progress in the understanding of persecutory delusions and paranoid beliefs that has been achieved since the early days of psychiatry. This progress has accelerated dramatically since the final decade of the past century, largely because of the pursuit of systematic psychological research programs. We ended this chapter by reviewing recent psychological models. Rather than focus on the disagreements between these models, we think it would be more helpful to conclude by summarizing what is now agreed on in terms of the processes and mechanisms that lead to paranoid thinking.

First, the idea that paranoia should be considered a phenomenon in its own right, and one that encompasses a continuum between persecutory delusions and ordinary mistrust and suspiciousness, has been extraordinarily fruitful. Although questions remain about this continuum, it is notable that many findings from psychological research have been replicated both with patients who have persecutory delusions and with nonpatients who score high on measures of paranoid belief.

Second, it is now widely agreed that adverse experiences, especially in childhood, play an important causal role in psychotic experiences (Bentall 2021), and this seems to be true for paranoia. In particular, disrupted early relationships with caregivers, exposure to harsh environments, and experiences of victimization seem to be important risk factors for the later development of paranoid states.

Third, there is consistent evidence that paranoia is associated with specific psychological-emotional processes: an exaggerated self-serving attributional bias, negative self-schematic processes, insecure attachment styles, and a tendency to mistrust. Fourth and finally, the most extreme form of paranoid belief—persecutory delusions—also seems to be associated with more general cognitive biases in the ability to integrate information and test hypotheses.

These findings provide many indications for how psychological treatments might be designed for patients with persecutory delusions. There is already evidence that cognitive-behavioral therapy can be effective for such patients, although effects are modest and may not exceed those achieved with other kinds of psychotherapeutic approaches (Mehl et al. 2015). At the time of this writing, considerable effort is being directed to enhancing the therapeutic effectiveness of cognitive-behavioral therapy for psychosis by focusing on some of the specific cognitive and emotional mechanisms highlighted in this review, such as reasoning biases (Eichner and Berna 2016) and negative beliefs about the self (Forkert et al. 2022), or on putative causal factors such as insomnia (Freeman et al. 2017) and trauma memories (de Bont et al. 2016). Throughout much of the past century, the psychological needs of patients with psychosis were neglected (Bentall 2009). We hope that an understanding of the causal mechanisms involved in paranoia will lead to better and more humane psychiatric care for patients in the future.

Questions for Discussion

1. In light of the evidence reviewed in this chapter, what factors should be considered when conducting an assessment of a paranoid patient?

2. Why have psychological interventions thus far shown only modest effect sizes in clinical trials?

3. How would you prioritize targets for psychological intervention for patients with paranoid beliefs?

4. What are the clinical implications of the association between paranoia and insecure attachment styles?

5. Is paranoia a public health problem?

KEY POINTS

- Persecutory (paranoid) delusions have often been viewed as symptoms of psychiatric disorders such as schizophrenia and delusional disorder, but there is evidence that they exist on a continuum with ordinary experiences of mistrust and suspiciousness.

- There is strong evidence that life experiences contribute to paranoid beliefs. People with these beliefs are likely to have had experiences of victimization and also to have experienced disruption of early attachment relationships with caregivers. These observations may help to explain why ethnic and sexual minority groups are at high risk for developing paranoid beliefs.

- A number of psychological models have been developed to explain the relationship between adverse life experiences and paranoia. These models have focused on anomalous perceptions, defensive processes, and cognitive and emotional biases. They indicate suitable targets for psychological interventions for paranoia.

References

American Psychiatric Association: Diagnostic and Statistical Manual: Mental Disorders. Washington, DC, American Psychiatric Association, 1952

American Psychiatric Association: Diagnostic and Statistical Manual of Mental Disorders, 3rd Edition. Washington, DC, American Psychiatric Association, 1980

American Psychiatric Association: Diagnostic and Statistical Manual of Mental Disorders, 5th Edition, Text Revision. Washington, DC, American Psychiatric Association, 2022

Axelrod SR, Widiger TA, Trull TJ, Corbitt EM: Relations of five-factor model antagonism facets with personality disorder symptomatology. J Pers Assess 69(2):297–313, 1997 9392892

Baas D, van't Wout M, Aleman A, Kahn RS: Social judgement in clinically stable patients with schizophrenia and healthy relatives: behavioural evidence of social brain dysfunction. Psychol Med 38(5):747–754, 2008 17988413

Barreto Carvalho C, Sousa M, da Motta C, et al: Paranoia in the general population: a revised version of the General Paranoia Scale for adults. Clin Psychol 21(2):125–134, 2017

Bebbington P, Freeman D: Transdiagnostic extension of delusions: schizophrenia and beyond. Schizophr Bull 43(2):273–282, 2017 28399309

Bebbington PE, McBride O, Steel C, et al: The structure of paranoia in the general population. Br J Psychiatry 202:419–427, 2013 23661767

Beckett S: Murphy. London, George Routledge, 1938

Bell V, O'Driscoll C: The network structure of paranoia in the general population. Soc Psychiatry Psychiatr Epidemiol 53(7):737–744, 2018 29427197

Bell V, Halligan PW, Ellis HD: Explaining delusions: a cognitive perspective. Trends Cogn Sci 10(5):219–226, 2006 16600666

Bell V, Halligan PW, Ellis HD: Are anomalous perceptual experiences necessary for delusions? J Nerv Ment Dis 196(1):3–8, 2008 18195635

Bentall RP: Madness Explained: Psychosis and Human Nature. New York, Penguin, 2003

Bentall RP: Doctoring the Mind: Why Psychiatric Treatments Fail. New York, Penguin, 2009

Bentall RP: The role of early life experience in psychosis, in Psychotic Disorders: Comprehensive Conceptualization and Treatments. Edited by Tamminga CA, Ivleva EI, Reininghaus U, van Os J. New York, Oxford University Press, 2021, pp 406–414

Bentall RP, Fernyhough C: Social predictors of psychotic experiences: specificity and psychological mechanisms. Schizophr Bull 34(6):1012–1020, 2008 18703667

Bentall RP, Kinderman P, Kaney S: The self, attributional processes and abnormal beliefs: towards a model of persecutory delusions. Behav Res Ther 32(3):331–341, 1994 8192633

Bentall RP, Corcoran R, Howard R, et al: Persecutory delusions: a review and theoretical integration. Clin Psychol Rev 21(8):1143–1192, 2001 11702511

Bentall RP, Rowse G, Shryane N, et al: The cognitive and affective structure of paranoid delusions: a transdiagnostic investigation of patients with schizophrenia spectrum disorders and depression. Arch Gen Psychiatry 66(3):236–247, 2009 19255373

Bentall RP, Wickham S, Shevlin M, Varese F: Do specific early life adversities lead to specific symptoms of psychosis? A study from the 2007 the Adult Psychiatric Morbidity Survey. Schizophr Bull 38(4):734–740, 2012 22496540

Berry K, Wearden A, Barrowclough C: Adult attachment styles and psychosis: an investigation of associations between general attachment styles and attachment relationships with specific others. Soc Psychiatry Psychiatr Epidemiol 42(12):972–976, 2007 17932610

Blanchard JJ, Andrea A, Orth RD, et al: Sleep disturbance and sleep-related impairment in psychotic disorders are related to both positive and negative symptoms. Psychiatry Res 286:112857, 2020 32087449

Blashfield RK: The Classification of Psychopathology: Neo-Kraepelinian and Quantitative Approaches. New York, Plenum, 1984

Borsboom D, Cramer AOJ: Network analysis: an integrative approach to the structure of psychopathology. Annu Rev Clin Psychol 9(1):91–121, 2013 23537483

Bosqui TJ, Hoy K, Shannon C: A systematic review and meta-analysis of the ethnic density effect in psychotic disorders. Soc Psychiatry Psychiatr Epidemiol 49(4):519–529, 2014 24114240

Bowlby J: Attachment and Loss, Vol 1: Attachment. London, Hogarth, 1969

Brown P, Waite F, Freeman D: "Twisting the lion's tail": manipulationist tests of causation for psychological mechanisms in the occurrence of delusions and hallucinations. Clin Psychol Rev 68:25–37, 2019 30617014

Brown P, Waite F, Freeman D: Parenting behaviour and paranoia: a network analysis and results from the National Comorbidity Survey–Adolescents (NCS-A). Soc Psychiatry Psychiatr Epidemiol 56:593–604, 2021

Brown TA, Barlow DH: Dimensional versus categorical classification of mental disorders in the fifth edition of the Diagnostic and Statistical Manual of Mental Disorders and beyond: comment on the special section. J Abnorm Psychol 114(4):551–556, 2005 16351377

Buck BE, Pinkham AE, Harvey PD, Penn DL: Revisiting the validity of measures of social cognitive bias in schizophrenia: Additional results from the Social Cognition Psychometric Evaluation (SCOPE) study. Br J Clin Psychol 55(4):441–454, 2016 27168196

Camerer CF: Behavioural studies of strategic thinking in games. Trends Cogn Sci 7(5):225–231, 2003 12757825

Černis E, Bird JC, Molodynski A, et al: Cognitive appraisals of dissociation in psychosis: a new brief measure. Behav Cogn Psychother 49(4):472–484, 2021 33446299

Chapman LJ, Chapman JP: The genesis of delusions, in Delusional Beliefs. Edited by Oltmanns TF, Maher BA. Hoboken, NJ, Wiley, 1988, pp 167–183

Cheesman R, Selzam S, Ronald A, et al: Childhood behaviour problems show the greatest gap between DNA-based and twin heritability. Transl Psychiatry 7(12):1284, 2017 29234009

Combs DR, Penn DL, Cassisi J, et al: Perceived racism as a predictor of paranoia among African Americans. J Black Psychol 32(1):87–104, 2006

Combs DR, Penn DL, Wicher M, Waldheter E: The Ambiguous Intentions Hostility Questionnaire (AIHQ): a new measure for evaluating hostile social-cognitive biases in paranoia. Cogn Neuropsychiatry 12(2):128-143, 2007 17453895

Combs DR, Penn DL, Michael CO, et al: Perceptions of hostility by persons with and without persecutory delusions. Cogn Neuropsychiatry 14(1):30–52, 2009 19214841

Conrad K: Beginning schizophrenia: attempt for a Gestalt-analysis of delusion (1958), in The Maudsley Reader in Phenomenological Psychiatry. Edited by

Broome MR, Harland R, Owen GS, Stringaris A. Cambridge, UK, Cambridge University Press, 2012, pp 176–193

Cooper AF, Curry AR: The pathology of deafness in the paranoid and affective psychoses of later life. J Psychosom Res 20(2):97–105, 1976 1271318

Corcoran R, Mansfield R, de Bezenac C, et al: Perceived neighbourhood affluence, mental health and wellbeing influence judgements of threat and trust on our streets: an urban walking study. PLoS One 13(8):e0202412, 2018 30114264

Couture SM, Penn DL, Addington J, et al: Assessment of social judgments and complex mental states in the early phases of psychosis. Schizophr Res 100(1–3):237–241, 2008 18255273

Dalenberg CJ, Brand BL, Gleaves DH, et al: Evaluation of the evidence for the trauma and fantasy models of dissociation. Psychol Bull 138(3):550–588, 2012 22409505

de Bont PAJM, van den Berg DPG, van der Vleugel BM, et al: Prolonged exposure and EMDR for PTSD v. a PTSD waiting-list condition: effects on symptoms of psychosis, depression and social functioning in patients with chronic psychotic disorders. Psychol Med 46(11):2411–2421, 2016 27297048

Dowbiggin I: Delusional diagnosis? The history of paranoia as a disease concept in the modern era. Hist Psychiatry 11(41 Pt 1):37–69, 2000 11624609

Dudley REJ, John CH, Young AW, Over DE: The effect of self-referent material on the reasoning of people with delusions. Br J Clin Psychol 36(4):575–584, 1997 9403148

Eichner C, Berna F: Acceptance and efficacy of metacognitive training (MCT) on positive symptoms and delusions in patients with schizophrenia: a meta-analysis taking into account important moderators. Schizophr Bull 42(4):952–962, 2016 26748396

Elahi A, Perez Algorta G, Varese F, et al: Do paranoid delusions exist on a continuum with subclinical paranoia? A multi-method taxometric study. Schizophr Res 190:77–81, 2017 28318838

Elahi A, McIntyre JC, Hampson C, et al: Home is where you hang your hat: host town identity, but not hometown identity, protects against mental health symptoms associated with financial stress. J Soc Clin Psychol 37(3):159–181, 2018

Ellett L, Freeman D, Garety PA: The psychological effect of an urban environment on individuals with persecutory delusions: the Camberwell walk study. Schizophr Res 99(1–3):77–84, 2008 18061407

Ellett L, Allen-Crooks R, Stevens A, et al: A paradigm for the study of paranoia in the general population: the Prisoner's Dilemma Game. Cogn Emotion 27(1):53–62, 2013 22731988

Ellis HD, Young AW, Quayle AH, De Pauw KW: Reduced autonomic responses to faces in Capgras delusion. Proc Biol Sci 264(1384):1085–1092, 1997 9263474

Faris REL, Dunham HW: Mental Disorders in Urban Areas. Chicago, IL, University of Chicago Press, 1939

Fett A-KJ, Shergill SS, Joyce DW, et al: To trust or not to trust: the dynamics of social interaction in psychosis. Brain 135(Pt 3):976–984, 2012 22366802

Fett A-KJ, Shergill SS, Korver-Nieberg N, et al: Learning to trust: trust and attachment in early psychosis. Psychol Med 46(7):1437–1447, 2016 26898947

Forkert A, Brown P, Freeman D, Waite F: A compassionate imagery intervention for patients with persecutory delusions. Behav Cogn Psychother 50:15–27, 2022 34078499

Fornells-Ambrojo M, Garety PA: Bad me paranoia in early psychosis: a relatively rare phenomenon. Br J Clin Psychol 44(Pt 4):521–528, 2005 16368031

Freeman D: Suspicious minds: the psychology of persecutory delusions. Clin Psychol Rev 27(4):425–457, 2007 17258852

Freeman D: The assessment of persecutory ideation, in Persecutory Delusions: Assessment, Theory, and Treatment. Edited by Freeman D, Bentall R, Garety P. New York, Oxford University Press, 2008, pp 23–52

Freeman D: Persecutory delusions: a cognitive perspective on understanding and treatment. Lancet Psychiatry 3(7):685–692, 2016 27371990

Freeman D, Garety PA: Comments on the content of persecutory delusions: does the definition need clarification? Br J Clin Psychol 39(4):407–414, 2000 11107494

Freeman D, Garety PA, Kuipers E, et al: A cognitive model of persecutory delusions. Br J Clin Psychol 41(Pt 4):331–347, 2002 12437789

Freeman D, Garety PA, Kuipers E, et al: Acting on persecutory delusions: the importance of safety seeking. Behav Res Ther 45(1):89–99, 2007 16530161

Freeman D, Pugh K, Vorontsova N, Southgate L: Insomnia and paranoia. Schizophr Res 108(1–3):280–284, 2009 19097752

Freeman D, Startup H, Dunn G, et al: The interaction of affective with psychotic processes: a test of the effects of worrying on working memory, jumping to conclusions, and anomalies of experience in patients with persecutory delusions. J Psychiatr Res 47(12):1837–1842, 2013 23871449

Freeman D, Dunn G, Murray RM, et al: How cannabis causes paranoia: using the intravenous administration of D9-tetrahydrocannabinol (THC) to identify key cognitive mechanisms leading to paranoia. Schizophr Bull 41(2):391–399, 2015a 25031222

Freeman D, Waite F, Startup H, et al: Efficacy of cognitive behavioural therapy for sleep improvement in patients with persistent delusions and hallucinations (BEST): a prospective, assessor-blind, randomised controlled pilot trial. Lancet Psychiatry 2(11):975–983, 2015b 26363701

Freeman D, Sheaves B, Goodwin GM, et al: The effects of improving sleep on mental health (OASIS): a randomised controlled trial with mediation analysis. Lancet Psychiatry 4(10):749–758, 2017 28888927

Freud S: Psychoanalytic notes upon an autobiographical account of a case of paranoia (dementia paranoides) (1911), in Collected Papers, Vol 3. London, Hogarth, 1950, pp 387–466

Furnham A, Crump J: A big five facet analysis of a paranoid personality disorder: the validity of the HDS Sceptical Scale of subclinical paranoia. J Individ Differ 36(4):199–204, 2015

Garety PA, Freeman D: Cognitive approaches to delusions: a critical review of theories and evidence. Br J Clin Psychol 38(2):113–154, 1999 10389596

Garety PA, Freeman D: The past and future of delusions research: from the inexplicable to the treatable. Br J Psychiatry 203(5):327–333, 2013 24187067

Garety PA, Hemsley DR, Wessely S: Reasoning in deluded schizophrenic and paranoid patients: biases in performance on a probabilistic inference task. J Nerv Ment Dis 179(4):194–201, 1991 2007889

Greenaway KH, Haslam SA, Bingley W: Are "they" out to get me? A social identity model of paranoia. Group Process Intergroup Relat 22(7):984–1001, 2019

Gromann PM, Heslenfeld DJ, Fett A-K, et al: Trust versus paranoia: abnormal response to social reward in psychotic illness. Brain 136(Pt 6):1968–1975, 2013 23611807

Gummerum M, Hanoch Y, Keller M: When child development meets economic game theory: an interdisciplinary approach to investigating social development. Human Development 51(4):235–261, 2008

Guze SB: Biological psychiatry: is there any other kind? Psychol Med 19(2):315–323, 1989 2762437

Haselton MG, Nettle D: The paranoid optimist: an integrative evolutionary model of cognitive biases. Pers Soc Psychol Rev 10(1):47–66, 2006 16430328

Hatzakis T: Towards a framework of trust attribution styles. British Journal of Management 20(4):448–460, 2009

Haut KM, MacDonald AW III: Persecutory delusions and the perception of trustworthiness in unfamiliar faces in schizophrenia. Psychiatry Res 178(3):456–460, 2010 20569994

Hemsley DR, Garety PA: The formation of maintenance of delusions: a Bayesian analysis. Br J Psychiatry 149(JULY):51–56, 1986 3779313

Hillmann TE, Ascone L, Kempkensteffen J, Lincoln TM: Scanning to conclusions? Visual attention to neutral faces under stress in individuals with and without subclinical paranoia. J Behav Ther Exp Psychiatry 56:137–143, 2017 27597173

Hoehne KA: Ernst Kretschmer's multidimensional psychiatry. J Pers Disord 2(1):28–35, 1988

Hooker CI, Tully LM, Verosky SC, et al: Can I trust you? Negative affective priming influences social judgments in schizophrenia. J Abnorm Psychol 120(1):98–107, 2011 20919787

Huddy V, Brown GP, Boyd T, Wykes T: An exploratory investigation of real-world reasoning in paranoia. Psychol Psychother 87(1):44–59, 2014 24497396

Humphrey C, Bucci S, Varese F, et al: Paranoia and negative schema about the self and others: a systematic review and meta-analysis. Clin Psychol Rev 90:102081, 2021 34564019

Kahn-Greene ET, Killgore DB, Kamimori GH, et al: The effects of sleep deprivation on symptoms of psychopathology in healthy adults. Sleep Med 8(3):215–221, 2007 17368979

Kaney S, Bentall RP: Persecutory delusions and attributional style. Br J Med Psychol 62(Pt 2):191–198, 1989 2751948

Kaney S, Bentall RP: Persecutory delusions and the self-serving bias: evidence from a contingency judgment task. J Nerv Ment Dis 180(12):773–780, 1992 1469376

Kasanova Z, Hajdúk M, Thewissen V, Myin-Germeys I: Temporal associations between sleep quality and paranoia across the paranoia continuum: an experience sampling study. J Abnorm Psychol 129(1):122–130, 2020 31343182

Kendler KS: The nosologic validity of paranoia (simple delusional disorder): a review. Arch Gen Psychiatry 37(6):699–706, 1980 7387341

Kendler KS: Kraepelin and the diagnostic concept of paranoia. Compr Psychiatry 29(1):4–11, 1988 3277769

Kendler KS: A joint history of the nature of genetic variation and the nature of schizophrenia. Mol Psychiatry 20(1):77–83, 2015 25134695

Kendler KS: The development of Kraepelin's mature diagnostic concepts of paranoia (die Verrücktheit) and paranoid dementia praecox (dementia paranoides): a close reading of his textbooks from 1887 to 1899. JAMA Psychiatry 75(12):1280–1288, 2018 30422155

Kesting ML, Lincoln TM: The relevance of self-esteem and self-schemas to persecutory delusions: a systematic review. Compr Psychiatry 54(7):766–789, 2013 23684547

Kinderman P, Bentall RP: Self-discrepancies and persecutory delusions: evidence for a model of paranoid ideation. J Abnorm Psychol 105(1):106–113, 1996 8666699

Kirk H, Gilmour A, Dudley R, Riby D: Paranoid ideation and assessments of trust. J Exp Psychopathol 4(4):360–367, 2013

Kong DT: Sojourners' ineffective sociocultural adaptation: paranoia as a joint function of distrust toward host nationals and neuroticism. Curr Psychol 36(3):540–548, 2017

Kramer RM: The sinister attribution error: paranoid cognition and collective distrust in organizations. Motiv Emot 18(2):199–230, 1994

Lee R: Mistrustful and misunderstood: a review of paranoid personality disorder. Curr Behav Neurosci Rep 4(2):151–165, 2017 29399432

Lewicki RJ, Brinsfield CT: Measuring trust beliefs and behaviours, in Handbook of Research Methods on Trust. Edited by Lyon F, Möllering G, Saunders MNK. Cheltenham, UK, Edward Elgar, 2012, pp 29–39

Lewicki RJ, Tomlinson EC, Gillespie N: Models of interpersonal trust development: theoretical approaches, empirical evidence, and future directions. J Manage 32(6):991–1022, 2006

Lewis A: Paranoia and paranoid: a historical perspective. Psychol Med 1(1):2–12, 1970 4948910

Lincoln TM, Salzmann S, Ziegler M, Westermann S: When does jumping-to-conclusions reach its peak? The interaction of vulnerability and situation-characteristics in social reasoning. J Behav Ther Exp Psychiatry 42(2):185–191, 2011 21315880

Longden E, Branitsky A, Moskowitz A, et al: The relationship between dissociation and symptoms of psychosis: a meta-analysis. Schizophr Bull 46(5):1104–1113, 2020 32251520

Maher BA: Delusional thinking and perceptual disorder. J Individ Psychol 30(1):98–113, 1974 4857199

Maher B: Anomalous experience in everyday life: its significance for psychopathology. Monist 82(4):547–570, 1999

Martinez AP, Agostini M, Al-Suhibani A, Bentall RP: Mistrust and negative self-esteem: two paths from attachment styles to paranoia. Psychol Psychother 94(3):391–406, 2021 33314565

McElroy E, McIntyre JC, Bentall RP, et al: Mental health, deprivation, and the neighbourhood social environment: a network analysis. Clin Psychol Sci 7:719–743, 2019

McIntyre JC, Elahi A, Bentall R: Social identity and psychosis: explaining elevated rates of psychosis in migrant populations. Soc Personal Psychol Compass 10(11):619–633, 2016

McIntyre JC, Wickham S, Barr B, Bentall RP: Social identity and psychosis: associations and psychological mechanisms. Schizophr Bull 44(3):681–690, 2018

McIntyre JC, Elahi A, Barlow FK, et al: The relationship between ingroup identity and paranoid ideation among people from African and African Caribbean backgrounds. Psychol Psychother 94(1):16–32, 2021 31742832

McLean BF, Mattiske JK, Balzan RP: Association of the jumping to conclusions and evidence integration biases with delusions in psychosis: a detailed meta-analysis. Schizophr Bull 43(2):344–354, 2017 27169465

Mehl S, Werner D, Lincoln TM: Does cognitive behavior therapy for psychosis (CBTp) show a sustainable effect on delusions? A meta-analysis. Front Psychol 6:1450, 2015 26500570

Melo SS, Taylor JL, Bentall RP: "Poor me" versus "bad me" paranoia and the instability of persecutory ideation. Psychol Psychother 79(Pt 2):271–287, 2006 16774723

Mikulincer M: Attachment style and the mental representation of the self. J Pers Soc Psychol 69(6):1203–1215, 1995

Mikulincer M: Attachment working models and the sense of trust: an exploration of interaction goals and affect regulation. J Pers Soc Psychol 74(5):1209, 1998

Mirowsky J, Ross CE: Paranoia and the structure of powerlessness. Am Sociol Rev 48(2):228–239, 1983 6859680

Mishara AL: Klaus Conrad (1905–1961): delusional mood, psychosis, and beginning schizophrenia. Schizophr Bull 36(1):9–13, 2010 19965934

Moutoussis M, Williams J, Dayan P, Bentall RP: Persecutory delusions and the conditioned avoidance paradigm: towards an integration of the psychology and biology of paranoia. Cogn Neuropsychiatry 12(6):495–510, 2007 17978936

Müller H, Betz LT, Bechdolf A: A comprehensive meta-analysis of the self-serving bias in schizophrenia spectrum disorders compared to non-clinical subjects. Neurosci Biobehav Rev 120:542–549, 2021 33148471

Murphy J, Shevlin M, Adamson G, et al: Memories of childhood threat, fear of disclosure and paranoid ideation: a mediation analysis using a nonclinical sample. J Aggress Maltreat Trauma 21(4):459–476, 2012

Murphy P, Bentall RP, Freeman D, et al: The paranoia as defence model of persecutory delusions: a systematic review and meta-analysis. Lancet Psychiatry 5(11):913–929, 2018 30314852

Murphy R, Goodall K, Woodrow A: The relationship between attachment insecurity and experiences on the paranoia continuum: a meta-analysis. Br J Clin Psychol 59(3):290–318, 2020 32227508

Myers E, Startup H, Freeman D: Cognitive behavioural treatment of insomnia in individuals with persistent persecutory delusions: a pilot trial. J Behav Ther Exp Psychiatry 42(3):330–336, 2011 21367359

Oosterhof NN, Todorov A: The functional basis of face evaluation. Proc Natl Acad Sci USA 105(32):11087–11092, 2008 18685089

Owen MJ: Implications of genetic findings for understanding schizophrenia. Schizophr Bull 38(5):904–907, 2012 22987847

Pickering L, Simpson J, Bentall RP: Insecure attachment predicts proneness to paranoia but not hallucinations. Pers Indiv Dif 44(5):1212–1224, 2008

Pilton M, Varese F, Berry K, Bucci S: The relationship between dissociation and voices: a systematic literature review and meta-analysis. Clin Psychol Rev 40:138–155, 2015 26117061

Pinkham AE, Hopfinger JB, Pelphrey KA, et al: Neural bases for impaired social cognition in schizophrenia and autism spectrum disorders. Schizophr Res 99(1–3):164–175, 2008 18053686

Qi R, Palmier-Claus J, Simpson J, et al: Sexual minority status and symptoms of psychosis: the role of bullying, discrimination, social support, and drug use—findings from the Adult Psychiatric Morbidity Survey 2007. Psychol Psychother 93(3):503–519, 2020 31343817

Raihani NJ, Bell V: Paranoia and the social representation of others: a large-scale game theory approach. Sci Rep 7:4544, 2017 28674445

Rankin P, Bentall R, Hill J, Kinderman P: Perceived relationships with parents and paranoid delusions: comparisons of currently ill, remitted and normal participants. Psychopathology 38(1):16–25, 2005 15714009

Reeve S, Emsley R, Sheaves B, Freeman D: Disrupting sleep: the effects of sleep loss on psychotic experiences tested in an experimental study with mediation analysis. Schizophr Bull 44(3):662–671, 2018 28981834

Renard SB, Huntjens RJC, Lysaker PH, et al: Unique and overlapping symptoms in schizophrenia spectrum and dissociative disorders in relation to models of psychopathology: a systematic review. Schizophr Bull 43(1):108–121, 2017 27209638

Ringer JM, Buchanan EE, Olesek K, Lysaker PH: Anxious and avoidant attachment styles and indicators of recovery in schizophrenia: associations with self-esteem and hope. Psychol Psychother 87(2):209–221, 2014 23913519

Schreber DP: Memoirs of My Nervous Illness (1903). Translated by Macalpine I, Hunter RA. London, Dawson, 1955

Shaver PR, Mikulincer M: Attachment theory and research: resurrection of the psychodynamic approach to personality. J Res Pers 39:22–45, 2005

Shevlin M, McAnee G, Bentall RP, Murphy J: Specificity of association between adversities and the occurrence and co-occurrence paranoia and hallucinations: evaluating the stability of childhood risk in an adverse adult environment. Psychosis 7(3):206–216, 2015

Sieradzka D, Power RA, Freeman D, et al: Heritability of individual psychotic experiences captured by common genetic variants in a community sample of adolescents. Behav Genet 45(5):493–502, 2015 26049723

Simpson JA: Foundations of interpersonal trust, in Social Psychology: Handbook of Basic Principles, 2nd Edition. Edited by Kruglanski AW, Higgins ET. New York, Guilford, 2007, pp 587–607

Sitko K, Bentall RP, Shevlin M, et al: Associations between specific psychotic symptoms and specific childhood adversities are mediated by attachment styles: an analysis of the National Comorbidity Survey. Psychiatry Res 217(3):202–209, 2014 24726818

Sitko K, Varese F, Sellwood W, et al: The dynamics of attachment insecurity and paranoid thoughts: an experience sampling study. Psychiatry Res 246:32–38, 2016 27649527

So SH, Siu NY, Wong HL, et al: "Jumping to conclusions" data-gathering bias in psychosis and other psychiatric disorders: two meta-analyses of comparisons between patients and healthy individuals. Clin Psychol Rev 46:151–167, 2016 27216559

Spitzer RL, Fleiss JL: A re-analysis of the reliability of psychiatric diagnosis. Br J Psychiatry 125(587):341–347, 1974 4425771

Stefanis N, Thewissen V, Bakoula C, et al: Hearing impairment and psychosis: a replication in a cohort of young adults. Schizophr Res 85(1–3):266–272, 2006 16650736

Strand M: Where do classifications come from? The DSM-III, the transformation of American psychiatry, and the problem of origins in the sociology of knowledge. Theory Soc 40:273–313, 2011

Strauss GP, Lee BG, Waltz JA, et al: Cognition-emotion interactions are modulated by working memory capacity in individuals with schizophrenia. Schizophr Res 141(2–3):257–261, 2012 22968207

Sullivan PF, Kendler KS, Neale MC: Schizophrenia as a complex trait: evidence from a meta-analysis of twin studies. Arch Gen Psychiatry 60(12):1187–1192, 2003 14662550

Thewissen V, Myin-Germeys I, Bentall R, et al: Hearing impairment and psychosis revisited. Schizophr Res 76(1):99–103, 2005 15927803

Tiernan B, Tracey R, Shannon C: Paranoia and self-concepts in psychosis: a systematic review of the literature. Psychiatry Res 216(3):303–313, 2014 24630916

Todorov A, Pakrashi M, Oosterhof NN: Evaluating faces on trustworthiness after minimal time exposure. Soc Cogn 27(6):813–833, 2009

Trémeau F, Antonius D, Todorov A, et al: What can the study of first impressions tell us about attitudinal ambivalence and paranoia in schizophrenia? Psychiatry Res 238:86–92, 2016 27086216

Trotta A, Kang J, Stahl D, Yiend J: Interpretation bias in paranoia: a systematic review and meta-analysis. Clin Psychol Sci 9(1):3–23, 2021

Trower P, Chadwick P: Pathways to defense of the self: a theory of two types of paranoia. Clin Psychol (New York) 2(3):263–278, 1995

Udachina A, Varese F, Oorschot M, et al: Dynamics of self-esteem in "poor-me" and "bad-me" paranoia. J Nerv Ment Dis 200(9):777–783, 2012 22922239

van Os J, McGuffin P: Can the social environment cause schizophrenia? Br J Psychiatry 182(4):291–292, 2003 12668402

Varese F, Smeets F, Drukker M, et al: Childhood adversities increase the risk of psychosis: a meta-analysis of patient-control, prospective- and cross-sectional cohort studies. Schizophr Bull 38(4):661–671, 2012 22461484

Vassos E, Pedersen CB, Murray RM, et al: Meta-analysis of the association of urbanicity with schizophrenia. Schizophr Bull 38(6):1118–1123, 2012 23015685

Wickham S, Bentall R: Are specific early life adversities associated with specific symptoms of psychosis? A patient study considering just world beliefs as a mediator. J Nerv Ment Dis 204(8):606–613, 2016 27065105

Wickham S, Shryane N, Lyons M, et al: Why does relative deprivation affect mental health? The role of justice, trust and social rank in psychological wellbeing and paranoid ideation. J Public Ment Health 13(2):114–126, 2014a

Wickham S, Taylor P, Shevlin M, Bentall RP: The impact of social deprivation on paranoia, hallucinations, mania and depression: the role of discrimination social support, stress and trust. PLoS One 9(8):e105140, 2014b 25162703

Wickham S, Sitko K, Bentall RP: Insecure attachment is associated with paranoia but not hallucinations in psychotic patients: the mediating role of negative self-esteem. Psychol Med 45(7):1495–1507, 2015 25388512

Wicks S, Hjern A, Gunnell D, et al: Social adversity in childhood and the risk of developing psychosis: a national cohort study. Am J Psychiatry 162(9):1652–1657, 2005 16135624

Winokur G: Delusional disorder (paranoia). Compr Psychiatry 18(6):511–521, 1977 923223

Woodward TS, Buchy L, Moritz S, Liotti M: A bias against disconfirmatory evidence is associated with delusion proneness in a nonclinical sample. Schizophr Bull 33(4):1023–1028, 2007 17347526

Woodward TS, Moritz S, Menon M, Klinge R: Belief inflexibility in schizophrenia. Cogn Neuropsychiatry 13(3):267–277, 2008 18484291

Young HF, Bentall RP: Probabilistic reasoning in deluded, depressed and normal subjects: effects of task difficulty and meaningful versus non-meaningful material. Psychol Med 27(2):455–465, 1997 9089837

Zavos HMS, Freeman D, Haworth CMA, et al: Consistent etiology of severe, frequent psychotic experiences and milder, less frequent manifestations: a twin study of specific psychotic experiences in adolescence. JAMA Psychiatry 71(9):1049–1057, 2014 25075799

5

Linguistic Techniques for Clinicians Working With Patients With Delusions

Nazneen Rustom, Ph.D., B.A., GMBPsS
Gordon Turkington, M.Sc., B.Sc.

Patients who have firmly held beliefs are usually preoccupied with trying to understand their experiences and beliefs, even when interacting with others, including clinicians. Firmly held beliefs, or *delusions* as they are referred to clinically, are multifaceted; are laden with symbolism; and are often connected to a person's values, perceived identity, experiences, cognitions, emotions, and unmet needs. Complex delusional systems often coexist with formal thought disorder, including loosening of associations, knight's move thinking, and the use of neologisms. These act as a barrier to understanding, the formation of an alliance, and progress in cognitive-behavioral therapy (CBT). Therefore, when a clinician cannot understand a patient's speech, the multifaceted nature and deep meanings behind a firmly held belief can be lost. With patients themselves unable to fully understand their experience, communicating the experience and details of a delusion to another person is a true challenge. Some individuals who experience delusions may also have a schizophrenia spectrum disorder and may experience disorders of thought process that influence the clarity of verbal communication with clinicians. This chapter is written for clinicians who pose the following questions: How can I understand what my patients are saying in relation to their delusions? It seems important; I really do want to understand and try to help. What can I do?

The language used to describe delusions is highly meaningful and personal to patients. However, to better understand speech content, clinicians must engage in some decoding, which can be achieved using tools adapted from the discipline of linguistics, in particular, applied language and discourse analysis. First and foremost, every interaction and language exchange between the clinician and the patient should be approached with the aim of promoting recovery and healing and reinforcing understanding with care and compassion (Wright et al. 2014).

The aims of this chapter are 1) to help clinicians increase their own self-awareness when working with a thought-disordered and delusional patient, 2) to introduce to clinicians clinical linguistic concepts linked to clinical work with psychosis, and 3) to demonstrate three linguistic tools (adapted specifically for CBT approaches) for understanding a patient's speech that can make more sense of firmly held beliefs. These tools can allow the patient to make therapeutic progress with the help of an empowered clinician. In this chapter, fundamental learning points, clinical tips, and frequently asked questions and answers are presented.

After reading this chapter and applying the tools discussed, clinicians may experience an enhanced therapeutic alliance with their patients with chronic psychosis such that the patients feel respected and understood on a deeper level. In seeking to understand, clinicians may even promote a new therapeutic alliance where none had existed before. After reading this chapter, clinicians may be better able to organize treatment and care and to ask questions of the patient that are more directly helpful and relevant to a delusion.

Verbal Communication From Patients to Their Clinician: Ingredients of Understanding

When a language exchange goes well between a speaker (e.g., patient) and listener (e.g., clinician), there is seldom a problem. Both parties align, can rephrase each other's understanding, and draw similar factual conclusions from the conversation. When a language exchange goes well, there is more clarity than ambiguity, and both parties communicating can affirm, in their own minds, that a degree of understanding and agreement was achieved.

Conversely, when a language exchange does not go well, 1) a patient expressing a delusion may make statements that are not understood, either partially or fully, by the clinician, or the clinician 2) may abandon a line of questioning or may not know what to ask or 3) may terminate meeting the patient. When a language exchange does not go well, if statements made by the patient *sound* incomprehensible—in terms of sounds, words, the order of words in a sentence, repetition, inconsistent tone(s), difficulty with pronunciation, or intentional variation in enunciation—the clinician may not know how to address the statements and may abandon the meeting. Alternatively, the clinician may respond to incomprehensible speech and persist in asking questions unsuccessfully or may equally misinterpret the patient. Therefore, the clinician may inadvertently create a nontherapeutic experience for the patient. It may be a missed opportunity to understand the patient when the patient cannot communicate clearly. In some treatment settings, interactions that involve incomprehensible speech from patients may result in clinicians writing an all too familiar brief clinical note such as "Patient expressed delusional content with thought disorder" or "Modify dosage/change medication." Furthermore, it is likely that a clinician may not have the time to address a patient who expresses themselves in an atypical verbal manner. Thus, when clinicians lack skills to make sense of a delusion, this can potentially leave the patient feeling frustrated, invalidated, abandoned, misunderstood, and unhealed.

Personal Reflection: Clinician Orientation and Addressing Clinician Automatic Thoughts That May Impede Recovery

When I (N.R.) was a clinical trainee, I worked on a long-stay psychiatric ward with individuals who had medication-resistant schizophrenia. There were certain patients who were very talkative but were challenging to understand because of the form and content of the language expressed. I noticed a series of my own automatic thoughts and observations:

> This person has something they want me to know. I wonder if I have the skills to help? I wish I could understand what this person is saying more clearly and what they mean when they express themselves in such creative and figurative language. What this person is saying does not make sense; I can only understand some words that pop out. It is my job to try to help this person and make sense of things. I wonder if they are saying the same thing to me each time we meet. Am I missing something? I really don't know what I can do for this person if I cannot understand them, but I want to try so much. This person seems very passionate about specific topics, and I can tell because of the change in the tone of voice and shift to an improved positive affect.

On reflection, I had optimism, energy, hope, and genuine interest and wanted to spend time trying to understand patients. I recognized a need to invest time in helping patients and act on finding a way forward with atypical patient speech. I started to use some tools I had learned in applied language and discourse analysis many years ago to break down the language expressed by these patients. Also, I had a very experienced, systematic, and compassionate clinical supervisor who mentored and supported me in seeking to understand patients. I also noticed that my clinical supervisor invested time to understand patients and usually tried to make sense of incohesive utterances made by patients. Therefore, I recognized that my automatic thoughts as a clinician made a difference in how I approached patients with atypical speech.

Fundamental learning point 1: The clinician must assume that patients are doing their best to communicate, even if communication is difficult to understand. Although the patient's speech may be atypical, it may be wise for clinicians to be curious and (inspired by the lyrics of Diane Warren and Aerosmith) take the approach "I don't want to miss a thing" when listening to patients speak about their firmly held beliefs.

In contrast, I believe my clinical approach would have suffered had my automatic thoughts when I was listening to a patient with atypical speech expression looked something like this:

> I don't have time for this. This is not clinically relevant. I don't understand; my supervisor looks impatient, the staff are rolling their eyes at me for trying, and this person really is unwell and does not make sense. They cannot be helped and won't respond to me trying.

In this situation, although I may have wanted to help initially, these sorts of automatic thoughts would translate into a distanced and alienating style of interaction based on how the patient was expressing themselves. Clinicians need to feel they have some support to be willing to try to shift their approach and may be hesitant if their training background or mentors have taught them otherwise.

Fundamental learning point 2: Patients, through no fault of their own, may have difficulty expressing themselves because of illness, intellectual disability, formal thought disorder, head trauma, or cognitive difficulties. Clinicians need to keep in mind that the diagnosis and atypical communication style a patient adopts are not intentional, and the communication style is not always chosen. Even if it is chosen, there is a meaning behind why a simpler form of speaking is not adopted by the patient. *Taking an interest in and learning new ways to engage with patients who are challenging to understand is truly how clinicians can do their greatest work and service.* Therefore, being willing to learn—no matter the stage of career—and believing that it is possible to reach patients are the first steps on the clinician's pathway to being able to do so. Giving up on, excluding, or ruling out the potential to reach and understand a person whom a clinician has the privilege and opportunity to treat is a tragedy. Clinicians must view every interaction with patients as a privilege.

Frequently asked questions: What happens after clinicians begin to understand and take an interest in patients who are challenging to understand? What if a patient speaks for long periods of time and it is hard for the clinician to speak back to the patient (hard to interrupt)?

When clinicians are willing and show interest in investing time in a patient's recovery by starting to listen to the patient and make sense of the patient's world, this can lead patients (especially those who have strongly held beliefs) to speak passionately now that someone is finally listening. It can seem like an explosion of information, and a clinician may find it challenging to be able to speak back or respond. This is likely because the patient may have been very socially isolated and desperately wants to have the clinician understand the details of their experience. Our experience has suggested that after an alliance is formed and when the clinician is interested and perceived as such by the patient, the length of time for which the patient speaks will tend to gradually decrease In addition, clinicians can share with patients in advance that they may gently interrupt them to ask them questions. It is advised that this be done at the beginning of any meeting. For example, the clinician can express the following:

> In our talk today, there may be times I need to interrupt you. I don't mean to be rude—it's just that I would like to understand and may have questions that will help me along to take note of all the valuable information you are sharing with me. Sometimes I might ask that you slow down so I can catch the details. I'll try to keep up. I am hoping that this is OK with you.

It is recommended that clinicians adopt basic CBT skills (e.g., personal disclosure, guided discovery, Socratic questioning) to learn gentle ways to help patients express themselves and normalize the conversation. In our experience, clinicians may need to spend most of the time during the first four or five sessions listening rather than talking, asking only curious questions as an information gatherer. Clinicians who work in this area must show a degree of openness (e.g., taking extra time to conceptualize the patient), interest (e.g., being committed to understanding), and wise use of time (e.g., scheduling sessions when the clinician is typically energized and keeping the session structure flexible).

Limitations and Important Factors to Keep in Mind

1. This chapter is appropriate for individuals who 1) want to start to interview linguistically challenging patients, 2) use cognitive-behavioral

techniques to improve the therapeutic alliance, or 3) have an interest in using techniques in CBT to better understand language conveying firmly held beliefs.

2. Clinicians should have a working knowledge of and appreciate the importance of patient automatic thoughts (knowing what these are and how to elicit them). It is crucial to write these down in clinical notes and integrate them into a cognitive conceptualization and/or cognitive model.

3. Clinicians cannot expect to become skilled at using an adapted discourse analysis framework to decode delusions overnight; rather, it is a skill that takes time and practice to learn and time in the therapeutic session itself to adapt.

4. Clinicians who work with individuals who have been diagnosed with a psychotic disorder such as schizophrenia, schizoaffective disorder, or delusional disorder may benefit from the techniques described in this chapter.

In a Nutshell: Verbal Communication From Patients

Clinicians may need to keep the following assumptions and expectations in mind to optimize their clinical orientation and approach to decoding delusions:

- What a patient communicates, in whatever way it is said, should be considered important and valid. What a patient expresses has some critical meaning to them regardless of whether it makes sense to the clinician. Clinicians must avoid discounting what they do not understand and alternatively move toward a mutual understanding.

- The clinician should treat what the patient says with attention, kindness, and respect, exploring the content of what is expressed with gentle curiosity using classical Socratic questions and Rogerian counseling skills (Wright et al. 2014). A comprehensive list of clinical orientation elements in CBT for psychosis has been published (Morrison and Barratt 2010).

- An awareness of clinician negative automatic thoughts in relation to a patient's expressed language are rate-limiting factors to therapeutic progress. Negative automatic thoughts will need to be evaluated so that they enable a *curiosity* and *time investment*–oriented approach toward the patient. This is a fundamental first step in shifting a clinician's mental framework to one that enables recovery.

Toward a Common Language for Patients and Clinicians

Once the clinician orientation is in place (see section "Verbal Communication From Patients to Their Clinician"), the next phase of decoding delusions using a linguistic approach involves moving toward a common language between patients and clinicians.

Personal Reflection: Two Contrasting Language Experiences

Once, I (N.R.) was on a holiday in Holland and there was a rainstorm. I found myself clicking through television channels. I was looking for an English-language channel because English is my first language and I do not speak Dutch. I eventually came across a television show I had watched previously in English, but the show was in Dutch without subtitles. I decided to watch the show, and in my mind I tried to fill in the content on the basis of my memories and direct observations of the characters' nonverbal behavior. After about 10 minutes, I started daydreaming about something else. After about 20 minutes went by, I changed the channel in the hope of finding a program in English. I grew slightly frustrated but then returned to what I had been watching before. After that experience, *I noticed that my mind skipped over much of the content, and I took little interest in what I did not understand in the Dutch program.*

This contrasts with another experience. A few years later, on a holiday in Italy, I was keen to watch Italian programming because I had begun to learn words and basic phrases in Italian before the holiday. *I enjoyed recognizing and understanding Italian as I watched, even though I did not understand everything. I had some invested interest, but I also had tools (e.g., my dictionary and translations book) to increase my understanding of the content that was unclear.*

These two experiences were insightful and helped me appreciate the relationship among interest, ambiguity, and the need for a shared understanding of language to have meaning. Research can help answer why my experiences were different: minds tend to discount and skip over things not understood—people are more likely to lose interest and not invest time in figuring out something they do not understand in both passive and active contexts (Clark and Clark 1977). This has implications for clinicians who work with individuals with unmanaged or refractory psychosis (Rochester and Martin 1979). Thus, clinicians need methods to achieve a common understanding of language expressed in delusions and practical tools to help to decode language that is unclear. This necessitates a greater understanding of linguistics on the part of the clinician.

Best Practice Foundations in Clinical Linguistics

Linguistic Foundations

There are many subdisciplines in linguistics. The discipline of linguistics used in this chapter is that of applied language and discourse analysis. Indeed, applied language and discourse analysis is the subdiscipline that allows for the analysis of the exchange of meanings between a speaker and a listener. Within this, a framework can be defined:

1. In this chapter, it is assumed there are only two parties to a language exchange (clinician and patient). Clinicians are listeners (or recipients) in a language exchange with patients who are speaking or expressing language in an unconventional and complex manner.
2. Language can be written or spoken and can be interpreted in conjunction with nonverbal feedback by the listener. In this chapter, the focus is on language expressed in spoken form.
3. The linguistics of delusion in the context of psychotherapy is of central interest because language is at the heart of exchange in psychotherapy (Ridley and Kelly 2007), and the process of psychotherapy is primarily verbal (Ridley et al. 1998).
4. Language in schizophrenia has been researched and discussed primarily in the context of disorders of thought process (Rochester and Martin 1979), viewed as a component of dysfunction within a medical model framework. In contrast, in this chapter, linguistics is applied within a recovery model.
5. Clinicians must keep in mind that patients who experience thought disorder may have been excluded in the past from access to psychotherapy because of their inability to communicate coherently. Clinicians must assume that patients with disorders of thought process may have had negative and nontherapeutic experiences with other clinicians. Such patients may have been labeled (sometimes incorrectly) as being unamenable to psychotherapy.
6. It is expected that after reading this chapter, clinicians will not passively receive information from patients; rather, clinicians should be active participants in receiving language and be prepared to stop and check what it is that they do not understand, much like a language learner.

Best Practice Foundations

1. It is best practice to take written notes in a notebook (not on loose paper) during a therapeutic session, meetings, or interviews—whether the clinician is using linguistic tools or not. From the first session, seek the consent of the patient to do so. There may be certain content that a patient does not want the clinician to write down, especially if they express that they are telling the clinician something "secret" or something they have never shared before that increases paranoia. Be considerate and ask.

2. Practice note-taking skills while in the therapeutic session, and when possible quote what the patient says in the session. Clinicians should always have more notes for the patients who are more challenging to understand. To practice this, it may be possible to ask a colleague to role-play so you can practice taking notes to increase your confidence in this skill.

3. Avoid using a laptop or other device that creates a division between you and the patient, such as a computer screen, because this can be perceived by the patient as a barrier—and optics do matter. In addition, face the patient's direction because this can build rapport and trust in a clinician-patient relationship.

4. In certain circumstances, writing notes is better than using an audio recorder, or vice versa. When using an audio recorder, still take notes (for some clinicians, it is unrealistic to conceive there will be enough time to relisten to entire therapy sessions on a regular basis because of service demands and workplace responsibilities). As the patient observes the clinician taking notes, this will provide indirect nonverbal feedback to the patient that what they are saying is important. It may also help the patient slow the pace at which they are expressing themselves.

5. Pay close attention to repeated sentences that a patient expresses and write them down. If a patient says a sentence or phrase over and over, take note of how often this is repeated (e.g., "the house on the hill"×4). If it is difficult to quantify, place an asterisk in order to emphasize the repetition in your clinical notes. This will provide a good indicator as to what language should be targeted for adapted linguistic analysis.

6. Clinicians who work with electronic patient records and input notes into a computer-based system should still take written notes while facing patients. This is best practice even for clinicians who are not seeking to use linguistic analysis tools.

7. Always address affect and emotions as they emerge in language and nonverbal communication. This should be prioritized by the clinician. Write down expressed emotions, when they occur, what had been talked about, and topics or words they are connected to.

8. Use active listening to rephrase and summarize what the patient has said during interviews or therapy sessions, not just for patient validation and rapport but to intentionally slow down the session to take notes and catch important details about what the patient is expressing in language.

9. Pay attention to patient-expressed language that is suggestive of red flags—risks to safety of the patient or others—as in all good clinical practice consistent with the highest standards of care.

10. Avoid making assumptions or assuming links (e.g., a leads to b, which leads to c) between statements a patient may make. Inquire about what the patient is expressing, carefully verifying the details with the patient.

11. It is recommended that clinicians underschedule their calendars to make additional time for patients whose verbal language is challenging to understand.

Tools and Techniques for Making Sense of Complex Speech Expressions in Delusions

In this section, applied case examples and clinical tips are presented. Templates and exercises can be viewed in the chapter appendices.

Tool 1: Transitivity—Who Is Doing What to Whom, Where, When, and How?
An Introductory Adapted Clinical Tool for the Practitioner

CLINICAL TIP

When trying to apply an adapted transitivity tool with a new patient for the first time, *clinicians should always preface questions* by sharing with the patient something like this: "I have noticed that you have commented on X a lot, and I think it would be very important for me to try to understand this better so that I may be able to support you. I wonder if I could ask you some specific questions about what you have just said. As I have mentioned before, I will treat this information with discretion and view it with kindness because I recognize it could be hard to talk about."

Transitivity analysis is the name of a technique in systemic functional linguistics that asks the following key question: Who is doing what to whom, when, where, and how? This involves fragmenting phrases and sentences of what a patient says—questioning each noun, verb, adjective, and adverb. It is best practice to pick a sentence or phrase that seems to be frequently repeated or expressed with concern (perceived as a threat) by the patient.

Adapting concepts in transitivity within CBT can be done by following practical steps in which the clinician asks key questions linked to the expressed language of a strongly held belief. Clinicians often may not know what to ask in the initial phases of inquiry. Here an assumption is made that the clinician is feeling lost and may doubt their own abilities to make progress with the patient. Clinicians should be encouraged to gently tap into their curiosity to use transitivity effectively. An adapted transitivity tool can be used when traditional Socratic questions are not enough to understand a sequence of beliefs. Transitivity can be applied alongside the downward arrow technique or sequencing in CBT. Transitivity may also help clinicians who do not perceive themselves to be innately curious. To apply transitivity analysis in a clinical setting, approach a key example of speech of the patient using questions that involve the five Ws (who, what, where, when, and why) and the H (how) applied to fragments of a phrase.

Steps of Transitivity Analysis for Firmly Held Beliefs

A patient repeatedly says, "You don't understand, and I don't think you get it. The devil is going to kill me and wants me to score devil points for redemption for a chance at a new life." Use transitivity analysis to examine this statement by following these four steps:

- **Step 1: Write down what the patient says.** "The devil is going to kill me and wants me to score devil points for redemption for a chance at a new life."
- **Step 2: Split the sentence.** Break down the sentence vertically on the basis of nouns and verbs and their objects (objects refer to what the verb is referring to doing), adjectives, and adverbs:
    the devil
    is going to kill me
    wants me to score devil points
    for redemption
    for a chance at a new life
- **Step 3: Generate questions that are appropriate and sensitively formulated on the basis of each component using the five Ws and**

how. Questions can be generated in the session or generated after the session and followed up with the patient at the next session (Table 5–1).

- **Step 4: As the patient responds, write down the sequence of events using a downward arrow technique or sequencing in CBT.** Alternatively, use a brainstorming map for each component (see Appendix A in this chapter for an example). You can share a clean version with the patient, if they would like one, to serve as a visual aid for your analysis.

CLINICAL TIP

In a session, the clinician can select which fragments of a sentence to focus on, picking one or two, until the system of the delusion can be decoded enough to explain it logically in sequence to another clinician.

Alternatively, if a patient shares a few different sentences, shorter phrases can be used within the adapted transitivity tool. The clinician should check their understanding of the delusion with the patient in a separate session after the delusion has been decoded. This will ensure that the patient has reliably validated the clinician's understanding of the delusion.

The example in Table 5–1 provides a series of potential questions that can be asked of a patient when breaking down a sentence that reflects a firmly held belief. Through questioning, it is possible to derive which fragment, or part of the threat, is perceived as most threatening, with the aim of trying to make sense of the patient's reaction to this delusion and its various impacts. Most important, by asking questions, it is possible to break through the isolation and avoid making leaps in understanding. It is crucial to ask questions in a sensitive manner, only after a therapeutic alliance is well established. It is unlikely the patient will want to share this information with the clinician if the alliance is not strong or reliable. After some analysis, as a starting place for therapeutic interventions, clinicians may select beliefs among a series of expressed speech that, depending on therapeutic goals, could affect quality of life, occupational and social functioning, or delusions that are accompanied by a repetitive hallucination.

How Can Clinicians Respond to Each Component of Complexly Expressed Thought in This Example?

The questions noted in Table 5–1 all center on who, what, where, when, why, and how, and the list of questions is not exhaustive. You will also notice that when the patient expresses firm modalities (e.g., *is* or *will*), clinicians may express the statement back to the patient in the question with softer

TABLE 5–1. Adapted transitivity analysis: an applied example

What the patient says, separated into components	Examples of how to address the statement
You don't understand, and I don't think you get it.	• You are absolutely right. I do not understand your experience in this moment, but I am genuinely curious to learn more about your experiences and what has happened to you. You have said this to me [re: the devil] a lot. Is it OK with you if I ask you some questions about what you just said? I know that this could be hard, and we can do this slowly and take our time.
The devil	• Let me refer to my notes for a moment. Can you tell me about yourself and remind me whether you consider yourself to be religious?
	• *When* did the devil start bothering you or come into your life?
	• *How* do you sense or gather that it is the devil that is bothering you? *What* do you hear that tells you this is the devil? *What* do you see that tells you this is the devil?
	• In the spectrum of things you could have interacted with, *where* does the devil fall on a continuum? For example, may I ask, has anyone other than the devil ever bothered you the same as the devil? And *what* about people who have bothered you less than the devil? And *what* about people who have bothered you more than the devil?
is going to kill me	• Other than the devil, do you perceive anyone else I should know about *who* could be trying to harm you?
	• *What* do you think you can do to keep yourself safe?
	• *What* do you think I or the treatment team can do to support you in coping with this?
	• *Where* do you think the devil could harm you?
	• *When* do you think that the devil could harm you?
	• *How* do you think the devil could harm you? Can you tell me about this step-by-step if you can guess how?

TABLE 5–1.   Adapted transitivity analysis:
                  an applied example *(continued)*

What the patient says, separated into components	Examples of how to address the statement
wants me to score devil points	• *Who* can usually score devil points?
	• *What* are devil points?
	• If there is a location, *where* are devil points usually scored? *Who* keeps track of this?
	• Are there specific times *when* it is possible to score devil points?
	• *Why* or *how* do devil points help you?
	• Is there any reason *why* devil points could be unhelpful or unsafe?
	• Are you the only person *who* can score devil points? Is there any reason *why* you are the only person you know who has knowledge of devil points?
for redemption	• If redemption is possible, *who* has the power to grant redemption? Is it temporary or permanent?
	• *What* is your definition of redemption?
	• Is there a place in your mind or body *where* you feel redemption?
	• *When* do you think you expect to feel redemption in relation to the devil points?
	• Is there a reason *why* you think you need redemption?
for a chance at a new life	• *Who* do you think would be people in your current life who you would want to include in or who could be part of a potential new life?
	• *What* is it about your life that you feel would change if you had a new life?
	• *Where [location]* do you think you would be in your new life?
	• *When* do you think your new life would start after redemption?
	• *Why* do you think, in the back of your own mind, you may want a new life?

TABLE 5–1. Adapted transitivity analysis: an applied example *(continued)*

What the patient says, separated into components	Examples of how to address the statement
for a chance at a new life *(continued)*	• Have you considered the possibility of *how*, if even small things changed in your current life, there could be a new life or a new chapter for you now without having a new life?

modalities such as *could* or *may*. This acknowledges what the patient has said but does not unknowingly or unintentionally collude with the belief.

It is noteworthy that the words *helpful* and *unhelpful* are classic CBT clinician words. In asking questions, always remember to ask about what is helpful as well as what could be unhelpful (Wright et al. 2014).

Last, patient statements such as "You don't understand," "You don't get it," or "Never mind" are all signals that any clinician should take as a cue to get more curious, take more time, and be kind and compassionate to help the patient work through the firmly held belief. Some patients test clinicians to determine whether they are committed to the therapeutic relationship by making statements such as "You don't get it!" This is an opportunity to build the therapeutic alliance. Patients do not want to work with someone who may give up on them.

In a Nutshell: Adapted Transitivity Analysis Questions

An adapted clinical tool based on transitivity can help clinicians and patients derive more meaning from complexly expressed delusions by breaking down the components of sentences. It is posited that the more a clinician can make sense of what a patient is saying using an adapted transitivity tool, the greater the likelihood the clinician can 1) ask better questions that increase the therapeutic alliance while not missing out on key details of a delusion, 2) decrease isolation, and 3) possibly create doubt in the conviction in the strongly held belief enough to increase daily social and occupational functioning. See Appendix B in this chapter for real-life examples of the use of the adapted transitivity tool.

CLINICAL TIPS

Self-beliefs can be conceived as pillars of our identity. Self-beliefs may allow a person to derive a sense of purpose in the world. Therefore, the most complex of delusions are those that are tightly linked with the believer's identity, especially if the holder of the belief gains privileges or powers as a result of the belief. Maladaptive core beliefs, which can be threatening and resistant to CBT, are also tightly linked with identity. Therefore, it is suggested and optimal to focus on analyzing beliefs that are *not tied to the identity of the patient* until later stages in therapy when an alliance is at its strongest and the patient has adopted less intense adaptive beliefs.

1. If the clinician notices that a patient has made a statement that contains delusional content but also contains a recognizable fragment, such as a real person, the clinician should focus the five Ws line of questioning on this real-life component first before asking questions about other fragments of the sentence. This will help the clinician form a tangible starting place because it is an element of a shared common reality between the clinician and patient.

2. Clinicians can use their best judgment to determine whether they are asking too many questions or simply ask the patient, "I know I have asked lots of questions. Is it OK if I ask a few more, or shall we postpone these until our next meeting?"

Tool 2: CBT-Adapted Vocabulary Chains as Supportive Tools for Clinicians Who Work With Strongly Held Beliefs

Constructing vocabulary chains is a semiquantitative technique used in applied language and discourse studies that may aid in the categorization of themes that emerge from patient-expressed language. *This tool can allow clinicians to more easily focus and understand 1) what, if anything, is being protected in the patient's life by virtue of the patient holding on to a strongly held belief and 2) to which CBT category of core beliefs the strongly held belief might be linked.* Working with vocabulary chains is done after capturing an audio recording and typing a transcript. It can take about 20–30 minutes after a therapy session but can serve as a valuable tool and be worth the time investment, especially if the clinician is unsure in which direction to proceed. It is proposed that the adapted vocabulary chain analysis be uniquely composed for each of the three core beliefs (of helplessness, worthlessness, and unlovability) in CBT (Beck 1995). Further detail on this process is beyond the scope of this chapter.

In the present chapter, the vocabulary chains presented are applicable to patients with strongly held beliefs. The applied example presented herein centers on fear and threat, with the goal of analyzing the meaning behind a strongly held belief. This tool may also help monitor progress in reducing how strongly beliefs may be held across therapy sessions when attention is paid to the linguistic modalities expressed (e.g., *should, could, would, is, may, may not, do, try*).

Applied Example of a CBT-Adapted Vocabulary Chain

- **Step 1: Create an audio recording of the patient speaking uninterrupted that would fill up to one page, double-spaced.** This could be 2–4 minutes of free speech by the patient. It could be preempted by you asking the patient, "Can you please tell me about something that has gotten your attention today that is very important to you?"
- **Step 2: Type the transcript.**
- **Step 3: Read the transcript.**

> *Patient:* My brain is ill; I have a scientific body. I'm going to fall asleep in my bed and then I will evaporate. I don't think they're going to storm the hospital. I'm going to freak out, and I'm warning you now when the clock strikes 12 on Christmas day, I'm going to need to be isolated. It's my scheduled Pentecostal. I say the more devil points I earn, maybe it'll help me when I come back to life. I won't even remember anything. My parents don't believe me. The demon is older than me, he overruled me before. He told me I need to sacrifice myself and score devil points. Are you my friend? I know you're professional. I've lost my sense of childhood, dreamed of my emotion; I have no emotion whatsoever. I wouldn't cry if my parents died, even if I wanted to—only if I was tortured. Everyone in this town doesn't like me too much—there are nasty rumors going around about me, and everyone thinks it's their business. I was a violent young man and now I need to pay. I didn't know about devil points until crazy spice. I'll never go anywhere without my badges, otherwise people won't believe who I am, and I am a mastodon.

- **Step 4: Separate the sentences from the transcript into vocabulary chain fixed categories.** For an additional applied example and a blank example vocabulary chain worksheet, see Table 5–2 and Appendix C in this chapter.
- **Step 5: Count the content in each category and place this in the "frequency" column.** Some content can be placed in multiple categories.
- **Step 6: Count references to "I," "me," "my," or "self."**
- **Step 7: Count references to other people outside self, including delusional identities "you," "they," "their.**

Steps 6 and 7 in the vocabulary chain are meant only to distinguish and count references to the self (e.g., *I*, *me*, references to self in the third person)

TABLE 5-2. Example of a cognitive-behavioral therapy-adapted vocabulary chain

Category reference	Content	Frequency
Perception of illness or stigma	• My brain is ill; I have a scientific body. • I was a violent young man. • I didn't know about devil points until crazy spice.	3
Objects of value or worthlessness	• I say the more devil points I earn, maybe it'll help me when I come back to life. • I'll never go anywhere without my badges, otherwise people won't believe who I am.	2
Relationship, social acceptance or social rejection, belongingness	• Are you my friend? • Everyone in this town doesn't like me too much. • There are nasty rumors going around about me, and everyone thinks it's their business.	3
Weakness or helplessness, gaining of strength (compensatory), accomplishment, powerlessness or loss of control	• It's my scheduled Pentecostal. • He [the demon] overruled me before. • And score devil points. • I am a mastodon. • I'm going to fall asleep in my bed and then I will evaporate. • I'm going to need to be isolated. • I won't even remember anything.	7
Unreasonable or unrealistic strength, grandeur, or power	NA	0
Emotions or emotional reactions	• I'm going to freak out. • [I've] dreamed of my emotion; I have no emotion whatsoever. • I wouldn't cry if my parents died, even if I wanted to. • [I'd cry] only if I was tortured.	4
Safety behaviors that could maintain threat	NA	0
References to others (individuals who exist in reality)	• I'm warning you now. • I wouldn't cry if my parents died.	2

TABLE 5–2. Example of a cognitive-behavioral therapy-adapted vocabulary chain *(continued)*

Category reference	Content	Frequency
References to others (hallucinatory characters)	• I don't think they're going to storm the hospital.	1
References to protecting self from harm, defending self, anticipating protecting self from harm	• I don't think they're going to storm the hospital. • And now I need to pay.	2
References to protecting others from harm, defending others, anticipating protecting others (real or hallucinatory identities)	NA	0
Blame	NA	0
Loss of pleasure or gaining of pleasure (re: things, events, situations that would be pleasurable to an average person)	• Clock strikes 12 on Christmas day.	1
Need(s) suggestive of support, normalization, or validation	• My parents don't believe me.	1
Red flags, risk indicators	• He told me I need to sacrifice myself.	1
References to "I," "me," "my," or "self"	Step 6: Count	38
References to other people outside self, including delusional identities "you," "they," "their"	Step 7: Count	4

Note. NA=not applicable.

and others (e.g., *they, you, them*). These are excellent indicators of whether an individual views events and situations as centered on themselves (with varying intensities), is balanced in their views of situations or events, or views situations and events in an outwardly focused manner (with the number representing varying intensities).

The adapted vocabulary chain has been developed on the basis of fixed categories of references that are commonly found in individuals with strongly held beliefs, in particular in individuals with schizophrenia. The categories can be modified on the basis of the content of the transcript if particular themes are salient—in this regard, it is a flexible tool. The vocabulary chain here should be sufficient for an initial guide. The categories are informed by standard core belief categories that are part of CBT, those of helplessness, unlovability, and worthlessness (Beck 1995). The categories are also informed by CBT targets and common orientations (e.g., attention to threat, power, stigma, hallucinations).

Analysis: What Can Be Learned From This Example Using the CBT-Adapted Vocabulary Chain?

This specific example includes seven references to weakness or helplessness, compensatory gaining of strength, powerlessness, or loss of control and four references to emotion. This suggests new directions for questions from the clinician and identifies new therapeutic goals. There is a strong likelihood that emotional references are tightly linked with categories that appear most frequently expressed. In this example, therapy would shift to focus on ways to normalize experiences of existing, such as institutional power differentials and perhaps those within the therapeutic alliance. Asking the patient to share present or past examples of when fear, defeat, helplessness, weakness, powerlessness, or loss of control were experienced is likely to be therapeutic. Subsequently, coping strategies can be developed for areas in which the patient feels powerlessness and a lack of confidence. Alternatively, a therapy task could involve collaboratively listing areas (e.g., personal hygiene, activities outside the home, spiritual activities, activities to get my medication) or daily tasks (e.g., putting "clean room at 10:00 A.M." on my plan myself instead of staff or voices telling me to clean up) that could increase the perceived power and control the patient has in life. Indeed, reinforcing life domains or tasks for which a patient has control, influence, or responsibility is crucial to increasing perceived power. Targeting the areas of reference in the vocabulary chain within a therapeutic framework is likely to indirectly diffuse the intensity of fear and threat associated with strongly held beliefs, thereby weakening their strength and associated delusions. Therefore, by using this tool, the clinician decodes difficult-to-understand speech and unmasks therapeutic directions.

CLINICAL TIPS

1. If there is no quantitative distinction between categories, it is recommended that clinicians analyze a longer transcript.

2. Consistent with good therapeutic practice, addressing emotion and affect is critical and can strengthen the therapeutic alliance. Therefore, no matter the frequency, it is suggested that this be discussed with the patient first.

3. In this case, the vocabulary chain analysis can help the clinician who is stuck. The CBT-adapted linguistic tool can be used as a guide to focus on core themes expressed by the patient.

4. This tool can be helpful when the patient is expressing multiple ideas that are not systematic and are difficult for an average clinician to comprehend and when deriving therapy goals has been a barrier to commencing the therapeutic process and therapeutic change itself.

In a Nutshell: CBT-Adapted Vocabulary Chain Analysis

Constructing vocabulary chains is a linguistic analysis technique that can be used to compare transcripts of patient-expressed language that is challenging to address in a meeting or therapy session. Careful analysis can guide the clinician to meaningful areas of reference within a CBT therapeutic framework. Clinicians can move forward with increased confidence that the needs of the patient and intensely held beliefs can be addressed alongside risk, affect, and emotion. An incomprehensible transcript can be analyzed and therapeutic areas and core beliefs identified after application by clinicians.

Frequently asked question: How do you know when a problem or core belief has subsided when using this tool?

Comparing transcripts of the same patient over time may reveal interesting patterns reflective of a "moving target" of life goals and therapy. The ultimate goal is to see a reduction in the frequency of references in a specific category that would typically be addressed in therapy.

CLINICAL TIPS

1. Ensure you have the recorded verbal and/or written consent of the patient before making a recording on a protected or encryptable device.

2. Have a template of the vocabulary chain in the therapy session before recording that you can later fill in.

3. If you are unsure what a specific word or phrase of the patient refers to, ask the patient directly after the recording is made. Use the template categories as a guide to what category the word or phrase most accurately falls into. For example, it could sound something like this: "When you said X, do you think this relates more to blame or pleasure?"

Tool 3: Linguistic Modalities (Adverbs) Within Vocabulary Chains

The next tool allows clinicians to take CBT-adapted vocabulary chains further by analyzing *linguistic modalities* (in particular adverbs) while helping make "Swiss cheese" out of strongly held beliefs. If strongly held beliefs are analogous to a brick of cheddar cheese, beliefs that develop holes—reducing in intensity (to become more adaptive)—are analogous to Swiss cheese (Wright et al. 2014). In CBT for psychosis, sometimes all that is needed to make Swiss cheese out of strongly held beliefs (or automatic thoughts) is to introduce the possibility of doubt that the belief is 100% true. This becomes more possible when nuances in the language of the patient are noted.

One method of measuring this linguistically is in the realm of the analysis of linguistic or philosophical modality (Table 5–3). Here *modality* refers to a description of a likelihood of an event, person, place, or thing. In this regard, *keeping track of modals (adverbs) expressed by patients* is a potential semiquantitative and useful way of tracking therapeutic progress. A simple way of ascertaining shifts in modals is to track them in a list relating to a specific belief. Clinicians should be on the lookout for the use of adverbs by the patient that remark on how often a verb is mentioned. Simultaneously, clinicians can also naturally introduce modalities themselves in rephrasing what the patient has said to them (e.g., showing the patient a list of potential modal adverbs and asking the patient to select one when expressing a belief; see Appendix D in this chapter). In this regard, this technique can use bidirectional communication (patient to clinician as well as clinician to patient) in adverb exchanges. Accurate adverbs only enhance

TABLE 5–3. Linguistic modality (adverb) analysis table

Belief expressed before intervention	Modal adverb (how often)	Frequency	Modified belief expressed during or after intervention
"I will *never* ever go to the grocery store without my badges; I'd *never* be able to prove my ranks."	Never Rarely Seldom Occasionally Usually Generally Normally Frequently Often Sometimes Always	2 (preintervention) 1 (postintervention)	"I can *sometimes* leave the badges at home when I go to the grocery store; it is much easier to walk when my backpack isn't full of my badges, and I can actually carry the groceries home OK. No one has ever asked me to show my badges."

and align with objectives in CBT to describe and conceptualize experiences more accurately.

Tracking Patient Adverb Choice Over Time

It is recommended that clinicians pay close attention to the modal adverbs expressed by patients over time, especially noticing when patients naturally start using these in expressed language (such subtleties often can be overlooked). Such an analysis makes tracking shifts in beliefs possible. Shifts can be strategically tracked in relation to specific times in therapy when interventions are introduced.

A CBT Activity With Adverbs

When reality testing is undertaken to examine a strongly held belief, writing down the belief before and after transition and how this is expressed by the patient can be immensely helpful and serve as evidence of therapeutic improvement. When the clinician is conducting a reality testing experiment, an add-on activity could be to track the use of adverbs before reality testing and again after reality testing, especially in writing take-home points from the session. In conclusion, when modals are expressed in a manner that suggests that the patient has some doubt in relation to the strongly held belief, this may lead to improvements in functioning and quality of life.

In a Nutshell: Linguistic Modality Analysis

Three adapted linguistic tools have been presented. These tools can allow clinicians to decode patients' complexly expressed language. The tools have been designed and adapted for therapeutic progress to be established and achieved using CBT. Analysis of modals (adverbs) is a technique that allows for patient-to-clinician language feedback as well as clinician-to-patient feedback.

CLINICAL TIP

Sometimes it can be possible for patients to relinquish a strongly held belief altogether after therapeutic intervention. This would mean that the belief in question no longer appears in the content of patient-expressed language. This may indicate that the patient has moved on and the belief is no longer a signpost in their daily life. It may appear, in what seems out of the blue in therapy, that the patient no longer fixates on the strongly held belief. Therefore, reduced discourse on the delusion should be considered progress (when avoidance to discuss the belief can be ruled out by the clinician).

Chapter Summary and Considerations

Clinicians need a common language with patients to have a shared understanding of patients' unique and strongly held beliefs when presented in the setting of thought disorder and neologisms. Tools in applied language and discourse analysis, in particular those stemming from systemic functional linguistics, are presented here as methods clinicians can use to decode atypical patient-expressed speech. Using such tools can "reduce the room" to make assumptions about the meaning of what patients say about their delusions and any linked topic.

Clinicians should attend to their own automatic thoughts when they encounter uniquely expressed language from patients or styles of language they do not fully understand. They are encouraged to adopt the approach of a keen language learner. Clinicians have been provided a framework for linguistic foundations as well as clinical best practices to establish communication and rapport. Tools derived from systemic functional linguistics are available to pick apart language. A key assumption is as follows: what a patient says matters and holds meaning. In this chapter, we have presented a few selected adapted tools for the clinician from the area of transitivity, which asks who is doing what to whom, where, why, and how. CBT-adapted vocabulary chains as applied to clinical settings were also described. Last, we discussed the importance of modals, which are adverbs specifically in the domain of approximating the likelihood of an action (verb). These tools allow the clinician to increasingly understand and develop a therapeutic alliance with a patient who may present with several strongly held beliefs. The examples provided were adapted from real case examples of how verbal language is expressed in therapy by individuals with a primary diagnosis of schizophrenia. These tools allow for clues to be detected in a patient's speech that can later lead to specific intervention using the cognitive model. Thus, these tools can allow for a true starting point when a series of clinicians have not known in which direction to proceed.

The most difficult and challenging beliefs amenable to change are those that are linked with the identity of an individual. When working with an individual whose strongly held beliefs are ones that provide them power, it is crucial for the clinician to identify and build on the patient's strengths before addressing any strongly held beliefs related to personal identity. The reason for this is that the individual is likely to not engage or will withdraw from the therapeutic alliance if it is perceived that their identity is threatened, or, worse, they will engage in harm to self or others.

There is much potential for applied language and discourse analysis in the context of CBT and the treatment of medication-resistant psychotic disorders. Applying the novel adapted tools presented here will enable clinicians to better enhance their practice and promote the gradual recovery of their patients.

Questions for Discussion

1. What assumptions or automatic thoughts do you have about people you do not understand verbally in everyday life? What assumptions do you make about patients you meet who express themselves verbally in ways that are challenging to understand? How does this affect your empathy, perception of resources available and offered, and clinical confidence or doubt?

2. Do you shy away from writing or write minimally in a therapy session? What are the benefits of taking notes in therapy or patient meetings? What do you think you could get better at capturing or need to capture more of what a patient is telling you?

3. What are the strengths and limitations of using the adapted transitivity tool?

4. What are the strengths and limitations of using the CBT-adapted vocabulary chain tool?

5. Why are adverbs important in relation to making Swiss cheese out of firmly held beliefs?

KEY POINTS

- The clinician's automatic thoughts about the patient's use of language have a direct influence on the formation of a therapeutic alliance.

- Systemic functional linguistic techniques aid comprehension by helping the clinician to identify ideas, nouns, adjectives, verbs, and clauses used in relation to delusions for further therapeutic analysis and inquiry.

- Adapted transitivity analysis questions allow the clinician to understand the how, when, and where details in the language used about a delusion.

- Developing adapted vocabulary chains allows the patient's expressed language about their complex delusions to be organized in such a way as to make the patient's experiences and ideas more understandable and workable in relation to CBT targets.

- Analysis of the use of modals, specifically adverbs linked with likelihood of occurrence, can be used to track the intensity of strongly held beliefs.

References

Beck JS: Cognitive Therapy: Basics and Beyond. New York, Guilford, 1995

Clark HH, Clark EV: Psychology and Language: An Introduction to Psycholinguistics, Vol 10. New York, Harcourt Brace Jovanovich, 1977

Morrison AP, Barratt S: What are the components of CBT for psychosis? A Delphi study. Schizophr Bull 36(1), 136–142, 2010 19880824

Ridley CR, Kelly SM: Multicultural considerations in case formulation, in Handbook of Psychotherapy Case Formulation, 2nd Edition. Edited by Eells TD. New York, Guilford, 2007, pp 33–64

Ridley CR, Li LC, Hill CL: Multicultural assessment: reexamination, reconceptualization, and practical application. Couns Psychol 26(6):827–910, 1998

Rochester S, Martin JR: Crazy Talk: A Study of the Discourse of Schizophrenic Speakers (Cognition and Language: A Series in Psycholinguistics). New York, Plenum, 1979

Wright NP, Turkington D, Kelly OP, et al: Treating Psychosis: A Clinician's Guide to Integrating Acceptance and Commitment Therapy, Compassion-Focused Therapy, and Mindfulness Approaches Within the Cognitive Behavioral Therapy Tradition. Oakland, CA, New Harbinger, 2014

Appendix A

Adapted Transitivity Brainstorming Map

Applied Example

Delusion: "I'm half horse, half man; I'm not human. I'm the angel of white. The normal rules don't apply to me. The Cylons are after me."

- Step 1: Write a quote of the expressed delusion.
- Step 2: Label as "Delusion 1" and place in the center of the diagram.
- Step 3: Ask relevant five Ws (who, what, where, when, and why) questions.
- Step 4: Fill in details as they are expressed in session in point form.
- Step 5: Revise and reformulate in further sessions.

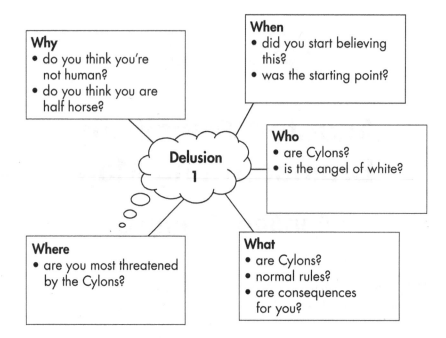

Appendix B

Adapted Transitivity Tool

Real-Life Examples

Applied Example 1

Context: Patient has been isolated for decades and has many complex delusions. Patient has not been able to speak with anyone to discuss delusions at length. Patient's affect is withdrawn and slightly agitated, and the patient is very preoccupied trying to work out details of a thought first thing in session. Patient is in the engagement phase of therapy and is a long-stay psychiatric patient. First thing the patient says in the interview: "I don't know, I don't know. Do you know Jane McBride? Are you sure you don't know her? She commit suicide? You know she's in the poppy…poppy good friends…did you hear it? I'm sure she committed suicide."

    Tip: In some cases, it is strategic to address phrases one at a time in order to attempt to resolve a situation coherently. *Note:* We have included a column in the table ("Real-life outcome: actual patient or clinician responses") to describe what happens when using this technique; this is not a column you would need to include in your table.

Phrases segmented	Clinician questions and actual response in session	Real-life outcome: actual patient or clinician responses
Do you know Jane McBride?	"I actually do not know of a Jane McBride. *How* do you think I should know Jane McBride? Is she a patient here, or someone *whom* you knew or know now?"	Patient: "She is a singer."
Are you sure you don't know her?	"I am sure I do not know her. The name does not sound familiar. Is there a reason *why* you think I should know her?"	Patient: "No, no...there isn't. I was just wondering."
She commit suicide?	"Because I do not know who she is, I am not sure what happened to her. Maybe we can find out if you tell me a little more. Does this sound OK?"	Patient: "Yeah, that's fine."
You know she's in the poppy...poppy good friends...did you hear it?	"I noticed that you said 'hear it'; is this a song you are referring to if she is a singer? *What* is the name of the music group? *What* is the name of the song? Roughly, *when*, as in *what* year, did you hear this song?"	Patient: "Yes, it's a song." Clinician looks up "Poppy Good Friends" on Google. Patient immediately recognizes song (nods). Observations: Moments later, the patient is crying intensely while listening to the song. Listening to the song, it is clear the lyrics relate to abandonment.

Phrases segmented	Clinician questions and actual response in session	Real-life outcome: actual patient or clinician responses
I'm sure she committed suicide.	"Thank you for listening to this song with me. It is OK to cry. This is a safe space, and I am not judging you at all." [Ask one or two of the following questions.] "*What* was it about this song that made you feel sad?" "*When* did you first hear this song?" "*What* does this song represent to you?" "It looks like the name of the singer is Susan Jacks in the group the Poppy Family. Can we look up some information together on *who* Susan Jacks was?" "Is suicide something that you have been thinking about now? Is this something you have thought about in the past?"	Clinician looks at biography of Susan Jacks with the patient in session. The biography confirms she is alive and does not seem to have attempted to end her life. Focus then shifts to the patient and risk assessment on suicidal ideation and the patient's history of suicidal ideation.

Applied Example 2

"I say Amandai but he says Amanda. Can you tell her about the book in a book? Not good, not good, it's a catastrophe. Alex Trebek told me."

Phrases segmented	Clinician questions and actual response in session	Real-life outcome: actual patient or clinician responses
I say Amandai but he says Amanda	"Let me see if I can help. *Who* is the "he" you are referring to? Are you asking about *how* to pronounce Amanda's name?"	Patient: "Alex Trebek. Yeah."
Can you tell her	"I am not sure if I will be able to speak with her, because she is no longer here; she's home now (discharged). *Why* might it be important for me to give her a message?"	Patient: "My brothers Christophe and Ben didn't have one and it wasn't good."
About the book in a book?	"*What* does it mean, a 'book in a book?' *What* is the main book you are referring to?"	Patient: "The Bible. You know, Matthew, John, Corinthians, et cetera."
Not good, not good, it's a catastrophe.	"This sounds very important and that it is upsetting you. Can you tell me more about *why* this is a catastrophe?"	Patient: "Amanda doesn't have a Bible; she doesn't know about the Bible. She needs to own a Bible. Can you please tell her 'I want you to know it is important to have a Bible in your house?'" Clinician: "If I have a chance one day sometime in the future, if this is a topic she brings up, I can talk to her about her religious beliefs."

Phrases segmented	Clinician questions and actual response in session	Real-life outcome: actual patient or clinician responses
Alex Trebek told me.	"I hate to tell you this, but I wanted to let you know that recently Alex Trebek from the TV game show *Jeopardy!* passed away from cancer. Is that *who* you are referring to, the man from that show? *Why* do you think he may have been talking with you about this?"	Patient: "Oh, that's sad. I'm sorry to hear that. I wonder why I'm hearing his voice messing with me and why he is telling me about Amanda and all this."
	How often do you have thoughts about people not owning a Bible? Is this a thought that preoccupies you and takes up a lot of time in the day, thinking about this?"	Patient: "It takes up all my time; I wish I could do other things, but I can't."

Appendix C

Cognitive-Behavioral Therapy–Adapted Vocabulary Chain Template

Category reference	Content	Frequency
Perception of illness or stigma		
Objects of value or worthlessness		
Relationship, social acceptance or social rejection, belongingness		
Weakness/helplessness, gaining of strength (compensatory), accomplishment, powerlessness or loss of control		
Unreasonable or unrealistic strength, grandeur, or power		
Emotions or emotional reactions		
Safety behaviors that could maintain threat		
References to others (individuals who exist in reality)		
References to others (hallucinatory characters)		
References to protecting self from harm, defending self, anticipating protecting self from harm		
References to protecting others from harm, defending others, anticipating protecting others (real or hallucinatory identities)		

Category reference	Content	Frequency
Blame		
Loss of pleasure or gaining of pleasure (re: things, events, situations that would be pleasurable to an average person)		
Need(s) suggestive of support, normalization, or validation		
Red flags, risk indicators		
Other:		
Other:		
Other:		
References to "I," "me," "my," or "self"	**Step 6: Count**	
References to other people outside self, including delusional identities "you," "they," "their"	**Step 7: Count**	

Source. Copyright © 2022 N. Rustom. Please email nrustom.cbt@gmail.com to disclose intention for clinician-patient use prior to use or photocopying. Please seek written permission for research use and citation/reference instructions.

Additional Applied Example of Cognitive-Behavioral Therapy–Adapted Vocabulary Chain

Patient: I had an intense feeling and vision watching television. There was a tightrope—one was 60 feet (mine), and the other 85 feet (my brother Christophe's). I pulled the card, and he fell. The tightrope walker fell and died...85 feet because he wanted to beat the record. Linda McCork ripped me off. I'm so down in the dumps, they say I don't have anything inside me.

Category reference	Content	Frequency
Perception of illness or stigma	NA	0
Objects of value or worthlessness	• Linda McCork ripped me off [money].	1
Relationship, social acceptance or social rejection, belongingness	NA	0
Weakness or helplessness, gaining of strength (compensatory), accomplishment, powerlessness or loss of control	• I pulled the card, and he fell.	1
Unreasonable or unrealistic strength, grandeur, or power	• I pulled the card.	1
Emotions or emotional reactions	• I had an intense feeling. • I'm so down in the dumps. • I don't have anything inside me.	3
Safety behaviors that could maintain threat	NA	0
References to others (individuals who exist in reality)	• *He* fell. • ...85 feet (*my brother Christophe's*) • *Linda McCork* ripped me off. • *They* say I don't have anything inside me.	4
References to others (hallucinatory characters)	NA	0
References to protecting self from harm, defending self, anticipating protecting self from harm	NA	0
References to protecting others from harm, defending others, anticipating protecting others (real or hallucinatory identities)	• There was a tightrope—one was 60 feet (mine).	1

Category reference	Content	Frequency
Blame	• I pulled the card, and he fell. • The tightrope walker fell and died.	2
Loss of pleasure or gaining of pleasure (re: things, events, situations that would be pleasurable to an average person)	NA	0
Need(s) suggestive of support, normalization, or validation	NA	0
Red flags, risk indicators	NA	0
References to "I," "me," "my," or "self"	**Step 6: Count**	8
References to other people outside self, including delusional identities "you," "they," "their"	**Step 7: Count**	6

Note. NA=not applicable.

Formulation

In this delusion, predominantly other people (four) tend to be responsible for the patient's emotional reactions (three). With further questioning, we were able to determine that the patient had made a bet on a real-life tightrope walker who had later fallen to his death. The patient indirectly blamed himself for the death because he had bet his brother and a woman named Linda and lost money (because the tightrope walker decided to try walking on a longer rope). The patient was concerned about his financial status and had experienced much grief and loss. The delusion was the tip of the iceberg that revealed these concerns. We targeted learning more about the patient's finances and discussing grief and loss in therapy.

Appendix D

Adverb Use Tracking Template

Likelihood-of-event adverbs:

- Never
- Rarely
- Seldom
- Occasionally
- Usually
- Generally
- Normally
- Frequently
- Often
- Sometimes
- Always

Patient initials _____

Date	Belief/automatic thought quotation	Adverbs

6

Assessing Delusions

Dimitri Perivoliotis, Ph.D.

Assessment is a critical component of cognitive-behavioral therapy (CBT) for delusions that is not a discrete phase of intervention but rather begins early and continues throughout the entire course of treatment as needed. The process of assessment serves multiple purposes. It allows the clinician to collect important information that will guide the therapeutic process, with an emphasis on inaccurate or maladaptive beliefs and behaviors that interfere with the patient's functioning and quality of life. The information collected via ongoing assessment is assembled into the case formulation in an iterative process, with the formulation serving as the clinician's working blueprint of the beliefs and behaviors that are maintaining the delusion and blocking the patient's recovery. Finally, conducting ongoing assessment in CBT helps the clinician and patient track progress throughout treatment.

There is no one prescribed way to assess delusions in CBT for psychosis. Clinical presentations can vary widely; for example, patients can exhibit different types of delusions and varying levels of insight, cognitive functioning, and ability or willingness to discuss their experiences. Depending on the type of CBT being conducted, the clinical emphasis and targets may vary somewhat as well; for example, some protocols target reasoning biases and cognitive distortions, whereas others emphasize behavioral activation and recovery goals. Regardless of the specific approach, assessment of delusions should be flexible and guided by what is most appropriate and feasible for each patient. Ideally, assessment is done in a multidimensional manner. The range of factors that can be assessed is illustrated in Figure 6–1, organized loosely in order from proximal to distal to the delusional belief itself.

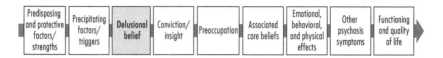

FIGURE 6–1.   Range of potential assessment targets in cognitive-behavioral therapy for delusions.

Assessment of delusions in CBT may occur both formally and informally. Formal assessment includes self-report questionnaires and structured clinical symptom interviews. Informal assessment includes natural questioning by the clinician; observations of patient behavior during sessions; and information derived from other providers, chart review, family members, or other loved ones. All of these sources of assessment can be useful, but informal methods should be favored at the beginning of treatment because premature or excessive formal assessment may trigger disengagement in certain patients; for example, someone with a persecutory delusion may be suspicious of the clinician, and a patient without insight might be triggered by a formal assessment that is obviously about symptoms of mental illness. Table 6–1 lists sample questions along with potential measures and tools that can be used to measure the different aspects of the delusional experience, which are discussed in detail later. With the exception of the interview-based Psychotic Symptom Rating Scales (PSYRATS; Haddock et al. 1999), the measures in the table are self-reports that are freely available online for ease of use in routine clinical settings, and all have been used in previous research involving people with psychosis.

The strategies contained in this chapter serve as a complement to routine elements of a standard mental health evaluation (i.e., history of present illness, current physical symptoms, family history, personal and social history, risk assessment, social circumstances), so I do not describe those elements here, except as they pertain to assessment of delusions. Delusions often do not exist in isolation and may be accompanied by associated symptoms such as hallucinations, depression, anxiety, trauma or PTSD, and substance use that also must be assessed, but in this chapter I focus primarily on assessment of delusions. Moreover, assessment should go beyond just symptoms and problems. Consistent with the recovery model, the patient is seen as a whole person who also has important strengths and abilities that must be recognized, channeled, and strengthened during treatment. Clinicians should assess for and keep these positive aspects in mind.

TABLE 6–1. Sample prompts, measures, and tools to assess delusions

Assessment target	Sample prompts	Possible measures or tools
Strengths and recovery goals	"What are your positive traits?"	SMART goals, QPR
	"What are you proud of?"	
	"What accomplishments have you made?"	
	"What is important to you? What are your values?"	
	"What are you like when you're at your best?"	
	"What are your life goals and aspirations (e.g., in areas of living, learning, working, socializing)?"	
Content of delusion	"Can you tell me more about this experience?"	PDI, R-GPTS
	"How do you make sense of it?"	
	"Do you have any guess about why this is happening?"	
	"Do you have any control over it?"	
	"What is bad/good about it?"	
Precipitating and protective factors	"When does it usually happen?"	Monitoring diaries
	"Are there times or places that make it worse?"	
	"Are there times or places that make it better?"	
Negative symptoms, functioning, and quality of life	"How does [delusion] affect your day-to-day life?"	CHOICE, RAS, PSYRATS, QPR
	"Does it keep you from working on things that are important to you? Does it help in some way?"	
	"How has it affected your relationships? What does [your loved one] say about it?"	
	"If this weren't happening, what would you be doing differently in your day-to-day life?"	

TABLE 6–1. Sample prompts, measures, and tools to assess
delusions *(continued)*

Assessment target	Sample prompts	Possible measures or tools
Emotional effects (distress)	"How does it make you feel? How strongly, from 0 to 10?" "Sounds like it makes you feel [emotion]?" "Do you ever get positive feelings from it?" [Show emotions chart for less verbal patients] "How much did [delusion] bother you in the past week, from 0 to 10?"	DASS-21, PHQ-9, PSWQ, PCL-5, PSYRATS, CHOICE
Behavioral effects (including safety behaviors)	"What do you do to cope with this? How well does that work?" "Many people with this experience tend to [safety/coping behavior]. Do you ever do that?" "Do you ever drink or take drugs to cope?"	PSYRATS, AUDIT, CHOICE, suicide risk assessments
Physical effects	"When it happens, what do you notice in your body?" "Where do you feel it in your body?" "Does it cause physical pain?" "How is your sleep?"	ISI
Preoccupation	"How much time and energy do you usually spend on it, from 0% to 100%?" "Do you ever find that you can't stop thinking about it?"	
Conviction/insight	"How much do you believe this is going on, from 0% to 100%?" "Could there be any other explanations for this experience?" "What do others in your life (family or medical personnel) think? What do you make of that?"	

TABLE 6–1.   Sample prompts, measures, and tools to assess delusions *(continued)*

Assessment target	Sample prompts	Possible measures or tools
Other psychosis symptoms	"When you have this experience, what happens to the voices? What do they say?"	PSYRATS, BAVQ-R
	"What usually comes first?"	
History and predisposing factors	"Tell me about when this all started."	LEC-5, personality assessments
	"What was going on in your life at that time?"	
Associated core beliefs	"What does it mean about you/others that this is happening?"	
	"What is it about you/them that would make people do that?"	
	"What would it mean if you found out this was really happening/not happening?"	

Note.   Addenbrooke's Cognitive Examination III (Hsieh et al. 2013) may be used to assess cognitive functioning. AUDIT=Alcohol Use Disorders Identification Test (Saunders et al. 1993); BAVQ-R=Beliefs About Voices Questionnaire—Revised (Chandwick et al. 2000); CHOICE=CHoice of Outcome In Cbt for psychosEs (Greenwood et al. 2010); DASS-21=Depression Anxiety Stress Scales (Lovibond and Lovibond 1995); R-GPTS=Revised Green et al. Paranoid Thoughts Scale (Freeman et al. 2021); ISI=Insomnia Severity Index (Bastien et al. 2001); LEC-5=Life Events Checklist for DSM-5 (Gray et al. 2004); PCL-5=PTSD Checklist for DSM-5 (Weathers et al. 2013); PDI=Peters et al. Delusions Inventory (Peters et al. 1999); PHQ-9=Patient Health Questionnaire–9 (Kroenke et al. 2001); PSWQ=Penn State Worry Questionnaire (Meyer et al. 1990); PSYRATS=Psychotic Symptom Rating Scales (Haddock et al. 1999); QPR=Questionnaire about the Process of Recovery (Neil et al. 2009); RAS=Recovery Assessment Scale (Giffort et al. 1995); SMART=specific, measurable, achievable, relevant, time-bound.

Beginning the Conversation

Patients with delusions may not be comfortable fully disclosing these beliefs early on in therapy, so do not push them. Having to talk about symptoms and other private experiences can be very difficult, frightening, or threatening. The critical goal of the first stage of therapy is to secure engagement and trust. Engage and befriend the patient through a discussion of topics such as current events and their interests and hobbies. Eventually, the conversation progresses to their recovery goals, such as school, work, relationships, housing, volunteering, and leisure pursuits. The patient's strengths (e.g., positive attributes, accomplishments) are discussed, as well as the issues and concerns that are interfering with their goals or causing distress—that is, why they have come to therapy. It is here that delusions usually enter the conversation.

How does one know if the experience a patient is describing is a delusion? This is a heavy label that carries stigma and can have serious implications, so it is important to handle this determination with a high level of responsibility and carefulness. DSM-5-TR defines delusions as "fixed beliefs that are not amenable to change in light of conflicting evidence" (American Psychiatric Association 2022, p. 101). Delusions fall under several categories, with the most common being *paranoid* (feeling that one is being persecuted by other people or entities), *grandiose* (believing that one has extraordinary powers not possessed by others), *reference* (believing that the environment consists of special messages directed at the individual), and *control* (believing that one's thoughts or behaviors are influenced by outside forces or that one's thoughts are being read or broadcast).

It is critical to consider the patient's beliefs in the context of their culture in order to avoid pathologizing very real experiences of discrimination or religious and cultural beliefs and practices. Asking the patient questions about their experience, conducting research on their culture and religion, speaking to their loved ones, and seeking consultation from outside experts are all useful methods of ensuring cultural sensitivity. Finally, just because a belief may be a delusion does not necessarily mean it needs to be the target of therapy. The *impact* that the belief has on the patient's life is paramount—CBT can be helpful if the belief causes distress and/or interferes with the patient's recovery, functioning, and quality of life.

When potential delusional beliefs emerge, the clinician maintains a calm, empathic stance and provides normalizing and destigmatizing statements as needed. Clinicians should not interrogate or push too hard for details. They should pay attention to the patient's emotional responses to questions and use these as their guide to topics that may be emotional hotspots. If a line of questioning appears distressing or the patient begins to disengage, backing off and switching to less distressing topics or taking a break are both good options. If the patient discloses multiple delusions, the clinician starts with the least emotionally charged one and works toward the others as the patient becomes more comfortable.

Delusions can be challenging to assess when the patient does not recognize that they are experiencing a delusion, or more broadly that they are having mental health challenges at all, as is often the case with grandiose delusions. The clinician must be careful to not come across as though they are assessing a symptom because this could invalidate and disengage the patient. Language is everything. Pathologizing terminology such as *symptom*, *psychosis*, and especially *delusion* or *paranoia* should be avoided. The word *experience* is typically acceptable to patients regardless of their level of insight. It is even better to use the patient's own terminology for their experience. However, note that sometimes patients will use a medical term such as *paranoia* or *schizophrenia* because other health care professionals have used it, even though the patients themselves do not ascribe to it, so the clinician should assess before adopting the term by asking questions such as "What does that term mean to you?" and "Do you agree with it?" A negotiation on the appropriate terminology then occurs.

Collecting a History

Assessing for the following three aspects of the history of the delusion can give the clinician clues about the case formulation as well as possible strategies for treatment.

1. *Onset*. The clinician asks about when the delusion began, focusing on the patient's life circumstances at the time, such as major stressors, fears, preoccupation with certain ideas, traumatic experiences, or onset of psychosis. In the case of delusions in patients with a high level of conviction, the clinician is careful to not call them "beliefs" (e.g., "When did you first start believing that you were being followed?" vs. "When did the experience of being followed start for you?"). It is especially important to assess for traumatic experiences, given their high prevalence in people with psychosis; administering a self-report measure such as the Life Events Checklist for DSM-5 (Gray et al. 2004) can help facilitate this discussion.

2. *Premorbid phase*. The clinician moves backward in time to collect more information about significant life events, beliefs, attitudes, fears, and so on that are relevant to the delusion. The question here is what occurred in the patient's past that could help the clinician understand—even if just partially—how the delusion may have come about? Were there any *predisposing factors*, such as experiences of trauma, social rejection, or failure? Was there anything notable about the patient's development or personality that seems to stand out? The clinician also should examine the premorbid phase for evidence of *strengths* and clues as to what may be harnessed or revisited now to facilitate the person's recovery, such as accomplishments, positive experiences and relationships, and past interests and activities that brought the patient meaning and purpose.

3. *Course*. The clinician assesses how the delusion has waxed and waned over time and tries to determine the reasons for these fluctuations, such as treatment, change of environment, activity level, and amount of social support.

Assessing Phenomenology

The content of the delusional belief is examined in sufficient detail; for example, if the patient is paranoid about being followed, the clinician finds out by whom, in what settings, the reason for it, how often, and so on. If hallucinations are present, how do they relate (if at all) to the delusion? For example, do the voices say things related to the delusion? Obtaining this level of information helps convey the clinician's concern and interest in the patient (patients are often not accustomed to clinicians examining details of their psychosis) while laying the groundwork for work on the delusion by exposing possible lapses in reasoning or other cognitive errors. See Table 6–1 for suggested prompts. Daily self-monitoring with simple diaries may be of benefit here.

Details about the delusion usually do not come out in a clear and linear matter, especially if talking about the belief triggers a high degree of negative affect or the patient has cognitive impairment or a thought disorder. It is not unusual to take several sessions to get a fairly full understanding of the experience. If the patient becomes highly activated, consider taking a break to practice an affect-regulating exercise together (e.g., soothing rhythm breathing, breath mindfulness, progressive muscle relaxation), engage the body (e.g., stretching), and/or change the setting (e.g., getting out of the clinic office to take a walk together) before returning to the conversation, if appropriate and productive. Sometimes just taking the "helicopter view" of a delusional experience is more feasible than getting every last detail and can still be useful; for example, it may be difficult to fully understand the paranoid delusion of a patient with severe thought disorder, but themes of powerlessness and vulnerability are clear.

Many patients with persecutory delusions experience intrusive, anxiety-provoking mental images with their psychosis (Schulze et al. 2013). Inviting the patient to describe or draw the images associated with their experience can also help to better understand the experience, especially if the patient struggles to communicate verbally. A patient once had difficulty articulating his experience of paranoia, but when asked to draw it, within a few minutes he produced an impactful drawing of himself inside a giant glass box, surrounded by large, bulging, veiny eyeballs, with the door to the room locked. He explained the eyeballs represented those who surrounded and watched him, and the box and door signified that he felt "trapped, with no way out." Other potential manifestations of mental imagery, including sounds, smells, tastes, and somatic feelings, should be assessed as well, if applicable (Hales et al. 2015).

Conducting Functional Assessments

Functional assessment of delusions is a method of collecting detailed information from specific occurrences in which the delusion is activated in order to inform the cognitive formulation and identify treatment targets. Put simply, it helps to understand how the delusion plays out in the patient's life. Functional assessments can also be therapeutic by helping patients better understand the delusional experience and its impact on their life, which is a first step toward managing it. It is important to pick specific instances in which a delusion is activated as opposed to asking the patient to explain "what typically happens," because the latter is a fairly abstract question and patients may have difficulty noticing and accurately recalling patterns in their emotions and behaviors across time. The steps of conducting a functional assessment of delusions are as follows:

1. *Identify precipitating and mitigating factors.* What situations, settings, or internal triggers set off the delusion or increase the distress or impairment it causes? Similarly, what seems to trigger the patient's preoccupation with the delusion or the distress or impairment it causes? Triggers for delusions often include hallucinations, stress-inducing thoughts (e.g., self-criticism, self-stigma), memories (e.g., of traumas), interactions (e.g., real or perceived looks from others, arguments), or places, but inactivity and social isolation can exacerbate delusional preoccupation and distress as well. To identify specific triggers, probe with questions such as "What was happening right before you had that thought/felt that way?" "What were you doing/thinking about/feeling right before it happened?" Pay attention to *mitigating factors* as well, such as situations, times of day, places, and people that tend to deactivate the delusion or reduce the distress it causes. Self-monitoring via diaries and speaking with the patient's loved ones (with their consent) can be helpful in collecting this information.
2. *Assess thoughts and beliefs.* The specific contents of the delusional belief that emerged in the situation are assessed, as described in the preceding section.
3. *Assess impacts on the patient's life.* The most important piece of information to collect is what effect the delusion has on the patient's life. The emotional impact of distressing delusions is often depression, worry, anger, and shame. The behavioral impact often manifests in the form of safety behaviors such as avoidance/isolation or hypervigilance, which the patient uses to cope with the belief; however, these behaviors ulti-

mately maintain the belief. Insomnia and suicidal ideation are also common. How do the patient's delusion and their response to it affect their recovery journey? Does the delusion prevent them from doing things they feel are important? Are they not acting in accordance with their values or postponing goals? Positive aspects of the delusion that may not be as obvious should also be assessed, as described in the next section.

Assessing Beliefs Associated With the Delusion

There are several types of beliefs surrounding delusions that should be monitored.

- *Conviction and evidence.* Events and experiences that the patient takes as evidence to support their delusional beliefs, along with percent conviction ratings. Assessing conviction throughout therapy is good way to measure progress and helps you to adjust your interventions accordingly. For example, you would be more careful and gentler when probing beliefs with 90%+ conviction ratings, or you may avoid them altogether until rapport is stronger or the patient's conviction is a bit lower.
- *Consequences of the delusion being true.* When the patient does not report complete conviction in a delusional belief (i.e., is not totally sure if it is true or not), asking about the consequences of the belief being true can help identify the implications of the delusion, the reasons why it may be distressing, and possibly the function that the delusion holds for the patient (see "Case Formulation"). The downward arrow technique of questioning can be helpful here. Sample questions may include the following: "What would it mean about you if you discovered that people really were monitoring your every move?" "If you found out that people really are reading your thoughts, what would you do/how would you feel?"
- *Consequences of the delusion being untrue.* Conversely, asking about the implications of the patient's delusions not being true could help to assess how much investment they have in their beliefs while at the same time planting the seed for cognitive restructuring. Be careful to use this questioning judiciously; the higher the patient's conviction, the more gently you should word the question (if you decide to ask at all). For example, "What would it mean if what your father said—that nobody is really monitoring you and that this is a sign of stress—were true? What would be good/bad about that, if anything?" "What would you think/how would you feel if you discovered that people are not reading your thoughts?"
- *Underlying nonpsychotic beliefs.* Delusional beliefs are typically maintained by maladaptive nondelusional core beliefs and schemata about

the self and others (henceforth referred to simply as *core beliefs* for brevity). Knowing what these beliefs are helps the clinician to select strategies and interventions to help disconfirm them, thereby helping to neutralize the delusion. In addition to functional assessments, a variety of other methods can be used to identify these underlying core beliefs:

- Gently questioning about the patient's reactions to significant life events (major losses, failures, traumas, rejection)
- Looking for recurrent patterns in automatic thoughts, delusional beliefs, or hallucination content (e.g., a patient who hears voices telling her "You're a loser" may think the same of herself)
- Examining beliefs about the delusional experience because these often mirror core beliefs (e.g., a patient who believes that he is totally powerless against others reading his mind and controlling his body may believe that he is generally a powerless and vulnerable person)
- Downward arrow questioning, as in the following example:

  Patient: They were sending thoughts into my head with telepathy.

  Therapist: What would make them want to do that?

  Patient: Because they want to wear me down until I end up in the psych ward or on the streets.

  Therapist: And what would it mean to you if you ended up being hospitalized or homeless?

  Patient: It would mean they were right, that I'm weak and a loser.

Case Example: Assessing a High-Conviction Delusion

Julie was referred to an outpatient veterans psychosis clinic for the treatment of long-standing persecutory and somatic delusions by her psychiatrist, who was concerned that she was barely leaving her apartment, had gotten into trouble with the landlord for yelling, and was at risk of being evicted. The psychiatrist noted that Julie had a long-standing somatic delusion of having a severe, disfiguring, and noticeable skin condition, but she actually had a mild form of eczema with occasional episodes, typically on parts of her body that were not visible. She also had a persecutory delusion that people would notice her skin and judge her for being unclean.

At the start of therapy, the clinician talked with Julie about her love of traveling and singing; they talked about their fond memories of the best places each had traveled to, and Julie even sang some of her favorite songs. When asked what new places she wanted to see, Julie became upset, stating she could not travel because "everyone defames me because of my skin." She was cryptic on details, so the clinician assigned logs to try to better understand Julie's experience of being defamed between sessions, but Julie would forget to complete them. A few sessions in, Julie came in very agitated, stating that she had been defamed again the previous day on the way to the grocery store.

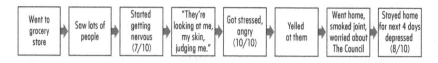

FIGURE 6-2. **Functional assessment of Julie's experience.**

The clinician started to conduct a functional analysis (Figure 6–2) to help break down the process of what occurred, but it was initially difficult because Julie was very emotional. The clinician guided her through a few cycles of soothing rhythm breathing and gradually drew out the entire cycle, drawing the boxes on a whiteboard and asking Julie for feedback and corrections along the way until she got it right. When asked why she thought people were defaming her, Julie described a shadowy organization called The Council that was orchestrating the whole thing, but she did not know why. She frequently used the term "my schizophrenia," but when asked what this meant and what she thought of the term, she said it was a word her doctors had used, and it meant she was a "basket case." Julie and the clinician agreed instead to use Julie's preferred term "defamation" as shorthand. Julie said she believed "100%" that the defamation was happening. She said that the worst part about it was the stress, depression, and anxiety it caused, so she agreed with the clinician's recommendation to start completing the Depression Anxiety Stress Scales periodically as a way of tracking these emotional effects. Julie and the clinician also broke down Julie's goals of traveling and singing into smaller steps and monitored her action toward these goals weekly.

Julie sometimes wondered whether it might be better to wake up dead, but she did not have thoughts or plans for ending her life. In terms of behavior, she coped by smoking cannabis, avoiding leaving the house, and sometimes yelling at neighbors whom she heard talking, presuming they were talking about her. The defamation seemed to ease off during the rare occasions when she had pleasant interactions with other people (one neighbor, her case worker, the therapist) and when she put on CDs and sang at home. When asked about the history of the experience, Julie explained that it had started when she left her parents' home in her mid-20s to enlist in the army. Her service had been difficult; she had felt different and ostracized, which was a consistent theme across her life because she had been bullied for her weight and for being a lesbian. She was medically discharged because of mental illness and subsequently experienced a number of social rejection experiences at work and in relationships. She described always having been socially awkward in her younger years, with few friends.

Case Formulation

Information that is collected about the patient is organized into a case formulation. The formulation is essentially a story of how past and present factors about the patient are believed to have influenced the onset and maintenance of obstacles to recovery, including delusions. Constructing and following a case formulation serves multiple important purposes in CBT for delusions. It helps the therapist maintain organization and structure to the therapy and prevents it from becoming aimless and random "Whack-A-Mole therapy," which is a risk with complex delusions. Formulation helps ensure that the therapy maintains its focus on the individual's recovery goals and that all interventions are selected accordingly. Interventions that are based on an accurate formulation therefore tend to be more effective. Also, by helping therapists be more strategic and effective in their decision-making, case formulation–informed treatment also boosts the therapist's sense of efficacy, which is especially important when working with people with challenging delusions that require longer treatment.

Case formulation is a tool for helping to decode the *psychological meaning* of a delusion, which includes its underlying core beliefs as well as the hypothesized function it may serve in the patient's life. Despite how distressing delusional beliefs may be, they can have certain reinforcing elements that can be viewed as serving a function for the patient. Identifying this function further allows the clinician to design effective interventions to neutralize the delusion by replacing the function it serves and can be particularly useful in making bizarre delusions more comprehensible. Examples of common functions of delusions include the following:

- *A means of avoiding pursuits for which the patient lacks confidence:* A man believes he is incapable of working but attributes this solely to his delusion-related experience. "How can I possibly work when I'm being followed and monitored everywhere I go?"
- *Compensation for low self-esteem (especially with grandiose delusions):* A man who feels ashamed and unintelligent for dropping out of school has the grandiose belief that he is a famous physicist and is invited to guest lecture around the world.
- *Punishment for perceived misdeeds:* A devout Christian woman who feels ashamed about past sexual encounters develops the somatic delusion that she has AIDS despite multiple negative tests and believes she deserves it as punishment.
- *A means of protecting oneself from a sense of extreme vulnerability:* A woman who experienced severe child abuse develops paranoia and avoids people because "it's better to be safe than sorry."
- *Stimulation or companionship:* A severely isolated young man is frightened by seeing covert messages just for him in license plates and TV broadcasts but also finds the phenomenon intriguing and stimulating, "like a puzzle to be solved."

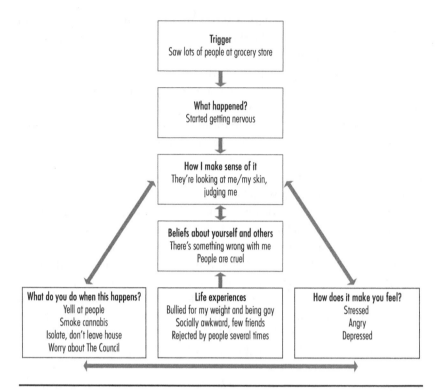

FIGURE 6–3. Longitudinal formulation for Julie.

In Julie's case, the clinician was able to develop a collaborative longitudinal formulation with her (Figure 6–3) (Morrison 2001) that connected the impact of her early experiences of social rejection to the development of her core beliefs about her being defective and others being cruel. These beliefs were believed to have manifested into her persecutory and somatic delusions over time. Her coping responses and safety behaviors of isolation and rumination maintained the delusion and blocked progress toward her recovery goals of singing and traveling.

Personal Reflection: Assessing Our Own Strongly Held Beliefs

How can we as clinicians apply some of the methods described in this chapter to assessing our own overvalued ideas and delusions? It is important for us to be able to recognize such beliefs because they can powerfully shape our emotions and behavior, often without our awareness and not always in a helpful manner. We have all had periods when we got wrapped up in a belief that seemed to consume us, despite plenty of evidence to the contrary. For me, this emerged at the beginning of my longest romantic relationship. When it started, I was excited and happy to have found a wonderful person with whom I connected strongly, yet at the same time, for the first few months I often believed quite strongly that my partner did not feel the same way about me. At times I would even become suspicious that my partner was still pining over a previous relationship and would inevitably lose interest in me and leave. My conviction would vary between 20% and 100% and was higher when we had tiffs, when I had had a particularly stressful day, and when I had not slept enough because of the demands of graduate school (precipitating factors).

I confided in some friends, who pointed out plenty of countering evidence that would help reduce my conviction for a while, but the effect would not stick for long. In terms of the emotional impact of the belief, my positive feelings of excitement due to our great connection and chemistry were yoked to fear and anxiety. Cognitive and behavioral effects included sometimes ruminating on my worries, especially when we were apart, and seeking reassurance from my partner (safety behavior). The belief would at times negatively affect my functioning by (as you might guess) irritating my partner, which would trigger my belief even more.

With time and introspection, I came to realize that the belief was likely related to difficult interpersonal experiences I had had earlier in my life; I was quite shy, was the shortest boy in the class, was bullied for several years, and on one occasion was betrayed by a close friend (predisposing factors). My belief about my partner seemed to reflect an old core belief of being unlovable or undesirable and was probably serving a function of ostensibly protecting me from getting rejected and hurt again. Somehow, if I could be hypervigilant about foreseeing rejection, it would not catch me by surprise when it inevitably happened. Thankfully, none of my fears came to pass; as I had more positive experiences with my partner (i.e., collected disconfirmatory evidence to my strong belief) and my attachment strengthened over the course of the next few months of the relationship, my fears began to fade, and I was able to be fully present and enjoy a positive relationship.

Discussion

Delusions can be complex, multifaceted phenomena that manifest in a multitude of ways across different patients. Assessment in CBT for psychosis is woven throughout the course of therapy and may be accomplished in a number of ways. The fundamental approach is to simply talk to the patient, using naturally curious questions couched in a calm, empathic, and destigmatizing style. Timing is everything, so the conversation should not be rushed or invasive, and the clinician must tread especially gingerly around delusions held with high conviction. Folding in emotion regulation strategies and paying attention to imagery and the body can help. Assessment of the patient's life aspirations, recovery goals, strengths, and protective factors is critical. Although good assessment of delusions is important, clinicians must be careful not to belabor it. Spending too much time excessively scrutinizing the patient's delusions runs the risk of reinforcing the excessive preoccupation that often accompanies and maintains delusions and perpetuating self-stigma from being in the patient role. An overarching goal of CBT is to help the patient out of their delusion and into their life. This activation also has a therapeutic effect on delusions because engaging in life shifts energy away from the delusions and toward successful, socially rewarding, and pleasurable experiences that provide powerful disconfirmatory evidence (Beck et al. 2020). When delusions do present as an obstacle to recovery, they can be decoded and understood using the strategies presented here and mapped into a case formulation that guides the treatment. An example of developing a formulation is shown in Video 8. For discussion of the video, see Chapter 20, "Decoding Delusions."

 Video 8: Formulation

Questions for Discussion

1. How should assessment be conducted when a patient has multiple complex delusions?

2. How should assessment be conducted when a patient is extremely guarded?

3. Can delusions ever be random, with no connection to underlying nonpsychotic core beliefs?

4. When should the formulation be shared versus not shared with the patient?

KEY POINTS

- Assessment of delusions is multidimensional and occurs throughout therapy via a number of methods as appropriate for the patient, but natural, gentle questioning in the context of a good therapeutic relationship is fundamental.

- Assessment of delusions and associated problems should be balanced with assessment of recovery goals and strengths.

- Tactfulness, flexibility, and creativity are key to maintaining engagement and navigating challenges that may accompany delusions, such as low insight, strong affect, and cognitive impairment.

- Functional assessments can be used to disentangle the chain of events that occur in specific instances of delusional activation.

- The information collected during assessment is assembled into a case formulation through an iterative process. The formulation helps to decode the psychological meaning and function of the delusion and guide the course of therapy.

References

American Psychiatric Association: Diagnostic and Statistical Manual of Mental Disorders, 5th Edition, Text Revision. Washington, DC, American Psychiatric Association, 2022

Bastien CH, Vallières A, Morin CM: Validation of the Insomnia Severity Index as an outcome measure for insomnia research. Sleep Med 2(4):297–307, 2001 11438246

Beck AT, Grant P, Inverso E, et al: Recovery-Oriented Cognitive Therapy for Serious Mental Health Conditions. New York, Guilford, 2020

Chandwick P, Lees S, Birchwood M: The revised Beliefs About Voices Questionnaire (BAVQ-R). Br J Psychiatry 177(3):229–232, 2000 11040883

Freeman D, Loe BS, Kingdon D, et al: The revised Green et al., Paranoid Thoughts Scale (R-GPTS): psychometric properties, severity ranges, and clinical cut-offs. Psychol Med 51(2):244–253, 2021 31744588

Giffort D, Schmook A, Woody C, et al: Construction of a Scale to Measure Consumer Recovery. Springfield, Illinois Office of Mental Health, 1995

Gray MJ, Litz BT, Hsu JL, Lombardo TW: Psychometric properties of the Life Events Checklist. Assessment 11(4):330–341, 2004 15486169

Greenwood KE, Sweeney A, Williams S, et al: CHoice of Outcome In Cbt for psychosEs (CHOICE): the development of a new service user-led outcome measure of CBT for psychosis. Schizophr Bull 36(1):126–135, 2010, 19880823

Haddock G, McCarron J, Tarrier N, Faragher EB: Scales to measure dimensions of hallucinations and delusions: the Psychotic Symptom Rating Scales (PSYRATS). Psychol Med 29(4):879–889, 1999 10473315

Hales S, Blackwell SE, Di Simplicio M, et al: Imagery-based cognitive-behavioral assessment, in Assessment in Cognitive Therapy. Edited by Brown GP, Clark DA. New York, Guilford, 2015, pp 69–93

Hsieh S, Schubert S, Hoon C, et al: Validation of the Addenbrooke's Cognitive Examination III in frontotemporal dementia and Alzheimer's disease. Dement Geriatr Cogn Disord 36(3–4):242–250, 2013 23949210

Kroenke K, Spitzer RL, Williams JB: The PHQ-9: validity of a brief depression severity measure. J Gen Intern Med 16(9):606–613, 2001 11556941

Lovibond SH, Lovibond PF: Manual for the Depression Anxiety Stress Scales, 2nd Edition. Sydney, Psychology Foundation, 1995

Meyer TJ, Miller ML, Metzger RL, Borkovec TD: Development and validation of the Penn State Worry Questionnaire. Behav Res Ther 28(6):487–495, 1990 2076086

Morrison AP: The interpretation of intrusions in psychosis: an integrative cognitive approach to hallucinations and delusions. Behav Cogn Psychother 29(3):257–276, 2001

Neil ST, Kilbride M, Pitt L, et al: The Questionnaire about the Process of Recovery (QPR): a measurement tool developed in collaboration with service users. Psychosis 1(2):145–155, 2009

Peters ER, Joseph SA, Garety PA: Measurement of delusional ideation in the normal population: introducing the PDI (Peters et al. Delusions Inventory). Schizophr Bull 25(3):553–576, 1999 10478789

Saunders JB, Aasland OG, Babor TF, et al: Development of the Alcohol Use Disorders Identification Test (AUDIT): WHO Collaborative Project on Early Detection of Persons With Harmful Alcohol Consumption-II. Addiction 88(6):791–804, 1993 8329970

Schulze K, Freeman D, Green C, Kuipers E: Intrusive mental imagery in patients with persecutory delusions. Behav Res Ther 51(1):7–14, 2013 23178174

Weathers FW, Litz BT, Keane TM, et al: PTSD Checklist for DSM-5 (PCL-5). National Center for PTSD, 2013. Available at: www.ptsd.va.gov/professional/assessment/adult-sr/ptsd-checklist.asp. Accessed February 22, 2023.

PART II
Treating Delusions
Types, Techniques, and Settings

7

Collaboration, Not Collusion

Befriending and Normalizing

Kathryn Eisen, Ph.D.
Melanie Lean, Clin.Psych.D.
Kate V. Hardy, Clin.Psych.D.

Collaboration is an essential feature of any strong therapeutic relationship. Fostering collaboration with a patient who has strong beliefs about reality that differ from those of the therapist presents unique challenges. At the same time, when working with a patient who is living with delusions, taking the time to build a trusting foundation from which to engage in productive therapeutic work is especially important. In this chapter, we describe key components of collaboration when working with individuals who are experiencing delusions, including befriending, normalization, curious questioning, shared goal setting, and avoiding collusion and confrontation. We explore the importance of considering cultural factors when building a collaborative relationship, and we use case examples to illustrate how collaboration supports therapeutic gains. Although we commence this chapter with normalizing and collaboration, these are not one-time events provided at the start of therapy and never again. Rather, they are an essential ethos at the core of the therapeutic relationship and process in cognitive-behavioral therapy for psychosis (CBTp), and arguably more so when working with delusions.

Befriending

Building a relationship, or *befriending*, is the cornerstone of any therapeutic interaction. The best advice I (M.L.) have been given in terms of commencing a therapeutic relationship and building rapport came from my systemic family therapy supervisor, who said, "Sit down and have a cup of tea with your patient." Although this frequently forms a key part of engaging when in the patient's home or in the community, it is less possible in other settings, such as the therapist's office or inpatient settings. However, the same principle still applies. Your demeanor should be warm, open, and friendly, interested but not intrusive. Especially when working with individuals who may struggle with paranoia or who may have had difficult experiences with the mental health care system in the past, establishing a sense of safety is essential.

In early sessions, much of the work in therapy may center on building trust in the relationship, which can take many forms. Befriending can take place when playing a card game, going for a walk, or discussing areas of interest to the patient, such as a favorite video game, television show, or hobby. Where appropriate, using humor judiciously can be a great way to build rapport. Through the engagement and befriending phase, information for a formulation can be gathered and developed that can help the clinician understand the development and onset of symptoms and their maintenance; this formulation can be shared with the patient. Befriending is not considered an active treatment but rather is the ground on which the foundation is built to move toward active formulation and intervention. However, information gathered during this phase can be helpful during the active phase of treatment, in particular because it gives the clinician a range of neutral and non-threatening topics that are known to be of interest to the patient to fall back on if there is evidence of a rupture in the therapeutic relationship or in the event the clinician needs to tactically withdraw from a topic if the patient is becoming distressed. An example of befriending a patient with a delusion is shown in Video 1, which is discussed in Chapter 20, "Decoding Delusions."

 Video 1: Befriending

Improving the therapeutic alliance when working with people with psychosis results in better outcomes (Goldsmith et al. 2015). Goldsmith et al. (2015) used structural equation modeling to show that when it comes to psychological therapies for psychosis, a good therapeutic alliance has a causal effect on symptomatic improvement, and, conversely, a poor therapeutic alliance has a detrimental effect. In fact, it has been demonstrated that therapy should proceed with caution if the therapeutic alliance is poor (Goldsmith et al. 2015). Furthermore, a qualitative analysis examining service user experiences of CBTp found that the therapeutic alliance emerged as a theme of critical importance (Mankiewicz et al. 2018). Establishing rapport through befriending is vital. Using a lot of explicit empathy can help build an effective therapeutic alliance by reducing the patient's anxiety and their need to defend their explanations of events. The assumptions and beliefs of therapists clearly influence interactions, and therapists should embody the therapeutic stance that delusions can be quite understandable (Morrison and Barratt 2010).

When working with individuals experiencing paranoia, a clinician should anticipate that it may take some time to build trust and should plan for this. This is especially true for individuals who may have had negative early experiences with the mental health care system, such as involuntary hospitalization or police involvement in a mental health crisis. In addition, if the patient comes from a group that has experienced systemic racism or marginalization and the therapist is a member of the majority group, it is understandable that it may take longer to build trust. We as providers must be careful not to mislabel understandable cultural mistrust as evidence of paranoia.

When there are challenges in establishing rapport, it is important to keep in mind that the pace and progress of interventions may need to be slowed down. In fact, the pace and therapeutic style should be careful, curious, and tentative and can be likened to a crab, approaching things not directly but by scuttling in sideways, looking out for open doors to push on. At times maintaining this sense of safety may require the therapist to take a step back from a particular area or topic when they observe that this topic heightens distress or conflict for the patient and to shift to neutral and nonthreatening topics that were identified during the befriending phase. This practice of gathering information and stepping back when needed is known as *tactical withdrawal* and may be called on throughout therapy, not just during befriending.

Normalizing

Normalizing is one of the most important components of effective CBTp. When used within the broader process of formulation, it was found to be a significant predictor of a good outcome (Dudley et al. 2007). The cognitive-behavioral therapy model of psychosis and delusions is inherently normalizing. By drawing links between what people think and what they subsequently feel and do, the clinician can highlight how beliefs emerge out of an attempt to make sense of our experiences and that anyone in a similar situation may come to the same conclusion. For instance, delusions or strong beliefs often function to provide structure to people's lives, often following trauma or loss, and paranoid-type thinking can actually be protective and functional in certain circumstances. The message we hope to convey is that we all experience negative thoughts, we all engage in unhelpful thinking, and we all use coping strategies that are not always the healthiest choice. This is no different for the patients we see with psychosis.

CBTp therapists also use normalization to demonstrate that experiences of psychosis exist within the range of "normal" functioning and can be experienced in the absence of distress or disability (Dudley et al. 2007). Evidence increasingly points to the existence of a range of psychotic-like experiences in the general population, which suggests that these experiences exist on a continuum. An important step in normalizing is sharing with patients data on the prevalence of symptoms of psychosis, including delusions, in the general population. Studies estimate the prevalence of psychotic-like experiences in the general population at around 7% (van Os and Reininghaus 2016), with at least 10%–15% of the general population regularly experiencing paranoid thoughts and persecutory thinking (Freeman 2007). A study of healthy volunteers from across 13 countries indicated that 93% of respondents had experienced an intrusive thought in the past 3 months (Radomsky et al. 2014). In addition, the intrusive thoughts reported by participants were no different from those reported by clinical populations and involved similar themes, such as doubt; harm; injury; aggression; and sexual, religious, and immoral intrusions (Radomsky et al. 2014).

Sharing the prevalence of these experiences in the general public can be an important normalizing process that demonstrates that psychotic experiences exceed the rate of diagnosed mental illness in the community (which suggests they can be considered part of the spectrum of "normal" or typical experiences). Normalization can also be achieved through sharing examples of well-known people (celebrities, lived experience advocates, scientists, authors) with psychosis as well as connecting with individuals with lived experience of psychosis. This can assist in renewing expectations of what is possible and can generate hope that people can and do live successful lives alongside experiences of psychosis, including having relationships, families, and friends. Working through these nonthreatening exploratory areas with patients prior to delving into their own symptomatology can be a useful way to forge connection and normalize experiences.

Normalizing helps reduce catastrophic thinking (e.g., "I'll never get a job," "I'll be on medication forever," "My life is over") because often this type of thinking is wrapped up in stigma and society's assumptions about mental illness and psychosis. Although normalization is an important counter to the catastrophic thinking that can accompany experiences of psychosis, therapists must be mindful not to normalize responses and behaviors to the extent that it minimizes the problem and the person does not see the value in change (Dudley et al. 2007). Furthermore, one must be careful not to invalidate the patient's experience in this process. Frequent feedback between patient and therapist while normalizing is important in order to assess how the patient is receiving and interpreting the information. For instance, if a patient holds beliefs that their experiences are due to an illness that makes the person experience "bad" thoughts, but then the therapist normalizes the symptoms so they no longer constitute a disorder or illness, then that person may start to believe that they are "bad," which may lead to shame and further distress (Dudley et al. 2007). Like all work in this area, it is about balance, and the focus of normalizing should be based on assessment, patient feedback, and formulation. An example of normalizing a patient with a delusion is shown in Video 2 (see Chapter 20).

 Video 2: Normalizing

Personal Reflection

It can be helpful at times to engage in judicious self-disclosure to aid in the normalization of psychotic-like experiences. The aim here is to demonstrate to the patient that psychotic-like experiences are varied and wide-ranging and occur in a number of different situations. For example, one day here in California, the sky turned a deep orange because of excess smoke from wildfires, and it was very dark despite it being early in the day. I (K.V.H.) noticed increasingly catastrophic thinking related to this experience, despite knowing that the phenomenon was due to the smoke. Surely something this extreme was due to something more threatening? Could it be a meteor? If it was a meteor on a collision course with Earth, it would make sense that it would get darker during the day, and obviously the authorities would not tell us this because it would lead to worldwide panic.

The more I thought about this, the more anxious I became, and the more anxious I became, the more catastrophic my thoughts became (as if the reality of millions of acres of wildfire was not catastrophic enough). However, this was a useful exercise in noticing the link between an extreme situation, my emotions, and subsequent thoughts, and it is something that I may share with patients as a means of normalizing the idea that it is common for people to experience catastrophic interpretations of events in extreme or unfamiliar circumstances.

Collaborative Empiricism

A collaborative relationship is one in which the patient and therapist are working together as a team to better understand how thoughts, feelings, and behaviors interact with one another to maintain problematic patterns and to explore how to change those patterns and move toward shared goals. The term *collaborative empiricism* refers to this process of shared detective work.

Shared Goal Setting

An important step in collaborative empiricism is identifying what goals the therapist and patient are working toward. Fortunately, developing shared goals does not demand that a patient give up a delusional belief that they may be unwilling or unable to relinquish. For example, an individual who believes he is being poisoned by a malicious entity may disagree with his therapist about whether his food is actually safe to eat. However, he may be able to identify as a shared goal that he would like to be able to eat a meal with his family without feeling unsafe. Being able to feel safer while eating would then be the shared goal. Once this goal is established, therapist and patient can work together to explore ways in which the patient might be able to feel safer while eating. This may entail cognitive techniques, such as questioning the evidence that he is being poisoned or developing a behavioral experiment that might test out the belief that the food is poisoned. However, it may also involve relaxation and stress management strategies or other interventions that have nothing to do with actually questioning the belief.

Curious Questioning

Curious questioning is another essential skill that supports the development of therapeutic rapport and facilitates the process of collaborative empiricism. At its most basic, this is simply the process of dropping assumptions and asking questions about an individual's experience. For many years mental health professionals were taught not to question individuals about their beliefs for fear that this would somehow make things worse. However, the wonderful thing about curious questioning is that it is an opportunity for the therapist to build rapport by expressing genuine interest in the patient's experience while also allowing the therapist to gather valuable information that will support formulation and the development of interventions.

Curious questions should be open-ended in nature, and the possibilities are endless. Without colluding with the patient's delusion, the therapist may express curiosity about any number of things: when the beliefs began, when they occur most frequently, when these beliefs are the most distressing, what assumptions the patient has about why things are occurring, how the patient copes with unusual experiences, whether any particular bodily sensations are associated with their unusual beliefs, and so on. This goes beyond an assessment of symptoms and embraces curious exploration of beliefs. By modeling genuine curiosity and dropping our assumptions, we as providers are inviting the patient to similarly engage in curious exploration. Supporting a patient to engage in this process requires a strong and well-established therapeutic rapport, which is one of the reasons why a strong therapeutic relationship is critical in working with strongly held beliefs.

Sitting on the Collaborative Fence: Collaboration Without Collusion

Building a strong therapeutic relationship with someone who is experiencing delusions often requires a provider to walk a tightrope of sorts: listening genuinely and with curiosity to the beliefs and experiences of the patient while avoiding both direct confrontation of the delusion and unhelpful collusion with the delusion. This delicate balancing act is sometimes referred to as the act of *sitting on the collaborative fence*. Sitting on the collaborative fence requires that we as providers drop assumptions and remain open to holding multiple explanations for a situation. We must leave the role of expert and instead join our patient on a journey of collaborative empiricism where, together, we explore the most effective way for the patient to navigate a challenging situation. Consider the following vignette, in which we explore a confrontational approach, a collusive approach, and, finally, an effective collaborative approach.

Case Example

Daniel is a 20-year-old single white man who lives at home with his parents. He is hoping to take classes at community college. He was enrolled in courses previously but has been unable to take classes the past year because he fears that others are able to hear his thoughts, including a number of sexually explicit and racist intrusive thoughts that are ego-dystonic in nature and therefore highly distressing. As a consequence, Daniel rarely leaves his home. He spends most of his time isolated in his bedroom, lying in bed or playing video games. Even when in his room at home, he worries that his neighbors can hear his thoughts, and he feels a great deal of concern about the distress that this must cause them, especially when he has sexual thoughts about a married female neighbor. Because of this, he prefers to sleep during the day and have his waking time occur overnight, when fewer people might be awake and able to read his thoughts. In order to stay awake at night, Daniel drinks large quantities of coffee throughout the night, although he also wonders whether his caffeine intake might actually be increasing his already high level of anxiety. Daniel is also aware that his nocturnal schedule will make it difficult for him to achieve his goal of attending community college.

Collusive Approach

Collusion occurs when the therapist joins in a patient's delusion, even though the therapist does not actually believe the delusion to be true. Again, this is often done with the most well meaning of intentions. However, a collusive approach has several clear disadvantages. First off, genuineness is a key element of any good therapeutic relationship. When the therapist is, in essence, lying to a patient by claiming to believe a delusion they do not believe, the entire therapeutic relationship is being built on an unstable foundation. Furthermore, by colluding with the patient, the therapist denies the patient the opportunity to learn how to practice cognitive flexibility and explore a belief from many angles (an important skill, not limited just to delusions). Consider what a collusive approach might look like in Daniel's case:

> After hearing Daniel's explanation of his symptoms, the therapist says to Daniel, "Well, we certainly don't want other people reading your mind! From now on, whenever you can feel people reading your mind, why don't you play some really loud music. That will certainly block them from being able to hear your thoughts."

Again, although Daniel might feel momentarily relieved by this suggestion, in the long term, the therapist's approach is likely to increase the strength of Daniel's belief in this distressing thought: if his therapist thinks he needs to be sure to cover his thoughts with loud music, then it must be very dangerous indeed to have these socially unacceptable thoughts! An example of collusion is shown in Video 3 (see Chapter 20).

 Video 3: Collusion as an Approach to Avoid

Confrontational Approach

We often think of confrontation as being an angry, critical approach that we, as thoughtful and empathic clinicians, would never engage in. However, it is entirely possible to find ourselves confronting a patient who is experiencing a distressing delusion with the most noble of intentions, out of a desire to alleviate suffering by convincing the patient that the belief causing them distress is simply not true or not possible. In cognitive-behavioral therapy, the term *challenging thoughts* is often used. However, the concept of *challenging* can inadvertently establish confrontation with the patient and automatically assumes that the clinician (who is doing the challenging) holds the correct view of the world and undermines the opportunity for a truly collaborative exploration of experiences. Consider how a well-meaning confrontational therapeutic approach might look with Daniel:

> After hearing Daniel describe the situation, the therapist tells him not to worry. "What you are describing is simply impossible. I am 100% certain that no one can hear your internal thoughts. Mind reading is impossible! Now, let's talk about changing your sleep schedule so you can go ahead and take some classes this fall."

Although the therapist is clearly well-intentioned in this case, Daniel is likely to be left feeling unheard. He shared with his therapist something that is deeply distressing, and the therapist dismissed it offhand. This is likely to echo feedback that Daniel already hears when he expresses his concerns to his parents or friends: everyone dismisses his concern, and no one is really hearing him or providing him with space to explore his fears. Alternatively, Daniel might feel momentarily relieved by his therapist's reassurances. However, the reassurance has come from an external source, and Daniel has not developed any skills to explore or question this belief on his own. As a result, when Daniel returns home and later that night feels very clearly that his neighbors are reading his thoughts, he may feel that he has been lied to by his therapist, who told him this was not possible. This in turn could have an impact on the therapeutic relationship between Daniel and his therapist and create a barrier to future work together. An example of confrontation is shown in Video 4 (see Chapter 20).

 Video 4: Confrontation as an Approach to Avoid

Collaborative Approach

A collaborative approach involves dropping assumptions and exploring the experience as a partner with the patient. Often, the first and most important step in this collaborative approach is to use the skill of curious questioning. As described earlier, when we as providers are genuinely curious, we are better able to explore and understand our patient's perspectives while neither confronting nor collaborating with the delusion. This shared understanding provides a foundation from which to build interventions collaboratively. The specifics of the intervention will depend on the details we learn during this period of curious questioning and will vary depending on the strength of the belief. Consider what curious questioning might look like in Daniel's case:

> **Therapist:** Are there particular times when you are most aware of this thought that people might be reading your mind?
>
> **Daniel:** Well, it seems that the thoughts I'm most embarrassed about are actually the thoughts that are broadcast the loudest. Like, if I have a sexual image come into my mind, the women who are around me get really uncomfortable and start giving me these dirty looks.
>
> **Therapist:** How have you coped with this in the past?
>
> **Daniel:** I hate to think that I'm making these women uncomfortable.... And I am super embarrassed about what they must think of me. So, I really just do my best to stay away from any situation where I would make someone feel bad. I figure if I'm asleep most of the day, at least if it happens at night, not too many people will be awake to receive the broadcasts.
>
> **Therapist:** Daniel, I wonder if you can tell me a bit about when you first had this concern that other people could hear your thoughts being broadcast?
>
> **Daniel:** Well, last year, back when I was going to school, the professor was lecturing when suddenly I had this image of a naked woman come into my head. Right when that thought came into my mind, I saw this girl who was sitting in front of me in class shift around in her seat. I knew that she knew what was going on in my mind, and she was totally disgusted with me. I felt like such a pig for making her feel uncomfortable. It was so embarrassing that I just got up and left class. I couldn't stop thinking about how upset she must have been, and I just never went back to that class.

Daniel and his therapist might take a number of different paths from this point, depending on the goals that they have identified for their work together. Daniel's therapist might focus on normalization by sharing research that shows the prevalence of intrusive thoughts, helping him to understand that many individuals have intrusive thoughts that are sexual or inconsistent with their own value system. The therapist might use cognitive approaches to explore alternative hypotheses for why the woman in Daniel's class shifted in her seat right after Daniel had the intrusive thought. They might use behavioral interventions to develop some experiments to help Daniel gather more evidence to assess whether his beliefs about this situation are accurate. Or they might work on relaxation or stress management techniques to help Daniel manage the distress associated with his strong beliefs about mind reading and thought broadcasting so that he might be more able to return to school and go out during the day, even if the strength of the beliefs does not change. The knowledge that Daniel's therapist gained by being curious and open when exploring Daniel's beliefs will be invaluable in terms of developing an idiosyncratic formulation and identifying the specific interventions that they will choose to use to support his movement toward his treatment goals. The time invested in building the relationship at the start of treatment is essential both for ensuring that Daniel trusts his therapist enough to share this information and for securing Daniel's buy-in that he and his therapist are working collaboratively toward shared goals. An example of collaboration is shown in Video 5 (see Chapter 20).

 Video 5: Sitting on the Collaborative Fence

We have highlighted in this chapter the need for a strong therapeutic relationship and ways in which to develop this relationship, including normalizing, befriending, and curious questioning. However, it is important to emphasize why this is so critical: As we as providers explore beliefs, how they were formed, and alternatives, we have to recognize that the stakes are incredibly high for the patient in terms of any changes in their beliefs. Consider the 2×2 grid in Figure 7–1 that demonstrates the potential positions in which individuals may find themselves in relation to their beliefs, using Daniel's belief as an example.

Three of the cells in the grid are associated with the potential for increased distress. Consider the possibility that Daniel stops believing that people can hear his thoughts (cell 3) and subsequently drops the behaviors that he perceived as keeping him safe (sleeping during the day, staying awake at night), only to discover that people could hear his thoughts all along—that would be a very frightening experience and potentially expose him to any risk associated with this. Similarly, consider what would happen if Daniel continues to believe that people can read his thoughts but discovers they cannot (cell 2). Depending on Daniel's cultural background, messaging he has received regarding psychosis, and experiences of stigma, this might also be a scary and frustrating cell to land in and might be associated with beliefs of being "crazy," a term that is typically used pejoratively in society. Exploration of Daniel's perception of mental health problems, internalized stigma, and reframing from "I am crazy" to "These experiences are understandable reactions to extreme circumstances" may be beneficial. By contrast, if Daniel no longer believes people can hear his thoughts and determines that this is true (cell 4), we might consider this to be symptom remission. As clinicians, it is important for us to recognize the risks patients take in undergoing this exploration with us. We are repeatedly humbled by the resiliency of patients as they walk along this path.

1. True positive	2. False positive
I believe that people can hear my thoughts, and they actually can hear them.	I believe that people can hear my thoughts, but they actually can't.
3. False negative	4. True negative
I don't believe that people can hear my thoughts, but they actually can hear them.	I don't believe that people can hear my thoughts, and they actually can't.

FIGURE 7–1.   Belief: People can hear my thoughts.

Cultural Considerations

When the therapist and patient come from the same cultural background, a backdrop of shared experiences, culture, language, and so on can make it easier to build rapport and trust. Conversely, if patient and therapist come from very different cultural backgrounds, it is understandable that it may take longer to build rapport. It is important for therapists to be aware of their own implicit and explicit biases, in particular when working with individuals from historically marginalized groups. We recommend that clinicians undertake their own work that examines these implicit biases and the intersection of their positionality (how one's own position of privilege related to race, class, gender, and sexuality influences how one understands and experiences the world) in order to be aware of how their biases influence the therapeutic relationship. As noted previously, it is also important that therapists not pathologize mistrust that patients may have based on real-world experiences they have had. When exploring whether a belief is based in reality, it is essential that therapists consider what their patient's reality looks like. Too often in the history of mental health care, behaviors that are understandable in the context of a challenging situation have been misinterpreted as evidence of pathology. One study that looked at responses on the Structured Interview for Psychosis-risk Syndromes found that elevations on measures of suspiciousness were correlated with neighborhood crime rate, which suggests that what was being called "suspiciousness" was in some cases an accurate awareness of dangers in one's community (Wilson et al. 2016). A Black man may have had real-world experiences with police officers that have led him to be suspicious of those in authority; this is understandable and should not be labeled as paranoia. A young man of Middle Eastern descent may have reality-based worries about being targeted or stared at when walking through the airport. Although we as providers can support our patients in managing anxiety around such real-world concerns, we should take care not to minimize or dismiss these concerns.

In addition, certain experiences that may sound delusional to one cultural group may actually be culturally normative to members of a different cultural group. Beliefs about spirits, talking to God and/or hearing God talk back, or seeing ghosts or deceased loved ones may all be culturally appropriate depending on the patient's cultural background. Excellent use of curious questioning, collaboration with family members or others from a similar cultural background, and use of semistructured tools such as the Cultural Formulation Interview (American Psychiatric Association 2022) can be helpful when trying to tease out whether a belief that seems unusual is more likely to be a culturally relevant belief or a delusional one.

Questions for Discussion

1. What are some strategies that you have used to support engagement and befriending with your patients? How have you needed to adapt these when working with patients from different cultural backgrounds?

2. What experiences have you had that you might be able to draw on in your sessions to support normalizing of symptoms? How would you share these and when?

3. Sitting on the collaborative fence can at times be tricky. What can you do if you find yourself being confrontational or colluding more than you intended?

KEY POINTS

- Developing a strong therapeutic relationship is a critical step in addressing delusions. This can occur in the initial sessions and may take varying amounts of time depending on a number of factors (e.g., patient presentation, patient previous experience with services). It may also be something the clinician needs to return to periodically throughout therapy.

- Befriending is considered an initial phase in treatment during which no active formulation or intervention occurs. However, it can support the development of therapeutic rapport and provides the clinician with an understanding of neutral, nonthreatening topics that are meaningful to the individual and that can be drawn on later in therapy as needed.

- Befriending can include normalizing, which allows the patient and clinician to decatastrophize symptoms and explore the prevalence of these experiences in the population while also examining different conceptual frameworks for the development and maintenance of these experiences.

- Curious questioning allows the clinician to engage in further exploration of symptoms with the patient. It requires the clinician to demonstrate genuine curiosity and to drop assumptions during this discourse. In doing so the clinician models to the patient the benefits of being curious regarding one's beliefs and gently encourages the patient to engage in the same process.

- Each of the elements described in this chapter should be conducted through a lens of cultural humility, and the clinician should encourage feedback from the patient and engage natural supports in understanding the cultural context in which beliefs have been formed.

References

American Psychiatric Association: Core Cultural Formulation Interview (CFI), in Diagnostic and Statistical Manual of Mental Disorders, 5th Edition, Text Revision. Washington, DC, American Psychiatric Association, 2022, pp 864–867

Dudley R, Bryant C, Hammond K, et al: Techniques in cognitive behavioural therapy: using normalising in schizophrenia. Journal of the Norwegian Psychological Association 44(5):562–572, 2007

Freeman D: Suspicious minds: the psychology of persecutory delusions. Clin Psychol Rev 27(4):425–457, 2007 17258852

Goldsmith LP, Lewis SW, Dunn G, Bentall RP: Psychological treatments for early psychosis can be beneficial or harmful, depending on the therapeutic alliance: an instrumental variable analysis. Psychol Med 45(11):2365–2373, 2015 25805118

Mankiewicz PD, O'Leary J, Collier O: "That hour served me better than any hour I have ever had before": service users' experiences of CBTp in first episode psychosis. Counselling Psychology Review 33(2):4–16, 2018

Morrison AP, Barratt S: What are the components of CBT for psychosis? A Delphi study. Schizophr Bull 36(1):136–142, 2010 19880824

Radomsky AS, Alcolado GM, Abramowitz JS, et al: Part 1—You can run but you can't hide: intrusive thoughts on six continents. J Obsessive Compuls Relat Disord 3(3):269–279, 2014

van Os J, Reininghaus U: Psychosis as a transdiagnostic and extended phenotype in the general population. World Psychiatry 15(2):118–124, 2016 27265696

Wilson C, Smith ME, Thompson E, et al: Context matters: the impact of neighborhood crime and paranoid symptoms on psychosis risk assessment. Schizophr Res 171(1–3):56–61, 2016 26777883

8

Cognitive-Behavioral Therapy for Paranoia

Conceptualization, Process, and Techniques

Douglas Turkington, M.D.
Kate V. Hardy, Clin.Psych.D.

Paranoia is a term whose meaning has changed over the years but is accepted as describing a delusional state without thought disorder, negative symptoms, or auditory hallucinations. Paranoia is usually a persecutory delusion with linked anxiety but may include grandiose or somatic content. Delusions exist on a spectrum with "normal" beliefs (Kingdon and Turkington 1994). The spectrum stretches from "normal" beliefs through eccentric beliefs, overvalued ideas, and circumscribed delusions (paranoia) to primary delusions. Jaspers's (1913) definition of the primary delusion has stood the test of time, but the majority of delusions dealt with in clinical practice bear little resemblance to the classical phenomenology of the primary delusion he so clearly described. Delusional mood, delusional perception, bizarre content, and systematization with resistance to exploration of the evidence are certainly hallmarks of the primary delusion, which is a symptom of the first rank (Schneider 1959). Interestingly, such bizarre delusions are very often resistant to antipsychotic medication, including clozapine, but can partially respond to a prolonged course (of the order of 50 sessions) of expert cognitive-behavioral therapy (CBT; Turkington et al. 2015). Jaspers described *circumscribed paranoia* as a separate entity from schizophrenia, and circumscribed delusions are best recognized as new beliefs that can powerfully drive affect and behavior. Bentall et al. (2009) explored the underlying mechanisms contributing to delusion formation and found a number of contributory factors, including jumping to conclusions, intolerance of uncertainty, and externalizing bias. No clear pattern emerges across delusional causation (see Chapter 1, "Delusional Beliefs and the Madness of Crowds"), and this is true of the subgroup of circumscribed delusions (including paranoia).

It is certainly the case that increased levels of dopamine, whether due to ingestion of cannabis, amphetamine, or other such substances or genetic sensitivity to stress in the mesolimbic system, will lead to increased salience of perception. When the meaningfulness of experiences is increased, it is easier to jump to conclusions and form new beliefs. Such delusions will be likely to respond to antipsychotic medication, and when this happens, the delusion becomes submerged, but, being unprocessed and untested, the delusion will reemerge as soon as the antipsychotic medication is discontinued. Relapse is therefore inevitable once the medication is stopped (Kapur 2003).

However, paranoia is not always the result of increased dopaminergic tone and can be triggered by conflict (including trauma), bereavement, and the inability to express painful emotion. The content of paranoia very typically moves with the times and goes with the flow of current events, environmental threats, and technological breakthroughs much more than do primary delusions (see Chapter 1). Typically, paranoia will be about issues pertinent to current culture, such as terrorist groups, climate change, the Knights Templar, social media, alien abduction, and satellite surveillance. Thus, paranoia is closer to "normal" beliefs held across society than to the primary delusions of schizophrenia. Such delusions also can be culturally and spiritually syntonic. Being cursed, the victim of witchcraft, or the victim of possession by a jinn are examples of paranoia in certain cultural and religious groups. However, for the clinician to address the delusion as such, a faith leader (e.g., an imam) or an expert within the religious community would have to declare that the delusion is not recognized as a normal belief within that faith. Thus, the ability of the clinician to hold a position of curious neutrality during clinical interaction requires a basic knowledge of such emergent belief changes, and the clinician must be open to consultation with experts in that subject area.

Personal Reflection: Acknowledging and Investigating Our Own Strongly Held Beliefs

If we as clinicians are hoping that our patients will give up their delusions when working with CBT, are we prepared to face our own overvalued ideas and simple delusions? Conspiracy theories usually exist at the level of overvalued ideas and have the potential to become delusional. Recent examples include the following: Who assassinated President John F. Kennedy? Was Princess Diana's death an accident or something more sinister? Is there a secret society (the Illuminati) behind all world governments? All of these could be presented at the level of conspiracy theory or as delusion. I (D.T.) have never entertained the first or the last of these overvalued ideas. I was too young to have been affected by President Kennedy's death. In relation to the Illuminati, I believe that any such secret society would have been outed by now purely to get an insider a very large payoff. However, the death of Princess Diana had an emotional aspect for me, as it did for many people around the world. I never knew her, but I sympathized with her struggle within the establishment and what I saw as her humility and honesty. I felt profound and surprising grief at the time of her death and for a period entertained the belief that the death was not an accident. Often, an emotional component is crucial in the emergence and maintenance of paranoia. Considering Diana's death in relation to the Morrison (2001) maintenance model (Figure 8–1), there was a clear trigger for the emergence of this new belief. I felt an emotion not only of sadness but also of anger. I also experienced rumination and an increasing search for the "real" story—the evidence had to be there. I felt a deeper belief that this event resonated with: that the people's champion would always be at risk from the establishment. This belief was informed by my own childhood experiences of being criticized for speaking up for what I believed in at school. These factors, as we shall see, are the typical elements maintaining delusions and preventing recovery. However, the conspiracy theory and paranoia I felt around Diana's death never took hold. I was able to deal with the emotions and realized that I was biased in searching for confirmatory evidence. Once I considered all the available evidence, my eventual conclusion was that the event was a tragic accident. Thus, people can do their own CBT, and perhaps we are all doing so on a regular basis. We all know that this is easier at certain times and that all beliefs seem to fluctuate in terms of conviction. The question then is why do some overvalued ideas get stuck, develop into paranoia, and not recover?

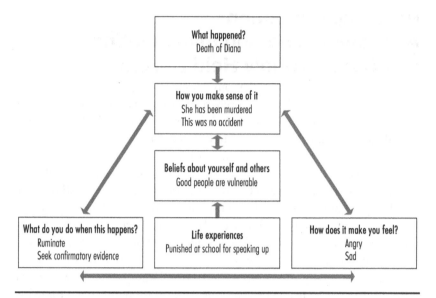

FIGURE 8–1.   **Idiosyncratic formulation.**
Source.   Based on Morrison (2001).

Changing Beliefs and Recovery From Delusions

The natural tendency for all episodes of persecutory paranoia is recovery with adequate treatment (Freeman et al. 2021). However, they are maintained by safety behaviors, underlying personal beliefs (schemata), and unprocessed affect. It can be important to normalize with the individual the fact that new beliefs are being formed all the time and old ones are gradually given up. An important aspect of belief formation and change is the understanding that new insights are crucial in terms of personal growth, scientific progress, and creativity. It is therefore normal to form new beliefs and to change them if they do not fit the evidence or are unhelpful. A normalizing example of this, drawing on the evolution of the treatment of delusions, can be seen in the early belief that psychoanalysis could not be used in the treatment of delusions because of the likelihood of the patient being overwhelmed by the psychosis from which the delusion was protecting the person (Freud 1911/1958). Freud described the delusion as "a sticking plaster over the unconscious" (Freud 1911/1958, p. 382). This was a very interesting idea, but only partially true, and led to talking therapies being overlooked as a treatment option for individuals with strongly held beliefs for many years. Different models of delusions are now accepted that allow psychodynamic therapists to work with delusions with safety and benefit (Garrett and Turkington 2011). Beliefs need to be voiced, tested, and then refined as need be. We therefore need new beliefs, and we need to be able to let old beliefs go. Unfortunately, letting cherished beliefs go can be a painful matter. This is particularly so if the belief is functional (e.g., it is potentially better to believe that you are related to royalty than to accept the stigmatizing label of schizophrenia) and when the belief has social value. It is always easier to move from one belief to another when there is a functionality for the new belief.

Case Example 1: Working With Acute Paranoia

Alex was an inpatient on an acute psychiatric ward, and he was terrified and agitated. He had been admitted for 6 weeks and was not improving. He spent a lot of his time hiding on the ward and asking people to check whether the two vans he could see out of his bedroom window were still there. He had ideas of reference thinking that certain television presenters were talking about his imminent death. Alex had been using cocaine and amphetamine prior to admission and had become increasingly paranoid.

An example of wellness planning is shown in Video 15 (see Chapter 20).

 Video 15: Maintaining Change

Phase 1: Open-mindedness and curiosity. In this phase, which is of variable length, the clinician shows the patient that they are humane, interested, and able to accept the patient's level of distress. This is done through using standard opening gambits to establish trust. Early discussion might be about the area they live in, family, or hobbies and involves a degree of self-disclosure. In Alex's case, it was discussion about the history of the local area and the personalities who lived there.

Phase 2: Exploring the delusion. This phase is characterized by gentle exploration and listening to the patient's account of the delusion and its various ramifications and impact on social functioning. In Alex's case, this helps the clinician begin to develop a maintenance formulation through understanding the impact of the beliefs and subsequent behaviors that Alex uses to maintain his self-perceived safety. This collaboratively developed formulation supports Alex in beginning to make links between his thoughts, feelings, and behaviors and in identifying how these behaviors may inadvertently maintain the problem (Figure 8–2).

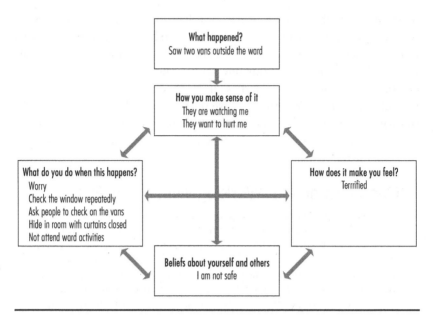

FIGURE 8–2.   **Maintenance formulation for Alex.**

Phase 3: Peripheral questioning. Questions of fact can then be asked around the periphery of the delusion.

> The clinician asked Alex the following questions: Is there a particular make of van that you are watching for? Is the color of the van relevant? Would the vans have signs on the sides or be plain? Would the vans have people inside or guarding them? In relation to the television and radio, are there any particular programs or personalities who you believe are talking about you? In response, Alex suggested that the vans would be plain colored, would have people inside, would possibly be guarded, and would be second-hand or stolen.

Socratic questions are used only sparingly; an example of the distress they can cause is shown in Video 7, which is discussed in Chapter 20.

 Video 7: Socratic Questioning

Phase 4: Reality testing homework. Shared homework can aid engagement and increase the patient's motivation to collaboratively explore the beliefs through reality testing.

With the information provided by Alex, it was agreed that the clinician would go out and locate the two vans Alex could see and bring back information. Alex agreed to keep a diary beside his bed to note the program that he believed was referring to him.

The clinician took pictures of the two vans (making sure to carry identification in case his actions raised suspicion) and brought them back to the ward for discussion with Alex. Alex decided that one of the vans was "too new" and had advertisements on the side, and the other was actually in someone's driveway and up on bricks being repaired. Alex concluded that one of the vans was too new, and the other too old, to be a threat. His anxiety level diminished, and he started to have escorted leave on the grounds.

Phase 5: Generating alternative explanations. The clinician can use evidence to strengthen the development of alternative explanations. In Alex's case, the clinician could obtain more van photographs and continue the discussion.

Together, Alex and the clinician postulated that there were many reasons for vans to be parked near the hospital. The vans might be owned by staff or by parents taking children to and from the local nursery school. They might be from a local business or from a service provider, such as the ambulance service or a local supermarket delivery service.

Phase 6: Anxiety reduction. The clinician then works with the patient to treat anxiety resulting from delusions.

It was clear that Alex's anxiety was lower, and his perpetual worry regarding the vans was reduced. However, Alex noted that anxiety did continue to be a problem for him, and he decided to work on reducing anxiety by taking the exercise class on the ward and by doing relaxation exercises. He disclosed that he had not been taking his medication previously because he had been too scared that it would sedate him and that he would not be able to escape when the people in the van jumped out to assault him. He started to take his medication rather than disposing of it.

Phase 7: Working with personal beliefs. The clinician explores the origins of the patient's beliefs and discusses the effects of events in the patient's life on these beliefs.

Alex went on to say that he had always thought that his area of town was very dangerous and that a friend who had not paid a drug debt had been jumped by people hiding in a white van. Further discussion revealed that safety depended on what part of this area you went to and who your friends were. Research in the local papers showed that there had been an assault as described, but it related to a much more complex situation than a drug debt. Alex's own family had actually paid off his drug debt.

Relapse prevention: So far so good! Alex's conviction in his beliefs was reduced, and he was discharged to his family with input from a home treatment team. He needed to tackle his substance use and maintain coping strategies, find work, and avoid drug-taking triggers. This required voluntary attendance at a drug support agency, which he successfully achieved.

Case Example 2: Paranoia Linked to a Bereavement

Bob had always lived with his mother. They were inseparable. He had been married for a period, and he and his wife lived with his mother prior to their divorce. Eventually, his mother had to be moved into a care home because of general frailty and two mini-strokes. Bob had long discussions with the general practitioner about giving up his work to care for his mother at home, but it was decided that it was not financially possible to do so. He was ambivalent and felt very guilty about the decision. His mother was in care for only a matter of weeks before he was contacted on his way to the care home after work with the news that his mother had died. He entered a state of shock and denial and was unable to deal with the feelings that arose. He blamed himself, he blamed the nurses at the home, and he developed the distressing delusion that his thoughts were being picked up by other people (thought broadcasting). He also developed the belief that he was shouting out obscenities in public. He refused medication and was treated in the outpatient clinic with the support of a community psychiatric nurse doing home visits.

Phase 1: Open-mindedness and curiosity. This phase provided a chance for personal disclosure by the clinician regarding difficulties around coping with the death of a loved one that helped to strengthen rapport and aid normalizing.

> Bob and the treating clinician agreed that the unexpected death of a loved one was a major stressor that would "knock anyone for six." It was no surprise that Bob's feelings were very raw. Had he ever experienced a death before, and how had it affected him?

Phase 2: Exploring the delusion. As with Case Example 1, exploration of the delusion included gentle questioning around the onset of the beliefs. Was Bob now avoiding public places such as shops and libraries? Did he have any coping strategies? How was this impacting his social and role functioning? Information gathered in this stage led to a maintenance formulation that was later used to develop a longitudinal formulation (Figure 8–3).

Phase 3: Peripheral questioning. In this phase, the clinician has to carefully monitor the patient's reaction to the questioning. Increased affect, disengagement, or shutting down would lead the clinician to take a different approach by potentially exploring the change in affect (if the patient is

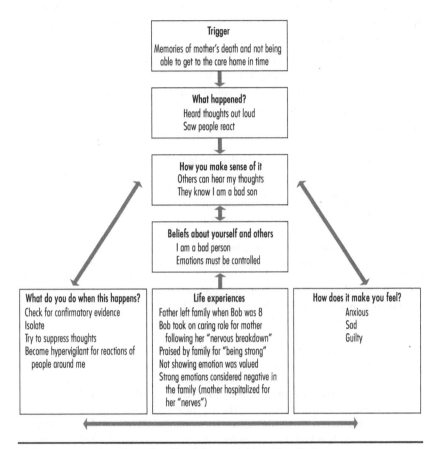

FIGURE 8–3. **Longitudinal formulation for Bob.**

willing), returning to befriending topics, or agreeing to explore a less emotionally charged and valent topic.

Once trust improved, Bob was open to more targeted questions in relation to his beliefs, including the following: How did he know that others were picking up his thoughts? Had anyone told him he was shouting obscenities in public? How often did he experience his thoughts being broadcast? Did he notice a reaction in other people at those times? Was it at times when he was thinking about what had happened to his mother and was distressed? How might that work? Was it something like the popular idea of telepathy? Had he ever noticed that kind of gift or experience before? Were there any particular types of thoughts that were more liable to seem as if they were being broadcast? Each of these questions helped Bob to consider his experience and to provide further information to the clinician, who was demonstrating genuine curiosity about Bob's experience.

It is important to note that the questions were not presented in an interrogative fashion but rather were discussed collaboratively and focused around mutual curiosity.

Phase 4: Reality testing and behavioral experiments. Following these questions, Bob became agreeable to finding out more. There were opportunities to collaboratively develop behavioral experiments to explore whether Bob had actually shouted out obscenities in the outpatient clinic when the clinician was present.

> Diary recording seemed to show that the belief about shouting out was related to Bob being in social situations. It was agreed that if someone did shout out an obscenity in a public place, the people present would look directly at the person shouting, would look afraid, and would probably move away. So it was agreed that Bob would go to a local café with the clinician for a cup of coffee, and together Bob and the clinician would watch to see if anyone behaved in the way predicted. No such reactions were seen, which introduced some doubt and reduced social avoidance. Bob practiced this activity and one day heard a passerby shouting outside and saw the reactions of those inside the café. This diminished his conviction in the belief and led him to consider a new belief: that he was frightened that he might shout out obscenities and that this was linked to his grief.
>
> In terms of his thoughts being broadcast, was this a similar mechanism? Did it happen in social situations? Could they test it out with the two secretaries next door? The experiment set up to test this included meeting the secretaries and asking them to write down any thoughts that came into their heads during the appointment. Bob was unsure whether his thoughts had "gone out" but had written down the key ideas on his mind: anger with the nursing home, fear about the bus trip back home, and concern about paying the rent. He was very interested to see what the secretaries had written. They wrote about a popular television program, not being able to understand the doctor's dictation, and a holiday that was coming up. Bob and the clinician agreed that telepathy did not seem to be a day-to-day experience but that speaking one's mind was important, and the clinician agreed to dictate more clearly. Further exploration regarding ways to collect additional data involved asking the nurse who visited Bob at home whether he could pick up Bob's thoughts. Data from these experiments helped to support the development of alternative explanations.

An example of a behavioral experiment is shown in Video 10 (see Chapter 20, "Decoding Delusions").

 Video 10: Behavioral Experiment

Phase 5: Generating alternative explanations. Through the application of behavioral experiments, Bob was able to consider alternative explanations for his experience, including 1) an intense reaction to grief, 2) telepathy, and 3) lack of sleep.

Phase 6: Anxiety reduction and linking emotions with the experience. This phase could not begin prior to further graded behavioral experiments because of Bob's level of anxiety about the shouting out in public and thought broadcasting delusions.

> Now that Bob had three possible explanations for his experience, he was more open to engaging in experiments that had initially felt risky. He was able to check further with the secretaries that they had not heard him shouting and had not picked up his thoughts. This gave him the confidence to look for reactions in other people in other social situations when he thought that he might have transferred thoughts or shouted out. Tracking this experience allowed him to make the link between his emotions and his experiences of telepathy or shouting out. These experiences happened when Bob was emotionally distressed and remembered the drive to the nursing home and receiving the call about his mother.

Phase 7: Working with grief and personal beliefs. With increased curiosity and openness to different explanations for Bob's experience, the clinician was able to develop a collaborative longitudinal formulation exploring the impact of early experiences on the development of Bob's beliefs in the context of significant bereavement (Figure 8–3). From this formulation it was agreed that Bob had not had an opportunity to fully grieve for his mother and that he was experiencing intense guilt surrounding her death.

> Bob disclosed that he did not believe he could live without his mother and that he could not let her go. He also said that strong emotions were dangerous and unbearable on the basis of narratives prevalent in his family when he was a child. Guided grief work began by looking at family photographs, and Bob decided to write a letter to his mother partly apologizing for not getting there on time and also expressing anger with himself and the nursing home. He asked for her forgiveness at the end of the letter. The telepathy belief and the belief about shouting out did not cause further problems. Medication was not needed in this case.

Discussion

Both cases in this chapter illustrate key principles in working with circumscribed delusions (paranoia). Time needs to be taken for trust to develop over a number of sessions. An inpatient ward, a day hospital, or a place where frequent visits are possible are ideal locations for this type of relationship building with the person with paranoia. Common ground needs to be found in the consideration of the delusion and curious questioning and open-mindedness need to be demonstrated. Clinicians need to walk the tightrope between confrontation and collaboration, and this is done by asking peripheral questions and gathering nuggets of evidence. It is appropriate to validate any components of the delusion that are jointly agreed to be true. Homework often initially has to be done by the therapist or clinician, and this is a crucial early phase. This type of CBT approach often facilitates improved medication adherence, and this is often a benefit. An appropriate therapeutic trajectory and formulation were utterly crucial to both cases described here. Both cases were ideally formulated in line with the Morrison model, but the question arises as to how much of the model should be shared with the patient. In these case examples, a maintenance formulation was used with Alex given the acuity of his delusion and the short-term inpatient setting. For Bob, a deeper longitudinal formulation was developed over time to help to make links between his early experiences, his recent bereavement, and the development of beliefs relating to thought broadcasting.

Working to drop safety behaviors, do graded behavioral experiments, and identify and process or reduce excessive affect is vital. If this approach does not result in a shift in the belief over 10–12 sessions (after the initial befriending period), then it may be that the paranoid delusion is not circumscribed and may have deeper roots that could become apparent following an exploration of the timeline (Kingdon and Turkington 2005). Systematization is typical of primary delusions, so if questioning leads to the emergence of new, secondary delusions, then the delusion is not circumscribed. For example, a primary delusion would have been considered if further exploration of Bob's experience had revealed that he believed his mother had been murdered by the government and that Bob was himself now being monitored through an unknown device, resulting in broadcasting of his thoughts (see Chapter 12, "A Bizarre and Grandiose Delusion," for a description of an intervention for systematized delusions). Similarly, delusions linked to underlying trauma will not respond to this approach, and more sessions will be required, which will include trauma reprocessing (see Chapter 16, "Trauma and Delusions"). The paranoid delusions described in these cases are very common in clinical practice, and the process of CBT as described here is viable when delivered by crisis and home treatment teams in acute and rehabilitation settings and in community mental health centers.

Questions for Discussion

1. Consider strongly held beliefs that you have held. Would others view them as not based in reality?

2. What about culturally syntonic beliefs that strongly and negatively drive behavior but do not fulfill criteria for delusion? How should these be defined and worked with?

3. Is there always a seed of truth at the heart of the delusion?

4. Is it more effective to work with the emotions investing the delusion or the maintenance factors?

KEY POINTS

- *Paranoia* is a term used to describe the majority of delusions seen in clinical practice, and the phenomenology is not typical of the complex primary delusions described by Jaspers (1913). Paranoia is a very viable target for CBT with or without the presence of antipsychotic medication.

- An engaging period will be needed to build a therapeutic alliance, with retreat into a befriending style of interaction if conviction and affect levels are very high.

- Curious questioning to guide the patient into an exploration of the evidence takes place from a position of neutrality (with the clinician neither colluding with nor confronting the delusion). This can be supplemented by the generation of homework exercises that may initially need to be completed by the clinician.

- Paranoia can be formulated in line with the Morrison (2001) model and usually has a clear proximal trigger. Social and evidential avoidance, rumination, and worry are key maintenance factors. With coping strategies in place, guided reality testing allows further exploration of the delusion and consideration of alternative explanations.

- Graded reality testing experiments are then done to test the various alternative explanations.

- After graded reality testing, the patient may be supported in holding a new belief and working with the emotional and behavioral implications.

References

Bentall RP, Rowse G, Shryane N, et al: The cognitive and affective structure of paranoid delusions: a transdiagnostic investigation of patients with schizophrenia spectrum disorders and depression. Arch Gen Psychiatry 66(3):236–247, 2009 19255373

Freeman D, Emsley R, Diamond R, et al: Comparison of a theoretically driven cognitive therapy (the Feeling Safe Programme) with befriending for the treatment of persistent persecutory delusions: a parallel, single-blind, randomised controlled trial. Lancet Psychiatry 8(8):696–707, 2021 34246324

Freud S: Psychoanalytic notes on an autobiographical account of a case of paranoia (1911), in The Standard Edition of the Complete Psychological Works of Sigmund Freud, Vol 12. Translated and edited by Strachey J. London, Hogarth, 1958, pp 3–82

Garrett M, Turkington D: CBT for psychosis in a psychoanalytic frame. Psychosis 3:2–13, 2011

Jaspers K: Allgemeine Psychopathologie. Berlin, Springer, 1913

Kapur S: Psychosis as a state of aberrant salience: a framework linking biology, phenomenology, and pharmacology in schizophrenia. Am J Psychiatry 160(1):13–23, 2003 12505794

Kingdon DG, Turkington D: Cognitive-Behavioural Therapy of Schizophrenia. New York, Guilford, 1994

Kingdon DG, Turkington D: Cognitive Therapy of Schizophrenia (Guides to Individualized Evidence-Based Treatment; Persons JB, series ed). New York, Guilford, 2005

Morrison A: The interpretation of intrusions in psychosis: an integrative cognitive approach to hallucinations and delusions. Behav Cogn Psychother 29(3):257–276, 2001

Schneider K: Clinical Psychopathology. Translated by Hamilton MW. New York, Grune & Stratton, 1959

Turkington D, Spencer H, Jassal I, Cummings A: Cognitive behavioural therapy for the treatment of delusional systems. Psychosis 7(1):48–59, 2015

9

At-Risk Mental State
Delusional Presentations

Mark van der Gaag, Ph.D.

Personal Reflection

It is strange to see how extreme ideas can become very prevalent during times of crisis and challenges to society. As these ideas are shared by large groups, we must consider the phenomenon a normal expression of fear. When glass was used more and more in the beginning of industrialization, some people experienced glass delusion: the conviction that their buttocks were made of glass and that excessive clothing was needed to prevent the glass from breaking. When trains were introduced, large parts of the general population were convinced that traveling faster than a horse would kill you. Microwaves were thought to poison the food with radiation. Conspiracy theories in politics are numerous and come and go. These are overvalued ideas that are shared among fearful groups; they are more obsessive and more upsetting by contradiction than delusions are, and the ideas are strongly defended and identified with. Yet they are difficult to distinguish from delusions and show overlap. An individual with delusions will probably shrug his shoulders if you do not believe him and conclude for himself that you do not understand at all what is going on, whereas people with overvalued ideas get very upset with people who dispute them. People who support QAnon share these characteristics. They are extremely convinced that Donald Trump fights the deep state; that the storm will come; and that after bloodshed, Trump will end injustice, repression, and democracy. In extreme cases, moral superiority will license the use of violence to defend overvalued ideas. Although overvalued ideas can result in much upheaval, they also disappear in the long run and demonstrate that we all are affected with odd ideas every now and then. A frequent theme in conspiracy theories is that the governing elite is trying to steal or fully control your personality.

Definition of the At-Risk Mental State

The at-risk mental state (ARMS) is a mental state with a heightened risk for developing a first psychotic episode. This condition is also referred to as *ultra high risk* and *clinical high risk*. It is also a severity marker in other disorders predicting long-term treatment trajectories with reduced success rates for therapy. It is not a homogeneous concept but a set of multiple risk factors composing a risk profile. Three subgroups can be distinguished on the basis of symptom profiles:

1. Familial or genetic subgroup with a help-seeking patient who either has had a quite severe decline in social and occupational functioning in recent months and has a parent (or first-degree relative) with a psychotic disorder or is classified with a schizotypal disorder and has had an associated severe decline in social and occupational functioning. This familial subgroup forms about 10%–15% of the ARMS group.
2. Brief limited interval of psychotic symptoms subgroup that has experienced an episode of psychosis in the past, shorter than a week, and has come into symptom remission without pharmacological intervention or intervention by a psychology professional. This group also makes up about 10%–15% of the ARMS group.
3. Subclinical psychotic symptoms and/or psychotic-like experiences subgroup. This subgroup has experienced psychotic-like symptoms but without delusional certainty, and multiple explanations are still considered possible. At moments the patient will embrace a delusional explanation, but there is still enough reality testing capacity to discard these delusional beliefs after some hours. This is the largest subgroup.

In clinical high risk, an additional subgroup is identified with basic symptoms. Basic symptoms are subjectively experienced disturbances of different domains, including perception, thought processing, language, and attention, that are distinct from classic psychotic symptoms in that they are independent of abnormal thought content and reality testing and insight into the symptoms' psychopathological nature are intact.

The subclinical symptoms have different appearances. A symptom can be a genuine psychotic symptom, such as an auditory hallucination, but it can also be short-lived, such as hearing a clear voice that is loud and has a distinct low-frequency tone for a few seconds but with only occasionally (e.g., about once a month). Or it can be a psychotic-like phenomenon, such as hearing one's own thoughts very loud within the head, sometimes so loud that it is hard to hear other people talk, with increased frequency but not continuously. Other examples of perceptual aberrations include seeing a face change when looking at a person or looking at oneself in a mirror; hearing things other people cannot hear, such as voices of people whispering or talking; or smelling or tasting things that other people cannot smell or taste. Most people with ARMS start with these perceptual experiences and then make a transition to psychosis with delusion formation related to these perceptual aberrations.

Other people with ARMS experience delusional mood, and in this chapter I focus on conceptualizing and intervening around these unusual beliefs. Some individuals may have the sense that some person or force is around, even though no one is present. Some patients speak of some loss of control over their own ideas or thoughts. Referential ideas can emerge, such as seeing special meanings in advertisements, in shop windows, or in the way things are arranged. These odd experiences are perplexing to individuals. They are still searching for an explanation for what is going on, and in general patients with ARMS are very eager to learn about rational and scientific explanations for their odd experiences. A transition to a first episode of psychosis occurs when the psychotic state lasts more than a week. If the person transitions to a first episode of psychosis, the conviction becomes a 100% delusional certainty, and the person starts to act on the delusion (behavior change). Very often the emotional arousal is diminished after the point of delusional certainty is reached. In many studies the emotional distress is higher for patients with ARMS than for those with first-episode psychosis.

The ARMS stage is characterized by doubt and despair. Almost all ARMS patients fear that they are slowly becoming crazy. As therapists, we can reassure patients that they are not crazy and that there are several non-psychotic explanations for their experience. This approach emphasizes the need for normalizing (see Chapter 7, "Collaboration, Not Collusion," for more on this). Part of therapy is to encourage ARMS patients to keep on engaging with other people and share their thoughts and feelings. Continued engagement with school and work is encouraged because it will be very hard in the future to regain school or vocational functioning if this is discontinued. Above all, one needs contradiction and opinions from friends and trusted fellow humans to stay within a shared reality.

Prevalence of the At-Risk Mental State in Help-Seeking Adults

The assessment of psychosis and high-risk state is done with the Comprehensive Assessment of At-Risk Mental States (CAARMS) or with the

Structured Interview for Psychosis-Risk Syndromes (SIPS), which are both gold-standard measures of this presentation. Screening with the Prodromal Questionnaire self-screen followed by a diagnostic assessment with the CAARMS detected 5.3% ARMS patients and 1.8% patients with undetected psychosis in the complete help-seeking population in The Hague in the Netherlands (van der Gaag et al. 2012a).

In the older literature, and in retrospect, it was noticed that psychosis is often preceded by depression. This is certainly true, but there is also much other psychopathology: In one study, 96% of help-seeking patients reported at least one psychotic-like event, and patients who were treated for ADHD, mood disorders, personality disorders, or PTSD reported more psychotic-like events than did patients experiencing other symptom presentations. No differences were found in the endorsement of different items among these diagnostic groups except for grandiosity, which was endorsed more than expected by people with ADHD (Rietdijk et al. 2014). No less than 87% of ARMS patients had experienced childhood trauma, as reported in a meta-analysis by Kraan et al. (2015b). ARMS patients with childhood trauma had higher levels of attenuated positive symptoms, general symptoms, and depression and lower levels of global functioning at 24 months follow-up (Kraan et al. 2015a). In a large European study, Kraan et al. (2018) found that in the ARMS stage, child maltreatment is a pluripotent risk factor for developing psychosis, depressive disorder, PTSD, panic disorder, or social phobia in adulthood. The ARMS group is thus heterogeneous in psychopathology and seriously impaired in social and vocational functioning, with depression, anxiety, PTSD, and ADHD dominating the clinical picture. Although the majority of ARMS patients are adolescents or young adults who still work or attend school, members of this group develop a complex psychopathology that predicts a long-term treatment trajectory. ARMS status has remained a specific predictor of psychosis, with an odds ratio of 13.8, and there are no differences from help-seeking control patients in terms of developing a nonpsychotic disorder (Webb et al. 2015). At baseline, ARMS patients already have many comorbid disorders that need therapeutic attention and therapy (Albert et al. 2018).

State Interventions for an At-Risk Mental State

An important thing to remember about treating ARMS is that it is not a disorder but a risk profile. In this way, it is comparable to metabolic syndrome, which puts an individual at risk for developing heart disease. Metabolic syndrome is characterized by high blood glucose, abdominal obesity, high cholesterol, and high blood pressure. All four conditions can be subclinical and nonsymptomatic, but they are associated with development of heart disease if not addressed. Heart attacks and cardiac death can be prevented by regular screening of these conditions by a general practitioner or primary care provider and diminishing of these risks through diet combined with exercise and medication to lower blood pressure. The same is done in ARMS. There is no psychotic disorder, but the aberrant experience may trigger delusional explanations. At the same time, these patients have many comorbid conditions that need to be addressed. For example, trauma-focused therapy is indicated in highly traumatized subjects with PTSD. Low self-esteem and depressed feelings are present in the majority of ARMS patients and can be addressed with competitive memory training and depression treatment (van der Gaag et al. 2012b). Many patients have panic disorder, and interoceptive exposure can be very helpful in mastering these episodes. Therefore, it is very important to explore all symptoms and comorbid conditions and the perceptual aberrancies and tentative delusional explanations to come to a comprehensive case formulation and multifocal treatment plan.

Omega-3 fatty acids are not helpful for all patients with ARMS, but supplemental omega-3 fatty acids can be preventive in patients with low levels of these acids (Amminger et al. 2020). Finally, most ARMS patients have trouble with theory of mind processing (van Donkersgoed et al. 2015). Very often they misunderstand the communications and behavior of others. This drives poor social skills and poor social and vocational functioning. Paranoid ideation is often the result of not understanding other people and misinterpreting social interactions and one's surroundings. Social skills training and learning to check one's interpretations with other trusted persons can be very helpful.

It becomes clear that the etiology of psychosis is understood as the unfolding of multiple accumulating problems, symptoms, and comorbid disorders that ends in the development of psychotic symptoms when the comorbid disorders persist. This is in accordance with the model in which psychopathology can be represented in one factor (Caspi and Moffitt 2018). In this model, prevention of psychosis includes the treatment of early problems, early symptom manifestations, and nonpsychotic symptoms. One has to go upstream for effective primary prevention. For instance, in psychotic disorders dopamine dysregulation seems to be a downstream problem (McCutcheon et al. 2020). The upstream processes in psychosis are probably deficits in the interneurons and the glutamate system. In the long run this deficit in the glutamate system dysregulates the dopamine system.

Therapy for ARMS patients also should focus on upstream problems and disorders to enhance functioning and result in a real gain in quality of life. Moving effective interventions to early adolescence or childhood might be hard to accomplish. Young people have more psychotic-like experiences, but these experiences are also more transient. Treating young people for ARMS would probably result in treating an excess of false-positive cases who would never have developed a psychotic episode. For the time being, the ideal candidates for treatment are help-seeking adolescents and young adults with ARMS and a comorbid disorder and social and vocational decline. The interventions in this group are effective and cost-effective (Ising et al. 2017; van der Gaag et al. 2012a).

Therapy Targets in Cognitive-Behavioral Therapy for Patients With an At-Risk Mental State

In the early years of treating people with ARMS, therapy was focused on preventing a first psychotic episode. Although early studies already showed efficacy for cognitive-behavioral therapy (CBT), CBT had no effect on social and vocational functioning, and many patients still experienced persistent anxiety disorders and depression at follow-up. Although ARMS patients do not have florid psychotic symptoms, they already have multiple disorders at the beginning of emerging psychosis, and a broad-spectrum approach is indicated (Albert et al. 2018).

The presence of multiple disorders that is characteristic of ARMS makes CBT for ARMS different from treatment for depression or anxiety. The case formulation has to be comprehensive, and all symptomatology must be formulated with identified treatment targets. Different treatment protocols need to be combined or sequenced. This means that trauma-focused treatment, emotion regulation training as in dialectical behavior therapy, self-esteem enhancement as in competitive memory training, and individual placement and support to enhance vocational functioning might all be indicated in a single treatment plan.

CBT for psychosis differs from CBT for ARMS in that the patient with psychosis is convinced of their psychotic explanations for what is going on, whereas the ARMS patient has multiple hypotheses to account for their experiences and seeks expert help to clarify things. The ARMS patient is eager for therapy and in need of psychoeducation. In the treatment protocol (van der Gaag et al. 2013), the therapist provides information to the patient and hands out written information on several of the patient's odd experiences. (Patient information can be downloaded from www.routledge.com/CBT-for-those-at-risk-of-a-first-episode-psychosis-evidence-based-psychotherapy/Gaag-Nieman-Berg/p/book/9780415539685, under "Support Material.") This means that the first sessions contain much education and normalizing. For most ARMS patients, it is an enormous relief to learn that some of their odd experiences are highly prevalent in the population and are not a sign that they are crazy. The therapist teaches the patient that many adolescents and young adults have a sensitized dopamine system that leads to heightened salience and pronounced cognitive biases. One of my patients finished the second session with the following remark: "So, it may be that there are no ghosts in my bedroom, and instead I have sudden dopamine releases." At the beginning of the next session, in quite a relieved mood, he reported that "I had two dopamine sensitizations last week and nothing happened."

The readiness for therapy and change of many ARMS patients makes them also willing early in treatment to test hypotheses with behavioral experiments. The information from psychoeducation is believed conditionally, but the real change comes with experiencing that real life is different from what is anticipated. Although the treatment of emerging psychotic symptoms is quite straightforward and time-limited, it is not simple. ARMS patients should be treated by a well-trained CBT therapist because their cases are complex, with varying symptoms and different developmental trajectories. Case formulations form the core of the approach, and treatment always involves the combination of different treatment protocols and stepwise addressing of multiple problems and pathologies.

Case Example 1: PTSD and Thought Broadcasting

Margaret was referred to me for therapy at age 28 for PTSD with reliving nightmares of assaults by her brother when she was a child. Her mother had never believed that when she was out at work, Margaret's brother Jim would take off Margaret's underwear and touch her genitals. Margaret often secluded herself in the bathroom to keep him out until their mother returned. Besides the disturbed family relationships, Margaret also experienced moments of salient experiences with a covariation bias or illusory correlations.

All people can experience the covariation bias, the experience that some contingent events and remarks by others are believed to be no longer coincidental. Covariation bias makes a person think that there must be a causal connection or a connection on the level of meaning. For example, in Wuhan, China, after 5G telephone poles were installed and started to operate, the first outbreak of COVID-19 occurred. A popular conspiracy theory emerged that 5G causes COVID-19 symptoms, and all over the world people with covariation bias started setting fire to 5G telephone poles. Experts calling this theory absolute rubbish resulted in a counterproductive response: "See, it is a conspiracy of the scientific elite!" In a similar manner, people with ARMS have stronger dopamine synthesis and experience more frequent dopamine releases in response to trivial stimuli that give rise to false moments of salience and stronger cognitive biases (Howes et al. 2020).

Margaret was shopping one day and was wondering where the cucumbers were stocked in the store. At the very moment this thought arose, a woman standing close to her asked an aide where she could find the cucumbers. For a moment, the thought flashed in Margaret's mind that her thoughts were known by the woman. At home she felt sad, and her boyfriend asked what had happened that she was in such a sad mood. Again she thought that her thoughts could be heard, this time by her boyfriend. This made her cautious, and she started to deliberately think about shopping lists or recite the alphabet to broadcast only neutral thoughts to others she met. Margaret also asked a friend whether he could hear her thoughts, and he laughed while denying it. She was concerned and thought he might have denied hearing her thoughts because it gave him an advantage in their relationship to hear her thoughts. Could he be trusted? Talking about these events with friends reassured her somewhat, but the thought of broadcasting her thoughts popped up at moments of salient experiences.

After a dozen or so times of her thoughts being expressed by other people, Margaret became quite firmly convinced of and concerned about this thought broadcasting. She and I agreed on two problems that needed attention in therapy: 1) the PTSD with recurrent nightmares and her disturbed relationships with her mother and brother and 2) the ideas about broadcasting her thoughts that interfered with her social and occupational life. A case formulation according to the referenced protocol (van der Gaag et al. 2013) is shown in Figure 9–1.

After a few sessions, we decided to start right away with eye movement desensitization and reprocessing (EMDR) sessions for the traumatic sexual experiences recurring in Margaret's nightmares. She was experiencing three recurrent nightmares, and these were the targets in EMDR therapy sessions. Margaret made quick progress, and after three sessions she experienced reduced distress with the memories of the sexual harassment.

Margaret's nightmares were inoculated, and fear was replaced by anger toward her brother. We decided that the anger could not be a target for therapy but was an existential issue that she had to settle with her brother.

Margaret agreed that the events of probable thought broadcasting could be a coincidence, and we designed a behavioral experiment to test the broadcasting in real life. Because of distrust, she could not do a collaborative experiment of sending thoughts and having another person guess them, so we needed a frightening involuntary exposure to her thoughts. The broadcasted thoughts had to be so alarming to the receiver that a behavioral response would almost certainly follow. Her mother had planned her birthday party for the next Tuesday, and on this occasion Margaret would send out thoughts such as "Your hair is on fire" while her mother lit a cigarette; "Your zipper is open" when her boyfriend got up from his chair; and "Your nose is bleeding" to her aunt when she started to talk and had all attention focused on her. Margaret was sure that her mother would immediately stroke her hair to extinguish the fire; her boyfriend would touch his zipper to check; and her aunt would use a hanky to stop the bleeding. Margaret sent out these thoughts repeatedly with the highest possible intensity, but nobody reacted. This encouraged her to expand the experiment to people in the streets. In the next session, she indicated that nobody had responded,

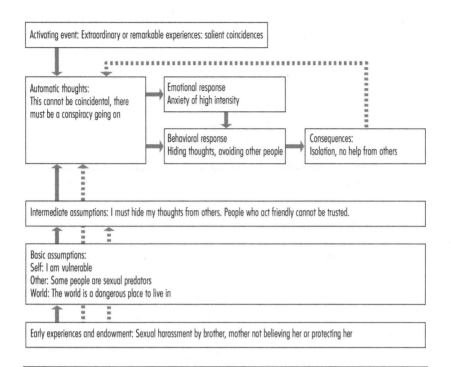

FIGURE 9–1.   Case formulation for Margaret on salient experiences and thought broadcasting.

and she was fully convinced that her thoughts were private. This was a successful part of the therapy, and it required relatively few sessions. The blocking of delusion formation only took one session and a single homework assignment.

Margaret decided not to talk with her brother because he had autism spectrum disorder and would not understand her feelings. She knew he would never regret what had happened or make apologies, but she decided to confront her mother about her denials. Margaret wanted her mother to sincerely acknowledge how much pain she had inflicted on Margaret by denying her call for help in past years. We planned a strategy of discussing this matter calmly, repeating the message as often as was needed to have her mother acknowledge the experiences and the despair of not being protected by one's mother. After a few failed conversations, Margaret's mother finally broke into tears, comforted Margaret, and asked for forgiveness.

Case Example 2: Haunted by Jinns

Ahmed was a young adult help-seeking patient with ARMS who was afraid of becoming possessed by a jinn. He had not finished school and worked as a warehouse clerk. He lived with his parents, brothers, and sisters downtown. He explained that jinns are creatures who live in the human environment, and most of them adhere to the Islamic religion as well. Their potential danger could not be put into perspective or downplayed. Ahmed had been drinking alcohol and was involved in dealing street drugs, and he had not been to the mosque for quite a while. Because jinns live in moist places like the kitchen sink, the toilet, or the bathroom, Ahmed had recently started to say a short prayer before pouring tea into the kitchen sink, just to warn the jinn and avoid burning the jinn with the hot water. He recited prayers before taking a bite from a sandwich to warn a jinn about being eaten, and he stopped using the toilet at night because he was afraid that a jinn might enter his body through his anus. Once a jinn is in your bowels you are lost and may become mad, he proclaimed.

Ahmed reported hearing sounds at night or seeing shadows while awake in bed, and he noticed that objects in the room had been moved. Ahmed interpreted these experiences as signs of a jinn who was out for him. To repel the jinn, Ahmed would recite Surah al-Falaq (113) and Surah an-Naas (114), in which the help of Allah is invoked to protect against an evil spirit.

Muslim patients may attribute voices, thought insertion, and experiences of alien control to jinns. In a study by Lim et al. (2018), 43% of patients interviewed thought their symptoms were caused by a jinn, and 31% were unsure. Jinns are invisible creatures, and the Quran was written for humans and jinns. It is important to understand that the existence of jinns is clear to Muslims, and denying their existence is sinful. In CBT it is key not to challenge the presence of the jinns in the life of the patient but to reason why the jinns are planning to do harm to the patient, whereas relatives experience no fear of harm by jinns.

Therapists should consider beliefs about intentions and powers of jinns not as delusional but as overvalued ideas. Delusions and overvalued ideas are both endorsed as being true. An overvalued idea has more obsessive characteristics in that the patient thinks about it all day long, whereas delusional subjects think about their delusions occasionally. Another difference between overvalued ideas and delusions is that overvalued ideas elicit strong emotions, and if another person doubts the idea, the person with the overvalued ideas can become angry. In extreme cases of overvalued ideas the person will identify with the overvalued idea and may even experience moral superiority that may result in violence against a nonbeliever. People with delusions are much less focused on their delusions, and they accept that other people disagree with them. The dominant thought of people who say the delusion is not reality is that the delusional subject will think that the other person has no idea what is really going on and is just not well informed.

Overvalued ideas and delusions cannot be disentangled completely. They overlap considerably. Delusions are idiosyncratic in single psychiatric

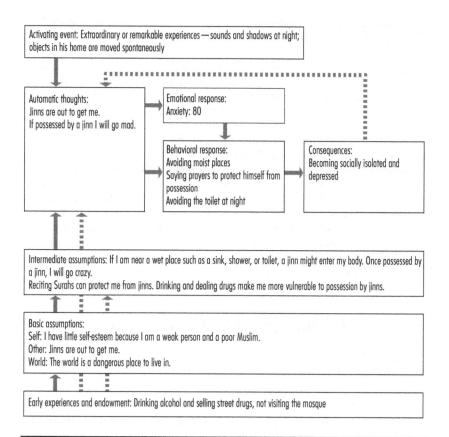

FIGURE 9–2.   Case formulation for Ahmed.

patients, and overvalued ideas are more prominent in master interpretive systems that include political ideologies and religious belief systems, which are highly resistant to challenge, are capable of generating considerable emotion, and are shared in groups (Bentall 2018).

It is important in discussing overvalued ideas to challenge not the content, such as the existence of jinns in the home, but the issue of being a victim of jinns while others in the home experience no threat at all. From a cultural perspective, it becomes clear that vulnerability to jinns is attached to guilt and shame over not being a good Muslim all the time. In Ahmed's case, he still lived with his parents and brothers and sisters. He was proud to be the oldest son, but at the same time he was ashamed that his little brother showed more bravery in dealing with wet and moist places in the home. The case formulation was written down in collaboration with Ahmed and is shown in Figure 9–2.

As with all anxiety disorders, exposure therapy with expectancy disconfirmation is an effective therapy. Ahmed understood that as long as he could not face the danger, it would haunt him, and avoiding all dark and moist places prevented him from learning whether the jinns would really harm him. A stepwise exposure was planned at the home. The first step was pouring the last of the warm tea in the pot into the kitchen sink without saying protective prayers. Ahmed succeeded and entered the next session with a smile. If there was a jinn living in the sink, he had not come out and hurt him. It was agreed that for the next step Ahmed would go into the bathroom in the evening all dressed and switch off the light for about a minute. He hesitated but agreed to the exercise. It took him 2 weeks of apologies before he succeeded in this accomplishment. He enjoyed the compliments from the therapist, and he evaluated himself as a braver person than he had anticipated being a few weeks ago. The final test was to go to the toilet at night, pull down his trousers, and sit on the toilet bowl for at least 5 minutes in the dark. After the previous successes Ahmed already had more confidence in his resilience to jinns, and he added another 5 minutes to the exercise. His conclusion was firm. He may not have been a true Muslim in recent times, but there were no jinns in the house to punish him.

Questions for Discussion

1. Are conspiracy theories delusions or overvalued ideas? Give two arguments.

2. Why are education and normalization of odd experiences so much easier to conduct in patients with ARMS than patients with an episode of psychosis?

3. Why is it important in ARMS to explore all psychopathology?

4. Why are behavioral experiments key in CBT with subjects with ARMS?

KEY POINTS

- In individuals identified as being at risk for developing psychosis, one can see the beginning of delusional explanations, with fluctuating conviction amid alternative explanations for what is going on.

- Perceptual aberrations are puzzling and often frightening, and attempts to explain these aberrations may result in either remission with normalizing explanations for the aberrations or full psychosis in the case of endorsing a delusional explanation for the odd experiences.

- Uncertainty and doubt are the hallmarks of ARMS, and they make people with ARMS open to new information, willing to search for evidence for explanations, and eager for therapy, in contrast to people with frank psychosis.

- A collaborative therapeutic relationship is essential and is enhanced by education, Socratic questioning, and behavioral experiments.

- Preventing transition to psychosis is a major goal, but most people with early psychotic symptoms have multiple comorbid conditions (including anxiety disorders and depression), and other treatment protocols are needed in the majority of cases.

Suggested Readings

Freeman D, Freeman J, Garety P: Overcoming Paranoid and Suspicious Thoughts: A Self-Help Guide Using Cognitive Behavioural Techniques. London, Constable and Robinson, 2006

French P, Morrison AP: Early Detection and Cognitive Therapy for People at High Risk of Developing Psychosis: A Treatment Approach. Chichester, UK, Wiley, 2004

van der Gaag M, Nieman D, van den Berg D: CBT for Those at Risk of a First Episode Psychosis: Evidence-Based Psychotherapy for People With an "At Risk Mental State." New York, Routledge, 2013

References

Albert U, Tomassi S, Maina G, Tosato S: Prevalence of non-psychotic disorders in ultra-high risk individuals and transition to psychosis: a systematic review. Psychiatry Res 270:1–12, 2018 30243126

Amminger GP, Nelson B, Markulev C, et al: The NEURAPRO biomarker analysis: long-chain omega-3 fatty acids improve 6-month and 12-month outcomes in youths at ultra-high risk for psychosis. Biol Psychiatry 87(3):243–252, 2020 31690495

Bentall RP: Delusions and other beliefs, in Delusions in Context. Edited by Bortolotti L. Cham, Switzerland, Springer International, 2018, pp 67–95

Caspi A, Moffitt TE: All for one and one for all: mental disorders in one dimension. Am J Psychiatry 175(9):831–844, 2018 29621902

Howes OD, Hird EJ, Adams RA, et al: Aberrant salience, information processing, and dopaminergic signaling in people at clinical high risk for psychosis. Biol Psychiatry 88(4):304–324, 2020 32430200

Ising HK, Lokkerbol J, Rietdijk J, et al: Four-year cost-effectiveness of cognitive behavior therapy for preventing first-episode psychosis: the Dutch Early Detection Intervention Evaluation (EDIE-NL) Trial. Schizophr Bull 43(2):365–374, 2017 27306315

Kraan T, van Dam DS, Velthorst E, et al: Childhood trauma and clinical outcome in patients at ultra-high risk of transition to psychosis. Schizophr Res 169(1–3):193–198, 2015a 26585219

Kraan T, Velthorst E, Smit F, et al: Trauma and recent life events in individuals at ultra high risk for psychosis: review and meta-analysis. Schizophr Res 161(2–3):143–149, 2015b 25499046

Kraan TC, Velthorst E, Themmen M, et al: Child maltreatment and clinical outcome in individuals at ultra-high risk for psychosis in the EU-GEI High Risk Study. Schizophr Bull 44(3):584–592, 2018 28666366

Lim A, Hoek HW, Ghane S, et al: The attribution of mental health problems to jinn: an explorative study in a transcultural psychiatric outpatient clinic. Front Psychiatry 9:89, 2018 29643820

McCutcheon RA, Krystal JH, Howes OD: Dopamine and glutamate in schizophrenia: biology, symptoms and treatment. World Psychiatry 19(1):15–33, 2020 31922684

Rietdijk J, Fokkema M, Stahl D, et al: The distribution of self-reported psychotic-like experiences in non-psychotic help-seeking mental health patients in the general population; a factor mixture analysis. Soc Psychiatry Psychiatr Epidemiol 49(3):349–358, 2014 24126556

van der Gaag M, Nieman DH, Rietdijk J, et al: Cognitive behavioral therapy for subjects at ultrahigh risk for developing psychosis: a randomized controlled clinical trial. Schizophr Bull 38(6):1180–1188, 2012a 22941746

van der Gaag M, van Oosterhout B, Daalman K, et al: Initial evaluation of the effects of competitive memory training (COMET) on depression in schizophrenia-spectrum patients with persistent auditory verbal hallucinations: a randomized controlled trial. Br J Clin Psychol 51(2):158–171, 2012b 22574801

van der Gaag M, Nieman D, van den Berg D: CBT for Those at Risk of a First Episode Psychosis: Evidence-Based Psychotherapy for People With an "At Risk Mental State." New York, Routledge, 2013

van Donkersgoed RJM, Wunderink L, Nieboer R, et al: social cognition in individuals at ultra-high risk for psychosis: a meta-analysis. PLoS One 10(10):e0141075, 2015 26510175

Webb JR, Addington J, Perkins DO, et al: Specificity of incident diagnostic outcomes in patients at clinical high risk for psychosis. Schizophr Bull 41(5):1066–1075, 2015 26272875

10

The Curious Case of Schreber

Kristin Lie Romm, Ph.D., M.D.
Douglas Turkington, M.D.

And the paranoiac builds it [his subjective world] up once more, not more splendid perhaps, but at least in such a way that he can live in it again. He builds it up through the work of his delusion. What we take to be the production of the illness, the formation of the delusion is in reality the attempt at a cure, the reconstruction.

Sigmund Freud,
Psychoanalytic Notes on an Autobiographical Account of a Case of Paranoia (Dementia Paranoides) (Freud 1911/1958, p. 60)

For more than 100 years, the Schreber case has been a puzzle and source of inspiration for mental health professionals who are interested in understanding delusional content. Sigmund Freud's analysis of the honorable German judge Daniel Paul Schreber's detailed accounts of his thoughts and experiences in asylums during the end of the nineteenth century, *Memoirs of My Nervous Illness*, saved Schreber from oblivion. Over the years, several

The authors would like to thank Dr. Anne Kveim Lie and Dr. Ketil Slagstad for their wise comments on the manuscript and for sharing their knowledge about the history of psychiatry in the nineteenth century.

theories of psychopathology have been applied to Schreber's case, most of which have focused more on psychoanalytical conceptions of psychosis and less on possible treatment approaches. It seemed important for a book titled *Decoding Delusions* to contain a chapter in which an attempt is made to decode the most famous and influential delusion of all time. Here we attempt to explore Schreber's case in light of cognitive-behavioral therapy (CBT) as a possible treatment option.

Schreber's delusions emerged at a key time in the history of psychiatry: during the emergence of biological psychiatry. At the time, European psychiatry was struggling with oversized asylums filled with "uncurable" patients. Insanity was seen as the product of degeneration and decay, not an illness per se. In Germany, the field of psychiatry followed another path. In the nineteenth century the understanding of disease was revolutionized when Wilhelm Griesinger, who was appointed professor of psychiatry in Berlin in 1865, placed the laboratory and the microscope at the center of research into mental disorders. He insisted that mental illness was an illness of the nerves of the brain. Detailed studies of the anatomy of the brain and spinal cord were conducted. However, German clinicians of the time had little interest in treating and curing patients (Scull 2015). They were more interested in dead tissue that they could observe under the microscope in the name of science. In line with this, Schreber may have considered that his psychiatrists were practicing a type of psychiatry without spiritual understanding. His psychiatrist attributed no meaning to his delusion and saw the delusional content merely as the emergence of a biological disease of the brain.

Half a century later, psychoanalysis emerged as another model for understanding mental disorders. Freud read the memoirs of Daniel Paul Schreber and postulated that the delusion was entirely meaningful in relation to his repressed and projected libidinal desires, which had become focused on his physician (Freud 1911/1958). He indicated, however, that the delusion was a sticking plaster over the unconscious and that psychoanalysis was not recommended because interpretation might lead to catastrophic psychotic decompensation. Thus, both psychoanalysis and the biologically based psychiatry of the time left Schreber without any opportunity for treatment.

The lack of focused treatment options persisted for many years, leaving patients like Schreber with grandiose delusional systems without much hope of recovery. However, this changed with the emergence of antipsychotic medication (in particular clozapine in 1972) and later the emergence of CBT. Would Schreber have responded to clozapine? Would he have even agreed to take it? Without early intervention, we consider it unlikely. Major delusional systems often show a low level of response, even to an optimal dose of clozapine. However, we do believe it would have been possible to engage Schreber in talking therapy because he was obviously a literate man with an urge to share his thoughts with those around him. Hence, in this chapter we consider a possible retrospective process of the use of a modified CBT intervention (in response to Freud's analysis done via reading the memoirs), here considering what degree of recovery may have been possible.

To introduce Daniel Paul Schreber to readers who are unfamiliar with his story, we start with the timeline that will eventually be part of the therapeutic work. We have based this summary on the writings of two major scholars on Schreber: William G. Niederland's (1984) *The Schreber Case: Psychoanalytic Profile of a Paranoid Personality* and Henry Zvi Lothane's (1992) *In Defence of Schreber: Soul Murder and Psychiatry*. The two scholars differ in their views of Schreber's father and his impact on his son's illness. However, both works contribute valuable information about Schreber's life.

Biography of Daniel Schreber

Family

Daniel Paul Schreber was born in Leipzig, Germany, on July 25, 1842, and was the third child of Daniel Gottlob Moritz Schreber and Louise Henriette Pauline Schreber. He was one of five children, with a brother and three sisters. The family had a substantial income and a wide social network.

The young Schreber grew up with a strict religious and moral upbringing. His father, Moritz Schreber, was a famous physician and orthopedist who wrote and published more than 20 books on orthopedics, anatomy, health, and childrearing. It is of interest that Moritz Schreber, like many of his contemporaries, vocally condemned masturbation and its potential to cause impotence and infertility. Voluptuousness, fertility, and masturbation are themes running through the memoirs. During Daniel's first 9 years, his father was the director of his own orthopedic institute and a founding member of the Leipzig Turnverein, an association of gymnasts that cultivated health and vigor through gymnastic exercise.

In 1878, Daniel Schreber married Ottilie Sabine Behr, the daughter of a singer and artistic director in various opera houses who later became a professor at the Leipzig School of Music. Sabine had several miscarriages.

Childhood

Moritz Schreber treated children with abnormalities of the musculoskeletal system, inventing different orthopedic supports to correct their postural problems. The family lived on the hospital premises, and Daniel and his siblings used to play with the patients. Between 7 and 15 children lived in the hospital at any time, and they were treated for scoliosis, kyphosis, club-foot, and paralysis, among other diagnoses. We must assume that the Schreber children were acquainted with both the pain and the suffering of these children, as well as the treatment methods used.

Over the years, there have been differing opinions as to what impact Moritz Schreber's childrearing and writings had on Daniel Schreber's illness. Moritz Schreber has been claimed to have been a tyrannical father and sadistic child abuser whose orthopedic methods were applied as instruments of torture on his own children. However, we must take into account that orthopedic medicine before the era of surgery was very much about inventing solutions to help straighten the body and treat deformities through the use of various machinery. Niederland (1984) described several of these inventions in his book on Daniel Schreber, with drawings that look horrifying compared with current surgical approaches. However, according to Lothane (1992), several statements from the writings of Moritz Schreber and quotes from relatives depict him as a moral and righteous man, one with a real interest in children, play, and physical fitness. He is not described as having been violent. Over the years, Moritz Schreber progressed from the use of mechanical devices toward more gymnastic-oriented methods, aiming to mold the body and gain posture and strength through exercise. It is unavoidable to think that the young Schreber's upbringing affected his eventual delusional preoccupation with his body being transformed.

Genetic Predisposition

In his early years, Moritz Schreber wrote about a young man with melancholia, and it has been speculated whether this was autobiographical (Lothane 1992). In 1851, he experienced a head injury, and both his personality and his life changed because of the headaches and bouts of depression that followed. He died in November 1861 after an acute intestinal illness. On the basis of statements from descendants of Daniel Schreber's sister Anna, several family members had depression and anxiety (Lothane 1992). Daniel Schreber's mother also had depression, and in 1877, his brother, Gustave, died by suicide by gunshot.

Career and Illness

Daniel Schreber was highly intelligent. He was described as a person with good social skills who was interested in politics, culture, and philosophy. In 1863, he passed his first bar examination with a grade of "excellent," and in 1869, he earned a doctorate in law. In October 1884, he was defeated as a candidate for election to the Reichstag. Because of "mental overstrain" he developed "severe (delusional) hypochondria" and met with Dr. Paul

Flechsig in November 1884 (Freud 1911/1958, p. 12). He was admitted to Flechsig's Psychiatric Hospital of Leipzig University from December 1884 to June 1885. During this period, he made two suicide attempts, and the episode seemed to have many features comparable with psychotic depression. Eventually, he fully recovered.

For several years, Schreber worked and prospered in his position as a judge, and in October 1893, he was appointed presiding judge of the Court of Appeals in Leipzig. This was the second-highest position in the courts of Saxony. At that time, he was the youngest person who had held this position, and he was responsible for judges far older than himself. This caused him a new period of "mental overstrain," resulting in severe insomnia in November 1893, with a subsequent suicide attempt at his mother's home. Schreber was then readmitted under the care of Dr. Flechsig in Leipzig. Except for a short stay at Hendrik Pierson's asylum, he was soon transferred to Dr. Guido Weber at the Royal Public Asylum at Sonnenstein in June 1894. By that time, he was clearly psychotic, with distressing commenting and command auditory hallucinations, visual hallucinations, persecutory and grandiose delusions, and episodes of catatonia. In the following year, he was detained in Sonnenstein, and an official instruction to institute permanent retirement was approved by the Ministry of Justice. During this period, he wrote his memoirs and ended up defending himself, arguing that his incompetency and guardianship orders should be rescinded. He finally succeeded and was discharged in December 1902.

The state of Schreber's mental health and social functioning following his release from the asylum is less well known. He published his memoirs in 1903. He and Sabine built a new house at Angelikastrasse 15 in Dresden. According to Lothane (1992), Schreber functioned well socially and did private legal work. He lived with his wife and adopted daughter until 1907, when his world fell apart. His mother died in May, and Sabine had a stroke in November of the same year. In November 1907, Schreber was admitted to Leipzig-Dösen Asylum, where he died on April 14, 1911, of cardiopulmonary complications at age 68 years.

Process of Retrospective CBT for Psychosis Intervention for Schreber

In the CBT model, the development of a systematized delusion is understandable, and the delusion is treatable (Moorhead and Turkington 2001). This is important to bear in mind as we move on and picture what a CBT approach to treating Schreber's illness could have looked like. There is postulated to be evidence of schema vulnerability in patients with delusions

(Samarasekera and Turkington 2005), in that underlying persecutory delusions tend to be compensatory schemata about the need for approval from others. This relates to core maladaptive schemata of failure, worthlessness, or unlovability. Therefore, the CBT therapist is keen to explore the life history of the person experiencing the delusion to understand the kernel of truth at the heart of the delusion and how the delusion was rooted in early experiences and then triggered by adult life events. Thus, the CBT therapist would spend time with Schreber and would be interested in learning about his experiences and beliefs without colluding with or confronting the veracity of the delusions. Schreber, we hope, would not have perceived the CBT therapist as "soul-less."

The following stages of CBT would have been pursued:

1. Engaging and forming a therapeutic alliance
2. Normalizing belief change and the links among stress, brain function, lack of sleep, worry, and anxiety
3. Generating an effective strategy for coping with distressing voices
4. Using gentle peripheral and Socratic questions in a guided discovery modality to understand the delusion and its emotional and behavioral impact; if necessary, agreeing to disagree about certain points
5. Developing scaffolding for the delusion by activating previous hobbies, interests, and areas of expertise
6. Exploring the pre-psychotic period using inductive questioning
7. Producing a timeline to understand key relationships and life events and how these led to the formation of key personal beliefs
8. Working on schemata and linked sadness and anxiety using schema-level techniques, such as the continuum, imagery, positive and negative logging, implications of negative constructs for daily life, and key personal meanings of specific life events
9. Tackling any goal conflict using focusing techniques

A Hypothetical Cognitive-Behavioral Therapy Approach

Engaging and Forming a Therapeutic Alliance

If we had been the mental health professionals on the ward at the time Schreber was there, we most likely would have used brief periods of regular personal interaction to introduce ourselves and explain our views of the nature of mental illness and the role of the asylum. There is no doubt that these early sessions would have been very difficult because of the degree of intensity, conviction, and preoccupation with the delusion and the distracting nature of the auditory hallucinations. There would have been times of stupor, periods of agitation, and times when all we could have done would have been to sit and listen to Schreber talk about the content of the delusion and voices. At times, patients in this position have referred to a regularly visiting mental health professional as "a sane reference point" with whom delusional ideas can be safely expressed and discussed in an accepting and non-stigmatizing way, and a dialogue begins to develop around some of the less distressing areas of content. Consistency, respect, humanity, and friendliness are all crucial elements of this engaging approach. This phase might take up to 10 brief sessions, by which time it is hoped the mental health professional is perceived not as an enemy but as a colleague in the midst of the emotional chaos of the delusion. In this early befriending phase, we would not have constructed a problem list, provided psychoeducation or produced a biological model, attempted to talk him out of the delusion, or asked questions that were too probing. This is a phase of absorbing and containing psychotic symptoms until an alliance has been formed and expectations of confrontation, humoring, and avoidance have all receded.

Normalizing

Normalizing is useful in that changing our beliefs is something we all do, and we can support this phase through personal disclosure of some of our own belief changes. One of us (D.T.) changed his career trajectory beliefs from primary care to psychiatry because he felt vocationally called to contribute to mental health. Schreber might have been interested in a psychiatrist who disclosed some personal information, especially given his documented criticism of his psychiatrist as being "soul-less." Times of belief change can also occur at times of upheaval and personal difficulty, and this might normalize his stress prior to belief change. When a belief changes, a person can feel different, euphoric, and empowered but also stressed and sleep-deprived. This normalizing approach might have helped engage Schreber further, especially around early treatment targets such as helping him sleep or reducing his anxiety and worry. Exercise and art therapy were available at that time. This phase would have lasted about five brief sessions.

Generating an Effective Coping Strategy

Generating an effective coping strategy is crucial because most people who struggle with hearing voices naturally develop unhelpful or counterproductive strategies that act to perpetuate voice-hearing (Howard et al. 2013). Schreber used his "bellowing cure" as a coping strategy to deal with distressing auditory hallucinations; this involved playing the piano loudly and bellowing while doing so. There are a number of problems with this approach because although it worked in the short term, it acted as a maintenance factor in the medium term. First, it was a pure distraction approach attempting to drown out the voices with loud noise. This precluded the use of selective listening or other types of focusing, which are much more effective in the medium term. Second, it was stigmatizing and frightening for those who saw the bellowing cure in action. This unusual coping strategy could have also acted to perpetuate his hospital stay because the approach might simply not have been acceptable in the society of the day. Finally, it was upsetting and anxiety provoking for him to have to do this, and what if there had been no piano nearby?

Within a CBT approach, Schreber would have been introduced to the list of 60 coping strategies for voice-hearing, of which about half are distraction approaches (Wright et al. 2009). Playing the piano is good because so much of the cortex is activated by the activity. How would the voices have reacted to different types of piano music? Would playing *Don Giovanni* have had a different effect than playing *Swan Lake*? What about reading Shakespeare aloud or in a whisper rather than bellowing? Doing so would have involved measuring voice intensity and having Schreber note his findings in a diary to scientifically generate a strategy that worked better (Turkington et al. 2016). Schreber would have likely been interested in self-reflection and tracking. We hope that together we would have found a better coping strategy than the bellowing cure. This would probably have taken about five brief sessions.

Using Questioning Styles and Scaffolding

During the questioning phase, we would have shown interest in the impact of the psychosis and its boundaries with Schreber's own personality. Questions might have included the following: Can we find the torture machines used against you by God, or are they spiritual? Can you draw them for us? Can you describe the rays that others don't see and how often they tend to appear? Is there any pattern to them? Are you in a different emotional state before, during, and after the experience? How much of your time do you use to fulfill the role as the "bride of God," and how much time do you have to spend for yourself? Are there any Old Testament prophecies referring to this role? How much of the time are you happy and euphoric, and how much of the time are you sad and frightened? Do you have periods of time each day to do previous hobbies and consider legal issues? Could you advise the hospital in relation to a (hypothetical) case being brought to reclaim some of the hospital grounds? Scaffolding predicts the receding of delusion and the need to reactivate previous hobbies and activities to fill the vacuum. Again, this would have taken 5–10 sessions but would have overlapped with the previous phases.

Exploring the Pre-psychotic Period

The couple of weeks leading up to the emergence of the psychosis are explored in detail to consider the impact of various life events and accumulations of stressors. This allows for an opportunity to catch key automatic thoughts and linked emotions. In Schreber's case, such thoughts might have been hypochondriacal ("I'm becoming ill; my stomach isn't working properly") or anxious ("I can't cope with this anymore; I am being overwhelmed with work") or sad ("This is me all over: a failure, no children and no job, and letting my father down. I will be a source of shame; there is no hope"). When the pre-psychotic period is explored in this way and key thoughts and emotions are explored, delusions and hallucinations are normally much less dominant in the conversation. Links can then be made between the very high levels of affect present and the emergence of the new belief, but the underlying high levels of affect cannot be interpreted as being causal to the new belief. This phase would have taken 5–10 sessions.

Producing a Timeline

The production of a timeline is usually a very therapeutic approach in the setting of a complex grandiose delusional system, such as that of Schreber. The therapist gradually works backward through the pre-psychotic period and all the way back through early adulthood, the school years, and then childhood. Family and friends are usually needed to fill in gaps and point out episodes of achievement and supportive relationships. Old photographs and reports are useful. The timeline can be done on a whiteboard, in a small diary, or, as in Schreber's case, in a book. It is likely that in Schreber's case, the writing of the book, the processing of the sadness and anxiety of the past, and the insights gained were crucial in his eventual recovery. Usually, explanatory causative connections (interpretations) between past events and the delusional content will not be accepted, and these should not be pursued.

Making Sense: Collaboratively Developing a CBT Formulation and Timeline

In the following timeline phase, 15–20 sessions would have been needed, and by this phase the sessions would have tended to be longer in duration and more readily tolerated. Some key background information was available from the hospital records, but in practice this would all have been produced collaboratively in discussion with Schreber as each key area of his life was explored, at which time the timeline information described previously would have been collected.

Predisposing Factors

Regarding predisposing factors, there may have been a genetic predisposition to mental illness in the Schreber family present in Daniel Schreber's father (who had also experienced a head injury, which may have caused some of his symptoms), his brother, and his mother. At the two first admissions, Schreber himself was well aware that his workload had been too heavy and that he was experiencing "mental overstrain." This was his own explanation for how it all started. The first episode was related to the stress of campaigning and being defeated during the election. On the second occasion, the stress became too high as a result of the level of responsibility in his post as presiding judge in Leipzig. We know that stress plays an important part in the development of psychosis. It is also worth mentioning that before the second episode, Schreber's wife miscarried for the last time. We do not know how this was handled in the family, but he wrote about the childlessness as a loss in his memoirs. We can assume that Sabine's inability to give birth was hard for both husband and wife.

Perpetuating Factors

Interestingly, Schreber considered lack of sleep one of the major obstacles to his recovery from the period of overstrain. It has been shown that correcting insomnia has the potential to reduce the intensity of paranoid delusions (Freeman et al. 2015). Dr. Flechsig approached the issue with medication that did not work and, according to Schreber, caused marked side effects. Another perpetuating factor may have been his isolation and long periods of coercion, in which he was forced to sleep in an empty cell in the basement because of his loud bellowing at night. He reported these events as being traumatic experiences. First, the isolation made it difficult for him to relate to other people and pursue his interests. His wife visited occasionally, but he did not feel any engagement with the other patients. Second, the isolation made it difficult for him to prove his capacity to organize his own life. Third, one could speculate whether the coercion made him violent because he felt misunderstood. The situation seemed to spiral when his resistance to treatment was interpreted as being a result of his illness, not a result of his fear and feeling of being misunderstood.

Protective Factors

Schreber had numerous protective factors that helped him eventually recover from his illness. He was extremely intelligent and was able to present himself well both verbally and in writing. We must assume that these qualities were compromised during his most psychotic periods, but before and after he seemed to be able to exert them. In addition, he was skilled in different cultural areas, such as music, philosophy, and politics, which made him able to participate in different kinds of social settings. He was married, and according to his adopted daughter, he was also very warm emotionally, even more so than his wife. The Schreber family was close, and they had a wide social network. Moritz Schreber's books also provided income for several years after his death. Schreber managed his affairs after he was discharged from Sonnenstein, and thus he had a reasonable income, even though he did not work as a judge after his second admission.

Contemporary concerns during his hospitalization. During the long period of hospital care, Schreber's concerns circled around his sleep, his tormenting experiences with the voices, and the "miracles." These were miraculous interventions by God damaging every limb and organ of his body. He was not able to concentrate, and he reported feeling physical pain when he was being "tortured." He had disturbing thoughts, of which the most concerning was that he was being transformed into a woman. He believed that God himself wanted to have intercourse with him to bring forward a new race that was destined to salvage the Earth. He reported feeling female nerves invading his body to make him attractive to God and observed how his body was changing. He believed that his breasts and hips were getting larger, and he cross-dressed according to what he viewed to be the will of God. In Schreber's mind, he knew this was not appropriate according to the standards he had grown up with, but he saw himself as the chosen one, the redeemer of the world, and as such he believed that he was not allowed to disobey. These transformations filled Schreber with different emotions, such as fear, anxiousness, omnipotence, distress, and sadness, and his behavior reflected this; he sometimes sat still in a stupor, relating to the content of his voices. At other times, he put on women's clothes or bellowed toward the sun as he was ordered to do. His preoccupation with his body resulted in periods of strong hypochondria, somatic nihilistic delusions of missing organs, panic, and anxiety in addition to sleeplessness.

Underlying concerns. It is tempting to think of Schreber as a man with an underlying insecurity manifesting in a concern about whether he was "good enough." He was the son of a famous published physician who was extremely preoccupied with body and posture. In addition, he grew up in a strict moral and religious environment in which childrearing and the ability to produce children had been worshipped. Even though he positioned himself among the best and brightest intellectuals in society, he may have had concerns about being worthless and that his or his wife's body was not good enough. It is possible that his childless marriage, his inability to win popularity and a position in the Reichstag, and his inability to lead the honorable judges had an incremental effect, resulting in the emergence of a delusional system to prevent any further increase in anxiety. Against this backdrop, it is possible to draw a diagram depicting a CBT formulation based on our fictitious assessment of Schreber and what we believe to be an anxiety psychosis. In an anxiety psychosis, an accumulation of unresolved stressful life events leads to escalating anxiety, delusional mood, and then the emergence of a delusional system that resolves the underlying anxiety (Figure 10–1).

Working on Schemata and Linked Sadness and Anxiety

Working on schemata and linked sadness and anxiety arises naturally from the work on the timeline. A change in mood might be detected as certain key life incidents are recalled, and then the beliefs linked to these events can be accessed and approached therapeutically. The following is an example of a dialogue that might have linked key life events and beliefs:

Therapist: You were talking about the machine your father used to help correct the children's posture, and you seemed a bit sadder. What thought was going through your mind?

Schreber: I was thinking that I wasn't good enough because my father always reminded me of how important a man's posture was. The machine was for children whose bodies weren't adequate, but maybe my father would have liked me to use it as well?

Therapist: Was there an image in your mind?

Schreber: Yes, I saw myself as a small boy left alone in the machine, crying and being ignored.

Therapist: What did that mean about you?

Schreber: It meant that I was damaged physically, and I would never make it.

Therapist: What do you mean by "make it"?

Schreber: [Tears up] Be approved and worthy of being his son.

Therapist: But were you actually physically unwell in any way as a child?

Schreber: Only standard infections, measles and colds, and hay fever.

Therapist: So how does this fit with your belief that you were physically damaged in some way? Maybe this belief is inaccurate. Could we do a list of all the things you can do physically? You are a talented walker, pianist, collector, tennis player, etc. Could we change the image of the crying child in the machine? What to?

Predisposing factors	Precipitating factors	Perpetuating factors	Protective factors

Strict upbringing
Father famous for several
  books on anatomy and health
Father religious
Genetic predisposition?
Brother died by suicide
	Was defeated during
	  election — depressed
	Got a high position with a
	  heavy workload and wife
	  miscarried
		Sleep problems
		Isolation?
		Trauma related to coercion?
		Understimulated?
			Intelligent and well educated
			Married
			Good economy
			Social network
			Good social skills/many
			  interests

Current concerns (large part of the time he was at the asylum)
1. Sleep   2. Experiences no rest from the psychotic symptoms 3. Not able to concentrate   4. Feeling pain when he is "tortured"

Thoughts	Feelings	Actions
I am turning into a woman My brain is softening God wants to have intercourse with me Female nerves have passed over into my body I will be the father of a new race I am in direct contact with God Flechsig wants me dead so he can examine me I am the redeemer of the world	Fear Anxiety Omnipotence Great distress Sadness	Sitting in rigid positions/stupor/voluntarily? Trying to do what the voices tell him Putting on women's clothes

Social	Physical
Gets visited by wife and some family Quite isolated, not much social interaction with the other patients	Insomnia Panic/anxiety Feels that his stomach is missing Hypochondria

Underlying concerns
I am not good enough as a person, I am worthless, my body is not good enough, I am a failure

FIGURE 10–1. Cognitive-behavioral therapy formulation for Schreber based on anxiety psychosis (Kingdon and Turkington 2005).

Schreber: *[Pause]* He has just broken out of the machine and smashed it and gone outside to play football in the sunshine.

Therapist: How do you feel now?

Schreber: Happier, not sad at the moment.

Therapist: Could we practice with the new image? It seemed in your legal career that you were driving yourself very hard for promotion.

Schreber: It felt good. I was thinking, "I'm a success. All the family will be proud of me."

Therapist: Would they have been proud if you had stopped at a slightly lower position?

Schreber: Yes. Before the final promotion I was working very effectively and had a good social life.

Therapist: So maybe this belief that you had to keep driving yourself pushed you over the edge. What would be a more viable belief? "I am good enough"? "I don't need to be the best in the world"? It seems that what came through your breakdown was a mixture of these two big beliefs that you were damaged physically and had to drive yourself forever.

Schreber: Maybe you are right.

Therapist: So we are going to do homework with this new image of the really strong Schreber child bursting out of the machine and running out into the sunshine and the photograph of you and your wife in your last job. You are going to write a letter to your father to tell him that you have made it in your career.

Working With Goal Conflicts

As you can see from the therapy account so far, we would have been asking Schreber to label and process some painful emotions. In so doing, there would have been schema shifts, but conflicts may have remained that would hinder recovery. One such goal conflict is "I want to be approved of by others and I want to tell the truth." The concern here is that if there is a mention of time in an asylum, or the word *schizophrenia*, then potential friends will walk away. Schreber dealt with this quite brilliantly by writing a book about his experiences with mental illness and publishing it. However, his intentions were not solely psychoeducational and oriented toward openness about mental illness; writing the book may have helped him to let go of some of the inner stress one experiences when important life events are suppressed. To deal with such a conflict, it is important to practice holding the conflict in mind; here, the mind itself will find a way to resolve the conflict. This may well result in becoming a peer support worker, setting up a support group, or lecturing on the subject. Resolution of the goal conflict often leads to altruism, which is a true hallmark of recovery.

Discussion

Schreber left the asylum without receiving any personal therapy as such and without access to effective medications. This shows that some degree of personal recovery is always possible. The question arises as to whether the modified CBT approach recommended here would have facilitated that recovery. It would seem that Schreber's recovery took many years and that he recovered in a state of isolation and by finding his own path. CBT, acceptance and commitment therapy, expert befriending, or structured psychodynamic therapy might all have been useful vehicles for recovery. The challenges of implementing a 16- to 20-session manualized CBT would have been that this powerful delusion would not have responded quickly to engagement and that goal setting would have been seen as confrontational. Also, Schreber clearly needed to have a psychiatrist who did not view him as a neurological disease process, with no meaning in his experience and no prospect of recovery. We are practicing psychiatrists who are humbled by studying Schreber's experiences, as written in his book.

Personal Reflection

Three main reflection points arise concerning alliance, diagnosis, and recovery. First, what would Schreber have thought of the therapeutic alliance within mental health care today? Are we really getting to know our patients in terms of the range and depth of their experiences? Are we allowing ourselves to be enriched by our relationships with our patients? Are we paying as much attention to their stories as we are to their symptoms?

Second, it is interesting to reflect on the futility of diagnosis in Schreber's case. His symptoms presumably met the criteria for a number of different diagnoses during the course of his illness. However, we believe that these diagnoses do not really help to facilitate treatment, so an individual formulation is crucial. By working on the formulation, we receive insight into the complexities and context and are better equipped to pick the right tools to achieve a positive outcome.

Third, Schreber entered a state of personal recovery. Schreber's ability to demonstrate the intricate relationship between insanity and sound reasoning through his memoirs is remarkable. Most people reading the memoirs will understand Schreber's ideas as delusional. However, he was able to defend himself as a lawyer in court, to manage his own affairs, and to plan and build a new house after he left the asylum—still in a delusional state but in personal recovery. User organizations have argued for a more holistic approach to facilitating recovery and argued that there has been too narrow of an approach to treatment.

We have too often disregarded the experiences and different explanatory models held by our patients. By being too narrow, we risk losing the alliance and might make things worse and recovery less likely. Schreber's feeling of acceptance as a person came when he was allowed to engage with the experts in normal conversations. We end this chapter with his own words and hope they will inspire our colleagues to engage in all aspects of their patients' lives:

> [T]he medical expert has only come to know me really well in the last year, that is to say since I have taken my meals regularly at his family table.... Before that time the medical expert only became acquainted with the pathological shell, as I would like to call it, which concealed my true spiritual life. (Schreber 1903, p. 365)

Questions for Discussion

1. Should we be recommending that all patients experiencing delusions attempt to write a summary or more detailed description of their experiences?

2. Who in our mental health services is best placed to deliver the longer-term interventions recommended in this chapter?

3. Is there always meaning at the heart of a delusion?

KEY POINTS

- The young Schreber may have formed a core schema of being a failure physically and formed compensatory schemata of needing to succeed both physically as a man and in his career to measure up to his father's very high standards of posture and performance.

- Schreber developed a grandiose and persecutory delusion that he had been turned into a woman, was married to God, was being tortured by machines, and had the role of producing perfect divine children to populate the world.

- Freud concluded that Schreber's case was understandable in relation to a repressed and projected homosexual impulse and that psychoanalysis was contraindicated because of the risk of psychotic transference and decompensation.

- A modified CBT intervention for Schreber might have consisted of up to 50 sessions, including the following stages: building a therapeutic alliance; normalizing through personal disclosure; practicing previous skills; generating a viable coping strategy; investigating the pre-psychotic period; and creating a timeline to access key memories, emotions, and schemata of failure and need for success.

- We believe that this CBT intervention would have led to reduced emotional investment and conviction in the delusion, allowing Schreber to live outside asylum conditions earlier and achieve a reasonable quality of life.

References

Freeman D, Waite F, Startup H, et al: Efficacy of cognitive behavioural therapy for sleep improvement in patients with persistent delusions and hallucinations (BEST): a prospective, assessor-blind, randomised controlled pilot trial. Lancet Psychiatry 2(11):975–983, 2015 26363701

Freud S: Psychoanalytic notes on an autobiographical account of a case of paranoia (1911), in The Standard Edition of the Complete Psychological Works of Sigmund Freud, Vol 12. Translated and edited by Strachey J. London, Hogarth, 1958, pp 3–82

Howard A, Forsyth A, Spencer H, et al: Do voice hearers naturally use focussing and metacognitive coping techniques? Psychosis 5(2):119–126, 2013

Kingdon DG, Turkington D: Cognitive Therapy of Schizophrenia (Guides to Individualized Evidence-Based Treatment; Persons JB, series ed). New York, Guilford, 2005

Lothane HZ: In Defence of Schreber: Soul Murder and Psychiatry. London, Routledge, 1992

Moorhead S, Turkington D: The CBT of delusional disorder: the relationship between schema vulnerability and psychotic content. Br J Med Psychol 74(Pt 4):419–430, 2001 11780791

Niederland WG: The Schreber Case: Psychoanalytic Profile of a Paranoid Personality. London, Routledge, 1984

Samarasekera N, Turkington D: Schemas, psychotic themes and depression: a preliminary investigation. Behav Cogn Psychother 33(1):115–117, 2005

Schreber DP: Denkwürdigkeiten eines Nervenkranken. New York, New York Review of Books, 1903

Scull A: Madness in Civilization: A Cultural History of Insanity, From the Bible to Freud, From the Madhouse to Modern Medicine. Princeton, NJ, Princeton University Press, 2015

Turkington D, Lebert L, Spencer H: Auditory hallucinations in schizophrenia: helping patients to develop effective coping strategies. BJPsych Adv 22(6):391–396, 2016

Wright JH, Turkington D, Kingdon DG, Basco MR: Cognitive-Behavior Therapy for Severe Mental Illness: An Illustrated Guide. Washington, DC, American Psychiatric Publishing, 2009

11

Erotomania and Sexual Delusions

Tania Lecomte, Ph.D.
Audrey Francoeur
Briana Cloutier

Erotomania

Erotomania is a person's strong belief that someone, at times a stranger, is in love with them and that this person is sending coded or discreet messages to the focal person that only the focal person can detect. Although erotomania is mostly found in women, who are often described as shy and lonely, men can experience it with at times insistent or even dangerous behaviors. Cases of celebrities being stalked (i.e., being followed, being sent messages, having their house illegally entered) by individuals believing they had a secret bond with them often come up in the news.

When working with people with psychotic disorders such as schizophrenia, it is possible to encounter individuals who believe their psychiatrist, for instance, is in love with them, or even that you, as their therapist, have strong feelings and desires for them. In these cases, the feelings are perceived as mutual, and the person can be extremely motivated to maintain this belief and imaginary relationship.

Case Example 1

Sophie was first hospitalized at age 14 with persecutory delusions and self-mutilation behaviors. She was treated at the hospital by a young psychiatrist who was very empathic and understanding. She soon became convinced that they were meant for each other and in love. To please him, she followed her treatment and recovered well. However, as soon as the treatment team told her she was ready to go home, she stripped off all her clothes and started running around the ward screaming that she was being attacked and her life was in danger. The staff felt she was too psychotic and kept her until she was better and was again ready to be discharged. Once she learned she would have to leave the hospital, Sophie had another "psychotic crisis." This circus lasted 19 years. Even when, as an adult, she no longer had contact with the psychiatrist (who specialized in treating children and adolescents at the institution), she did everything in her power to stay hospitalized in order to hopefully run into him and continue their "love affair."

How can we understand these beliefs? In terms of cognitive models, erotomania has not been studied extensively, but it is considered to essentially have the nature of a grandiose delusion, with elements of delusions of reference. First we consider the grandiosity aspect. When a person is convinced that someone—often someone important, someone famous, or an authority figure—is in love with them, this speaks of being chosen, somewhat like how someone would be chosen for a mission, although here they are chosen for love. A recent qualitative study from Isham et al. (2021) described how such grandiose beliefs offer meaning to the person, such as making them feel important, needed, or loved. Although possible harm can arise from erotomanic delusions (e.g., spending 19 years in a psychiatric institution as in Case Example 1, or being incarcerated in the case of stalkers), most individuals are happy to believe they are entertaining a secret love affair. As documented in many cases, the person who develops such delusions is often single and lonely, with few rewarding experiences in their life. The delusion acts as an uplifting feeling of being special, being loved, and being desired, whereas the person's reality is most often negative and lonely. Given that such an experience is linked to positive emotions and potentially is even protective of the person's self-esteem, the erotomanic belief is easily maintained without any apparent facts or external elements.

Knowles and colleagues (2011) proposed a cognitive and affective review to understand grandiose delusions that can also apply to a certain extent to erotomania. They proposed that grandiose delusions can be explained by one of two models. The first, by Freeman et al. (1998), speaks of delusion as defense, whereby the person develops a delusion to counteract a negative situation they are in and to protect their self-esteem from feelings of unworthiness and loneliness. The second suggests that grandiose delusions tend to develop in those who already have a heightened view of themselves (Smith et al. 2005). In the context of erotomania, and given the profile of those who tend to develop such delusions (single, lonely, shy), it appears that the former model (delusion as defense) seems a better fit. Furthermore, there is no attempt at a higher social status or need for power (as can be seen in those who already believe they are better than most) because the delusion is often kept secret.

Another aspect of erotomania is the presence of ideas of reference. People with these delusions see secret codes revealing the other person's love for them hidden in various ways (e.g., in songs, television shows, newspapers). Erotomanic beliefs can be sustained by various cognitive biases, namely, *confirmation bias* ("She wants to help me! She said so in her song"), *jumping to conclusion bias* ("The way he looked at me, I knew it was love"), and *rejection of disconfirmatory evidence bias* ("He had to get married, but I know it is just a front because he wants to be with me").

As with many delusions that bring more joy than distress, it is not a good idea to directly target erotomanic delusions in cognitive-behavioral therapy for psychosis (CBTp). In fact, it is often more useful to start by exploring the person's perception of self-worth and seeing whether their life (other than the secret relationship) is fulfilling to them. Specific goals, such as finding a satisfying job or developing friendships, which can lead to the person feeling proud, appreciated by others, and supported, have a more direct impact on the delusional thoughts than confronting the belief head-on. When things start looking up and the person is feeling desired by someone real who actually is interested in them, the delusion can at times go away instantly. One person once told me (T.L.), after developing a romantic relationship with an old boyfriend from her youth who had found her through social media (and who thought she was great and beautiful), that she decided to just "turn the page on all that." It is difficult to predict whether such delusions will ever come back should the person experience loneliness or adversity again, but for some, finding love in someone who is actually available and loves them back is the best cure.

Personal Reflection

During the Victorian era, Freud described forbidden sexual desires and past sexual trauma as being linked with mental disorders. Although most of his theories are no longer culturally valid, some of these realizations still hold true. On the one hand, we have not yet found a way to protect our young against sexual trauma—more work and education are definitely needed. Talking about sex is still taboo in many families and cultures, which can result in great distress for someone who feels different from the norm or has questions without answers. On the other hand, pornographic fantasies of every kind are easily accessible on the internet, but they do not represent reality. These contrasts can be confusing. Furthermore, lonely people with limited social cognitive skills can at times confuse sexual desire and love. Wanting to be loved is at the core of many desires. When asked, most patients mention wanting to be loved (romantically) as one of their top recovery goals. As a society, if we had more open and honest conversations about healthy romantic love and sexual relationships, while accepting diverse models of love and sex, we might see fewer sexual delusions.

Delusions of Sexual Aggression

Two types of delusions pertaining to sexual aggression are often found: that a person has been sexually abused and that a person has abused others. More commonly, the person mentions having been sexually abused. Sometimes the person can accuse a family member, a neighbor, or hospital staff of having sexually abused them. Other times the aggression is described in childhood or within a complex delusional and hallucinatory story. This type of belief is considered a delusion because the constructed belief is too complex to seem realistic. For instance, one patient believed doctors came to her house to rape her at night and filmed everything with hidden cameras. She made holes in all her walls to try to find the cameras but could not find any. Another patient believed she had been raped as a child by a satanic cult of pedophiles, including her father's famous friends. No such cult has yet been documented where she lived. Another patient told me (T.L.) that she was raped after being kidnapped by criminals who learned that she was a spy. She remembered clearly what happened, the criminals' faces, and her fellow spies explaining it was part of the job.

How can we understand these beliefs? We now know, thanks to retrospective and prospective studies (Bourgeois et al. 2020) and meta-analyses (Bailey et al. 2018; Varese et al. 2012), that childhood trauma, including sexual trauma, is quite frequent in people who develop psychotic symptoms, especially delusions and hallucinations with a sexual theme (Blom and Mangoenkarso 2018). Some authors explain this by the fact that strategies for posttraumatic stress emotion regulation (e.g., avoidance and numbing) are linked to the development of auditory hallucinations and related beliefs (Hardy et al. 2016). Sexual trauma is in fact considered a risk factor for psychotic symptoms (Lecomte et al. 2019). Figure 11–1 translates a model proposed by Beck and Van der Kolk (1987) that suggests that childhood trauma and PTSD create emotional turmoil and overstimulation, leading to a disorganization of thought processes. When the person is later confronted with sexual stimuli, this can trigger a high level of arousal that makes the

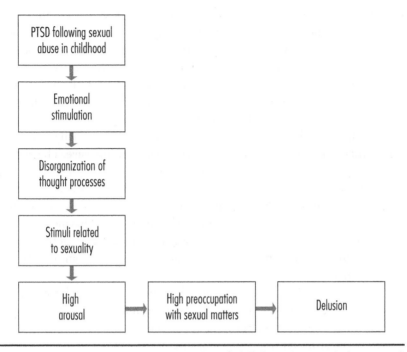

FIGURE 11–1. **Explanatory model of childhood sexual abuse and delusions.**

person become overly preoccupied with sexual themes and thus can lead to a sexual delusion.

Experts in the field strongly suggest that trauma-focused CBTp (including PTSD components) be offered to people with psychosis who have been sexually abused. The efficacy of such treatments comes from experiential reprocessing (or *exposure*), which means the person has to revisit the trauma, describe it, and eventually learn to talk about it without being over whelmed with symptoms and difficult emotions. Thus, the treatment involves developing emotion regulation strategies, such as relaxation techniques, breathing, or other coping skills, in order to separate the traumatic experience from its intense emotions. Many people with psychosis can talk openly about their trauma and could therefore benefit from such integrated treatments for PTSD/trauma and psychosis (Keen et al. 2017).

However, people with sexual delusions do not recall the actual event; their recollection, if a sexual trauma actually occurred, is distorted and transformed into something else, often with different actors. When asked, family members either deny any such trauma or think that "something might have happened" (e.g., with a neighbor) but are not sure. Thus, in the presence of a sexual delusion it is important to construct a timeline with collateral evidence included to identify any underlying sexual traumas. The patient who believed she had been abused by a cult of satanic pedophiles had seen a movie with such a theme while taking drugs (which precipitated her psychotic break) and kept on seeing images of the movie, with the strong sensation that the movie was really about her. Still, she had no real recollection of her own, only flashbacks from the movie and stories she read on the internet that such cults really existed.

It is also possible that the person has experienced not sexual trauma but some other form of trauma that was perceived as very intrusive. The person who believed she was a spy and raped by criminals, when feeling better, stated she was never raped in reality but was severely bullied as a child while attending a boarding school for girls. For example, a student shaved her eyebrows while she was sleeping. We can also suppose that having been sent to that boarding school while the rest of her family stayed together might have also created some attachment issues and perhaps also some experience of emotional neglect.

How do we help such patients who experience real pain and strongly believe they have been abused but whose story cannot be verified or recollected? They might wrongfully (or not) accuse someone of being their aggressor, creating tension and social distancing from caretakers or clinicians. There is no easy answer. One thing is for sure: the absence of facts will not lead the person to doubt. Here is an example:

> **Therapist:** So, if I understand correctly, you are convinced your dad let his famous friends sexually abuse you as a child. How can you be so sure?
> **Patient:** I have flashbacks. They are not precise, but I remember being on a table. I was so young, maybe four; that is why I can't remember.
> **Therapist:** How about your mom, did she say anything?
> **Patient:** She thinks something happened to me with a neighbor, never asked them to babysit again. But I think it was my dad's friends. I am so angry with him. He didn't protect me; he gave me to the wolves. You know that man who is being accused on TV with the #MeToo movement? Well, he was one of them.
> **Therapist:** You said you were four and don't remember much, yet you are convinced you know who the aggressors were. How do you explain that?
> **Patient:** You don't believe me. You think I am just psychotic like the rest of them. Let's give her drugs so she won't talk!

In CBTp, when we cannot verify the facts or propose another way of seeing the situation, we aim to decrease the distress. We need to help patients realize that they can survive this, that they can heal. Rationally, patients can be helped to realize that going to court or officially accusing someone without sufficient proof will not lead to anything and will not make the pain go away. Although we do not have the luxury of revisiting the actual traumatic event, we can talk about the pain and how it affects patients in their daily lives. It is then possible to start exploring emotion regulation strategies to soothe the person during moments of flashbacks or fear. Some might be open to metaphors, as used in acceptance and commitment therapy (ACT; Hayes et al. 1999) for instance, such as the idea that they have this really heavy luggage to carry, they cannot get rid of it, and they will not get anywhere if they just stare at the luggage (i.e., the trauma story). They have to learn to carry it with them, and with time it will become lighter as they become stronger. One patient once told me (T.L.) she felt like a crooked tree—her childhood did not help her grow straight, but she eventually was able to reach for the sun and survive through time. When working with patients with delusions of sexual aggression, our role is to be the person who believes that they have what it takes to move on and who tries to help the patient realize that their life can be much more than the trauma. It is not about whether the belief is linked to something real, it is about dealing with the pain linked to the belief.

Here is another vignette with the same patient:

Therapist: Sounds like you are constantly thinking about what happened to you as a child. Tell me how it feels.

Patient: Scary. I walk outside and keep on seeing scenes from the movie, but it's me who is in it. If someone says "Hi," I jump. I am getting scared of everyone, especially men. I refuse to talk to my dad. He says he doesn't understand; he thinks it is because he was so absent when I was a kid (he was always on tour). But he knows it's more than that!

Therapist: Must be hard, carrying these thoughts and images with you all the time.

Patient: Yes. I wish I could think of something else, but I can't. Not sure how I can go on now that I know what happened to me. My life stopped when I had this recollection a year ago.

Therapist: Sounds like it is hard to imagine having a life now. Would you want that? To have a life? Even if it meant still having these thoughts at times, but maybe not all the time? I'm not asking you to forget or pretend all is OK, but I am asking whether you think you would like to get to a place where your life is not scary and full of flashbacks?

Patient: Yeah, I would.

Therapist: OK, so would you like to start with seeing how we can cope with these flashbacks?

Patient: OK.

As can be seen in the vignette, by acknowledging the emotions, not confronting the story, we can bring the patient to consider that there can be more to life than the delusion. Coping strategies, such as grounding techniques, whereby the person learns to focus on concrete things (e.g., naming five furry animals, five television shows with groups of friends, five smells), can help them to snap out of the fear linked with the images or obsessive delusional thoughts. Positive imagery (e.g., imagining being in a safe place) or mindfulness strategies (e.g., focusing on the five senses) can also soothe the person during these impressions of flashbacks. In fact, merging strategies from CBT, ACT, and dialectical behavior therapy can be very helpful with these patients (Tai and Turkington 2009).

Once the person is able to cope with the distressful thoughts, we can work on trying to move on and find personal goals or objectives to reach. Delusional beliefs of sexual abuse can be so overwhelming that the person's life is on hold for a long time. Focusing on recovery, on surviving and healing, can be difficult at first but can start to make sense and have meaning once the person is able to not constantly think about the delusion. For instance, the person described earlier who used the metaphor of the crooked tree discovered that she wanted to learn about organic gardening and found solace in making healthy vegetables grow.

Another delusion of sexual aggression is wrongfully believing that *one is an aggressor and has abused others*. As in most cases involving delusions of sexual abuse, the first reflex is to consider that the person might have been sexually abused as a child. It is indeed possible that a person who was sexually abused has internalized the trauma and now confuses being a victim with being a perpetrator. Such a reversal of roles has been documented, for instance, in men who were sexually abused as children (and did not remember it) becoming pedophiles and abusing children as adults (Glasser et al. 2001). We also hear of victims of sexual abuse developing sexual fantasies of abuse (Shulman and Horne 2006). In order to psychologically tolerate what happened to them, they unconsciously transform the experience into something desirable. Therefore, it is possible that someone who was a victim could find that memory intolerable and transform it into a delusion of being an aggressor themselves. In this case, it is important to try to discover if there is any chance the person might have been sexually abused or victimized somehow. If so, then the treatment will resemble what was described earlier for those who believe they were sexually abused.

However, it is possible that the person was never sexually abused, or abused in any other way, and has never sexually abused anyone. Then what? How do we understand this?

Sexuality is a basic human need. It also comes with many taboos and mixed messages. For instance, one's church or parents might speak little of sexuality or mention only what is "bad" (e.g., sex outside marriage should be prohibited), whereas pornography might portray images that are very different and at times disturbing. Men with mental illness in particular tend to develop their first symptoms in late adolescence and early adulthood, during a developmental period when they would normally be dating and developing their intimacy and sexual skills. As a consequence, they are very often single for years and have difficulty developing romantic relationships that would allow them to express a healthy sexuality. This need for intimacy and sex can lead to the use of pornography, obsessive thoughts regarding sex, guilt regarding these thoughts, and sexual delusions of being an aggressor.

Case Example 2

Joey has been very down and depressed lately, convinced he has sexually abused his mother and sister-in-law. Both have denied he ever touched them, but he is truly convinced he has sexually abused them and feels so guilty that he asked the police to lock him up. His mother does not understand what he is going through or why he is having such thoughts. She describes him as having always been sweet. Joey has never hurt anyone, nor did he ever experience any trauma as a child or teen. He developed his first psychotic break at age 17 after taking Ecstasy at a party. His original beliefs and hallucinations have abated in the past 5 years, but he is now convinced that he is a sexual abuser. He is currently not working, has few friends, and has been single for the past 5 years. A look at his computer history shows he is regularly on a pornography website.

When a therapist is working with someone like Joey, Socratic questioning and checking the facts most often do not work. In fact, regardless of the number of times Joey's presumed victims say he never touched them, he still believes it happened. Probably, after watching pornography, he imagined doing some of the things he saw with the women around him. This mix of sexual images, sexual desire, and guilt (or shame) for thinking these thoughts created a great deal of distress and became a delusional belief of sexual aggression. His *thinking about it* became *having done it* in his mind.

There are a few ways we could work with Joey here. We could focus on the central emotion expressed, in this case shame or guilt. We could explore which of these two feelings he experiences more. We could ask whether he also feels the same way after watching pornography. We could have a discussion about pornography, what he likes about it and what he does not. This could lead to an exploration of images that stay in his mind or not after he watches pornography and trying to see how he feels about these images (e.g., disturbed, excited, ashamed). Realizing the link between these images and his feeling of shame or guilt, we could emphasize how sometimes a thought, especially a very strong one, can make us feel terrible. Working on this link, we could suggest that both pornography and Joey's believing that he sexually molested his mother and sister-in-law are linked with his feeling guilty and ashamed. Could there be a link between pornography, having those images, and believing he is a sexual molester? Maybe the images became so real that the thought became real in his mind?

Another approach could be to talk about sexuality up front, asking how his sex life has been in the past and recently. Normalizing sexual needs and desires could help Joey open up about his needs and his pornography use. We could also discuss difficulties meeting women and engaging in sex with someone. Maybe we could ask, if Joey did have a girlfriend, what would he imagine sex would be like? Would it be like in pornography or different? This could lead to a discussion about fantasy versus reality—whether Joey could picture himself forcing himself on his partner or whether he believes he would be respectful and have shared pleasure. Should Joey mention preferring reciprocity and caring to forced sex in his relationships, we could explore why he believes he could harm others. If, in contrast, he admits to fantasizing about forced sex, then we could explore how these thoughts make him feel (likely guilty and ashamed) and how these feelings are linked to the sexual thoughts, even if he does not perform any actual behavior. We could also offer some psychoeducation about how people can have sexual fantasies without them translating into real acts. The discussion might address whether it could be considered normal to have a fantasy that is "deviant" or involves doing something one would never wish to do in reality. The idea is to help Joey feel less guilty about having sexual desires and less ashamed about looking at pornography. If he feels pornography brings mostly negative thoughts about sexual acts he would not enjoy, we could discuss stopping his pornography use and considering meeting real women instead.

We could also consider talking with Joey about the power of a thought—that sometimes, just thinking about something, we start believing it is true. If I think I am an idiot because I made a mistake, I might actually believe I am an idiot and feel really bad about myself. Yet it is only a thought that, if I really think about it, could be circumstantial and not at all a reflection of who I truly am. It is possible to use such an example to demonstrate the power we can give to a thought, how it can start as an image in our mind, or an idea, and how, especially if we are not feeling 100% (e.g., if we are feeling lonely or tired or have not felt like we have accomplished much recently), it can turn into a horrible belief about ourselves. Yet a thought is just a thought; it has power only if we give it power. This discussion could help Joey take a step back from his belief and consider it only as a thought, not a reality.

As illustrated here, there are multiple ways of helping Joey with his current delusion of being a sexual abuser. It is difficult to say which of these strategies will work best; it really depends on how in touch Joey is with his emotions, whether he responds better to psychoeducation about sex, or whether a better understanding of the link between thoughts and emotions will help him make sense of his beliefs. A therapist can use any of these paths, or even all of them, when working with him. Given that the sexual abuser thoughts cause him a great deal of distress, Joey is likely going to be open to diminishing this distress and might respond well to these therapeutic approaches.

Conclusion

In this chapter, we have tried to illustrate how sexual delusions are not always what they appear to be. They might mask a grandiose delusion paired with a delusion of reference in a lonely person seeking love, as in erotomania. They might suggest a childhood trauma, of a sexual nature or not, transformed into a sexual delusion of having been molested. Or they might be linked to emotions of guilt or shame linked with desires for sexual relationships in some who believe they are sexual abusers. There are likely other possible explanations, such as fantasies of power for instance, because sexuality can be used or be perceived as powerful. The point is to keep an open mind and explore the meaning behind the belief while attempting to grasp where the distress lies because when there is a delusion, sexual or otherwise, there is always some form of distress. As CBTp therapists, we aim to help our patients diminish, or cope with, this distress in order to help them lead more satisfying and fulfilling lives.

Questions for Discussion

1. Have you ever been in a situation in which a patient seemed to have developed romantic fantasies about you, as a therapist? How did you deal with this?

2. How can you go about inquiring about past sexual trauma, while being careful to not retraumatize the patient?

3. Sex can be considered taboo in several cultures. Can you think of ways of talking about sexuality that could be normalizing and acceptable?

KEY POINTS

- Delusions can at times have a sexual or romantic theme.

- We can find at least three types of delusions in this category: a person's delusion that someone is secretly in love with them (erotomania) and delusional memories that someone sexually abused them or that they have sexually abused others.

- These three most common types of sexual delusions can be related to very different life experiences or meanings and are not treated in the same way with CBT.

- Recovery lies less in exploring disconfirmatory evidence and more in working to reduce distress, shame, and guilt.

- Techniques from CBT (normalization and reprocessing), dialectical behavior therapy (grounding and emotion regulation), and ACT (acceptance and metaphor) are all potentially important.

References

Bailey T, Alvarez-Jimenez M, Garcia-Sanchez AM, et al: Childhood trauma is associated with severity of hallucinations and delusions in psychotic disorders: a systematic review and meta-analysis. Schizophr Bull 44(5):1111–1122, 2018 29301025

Beck JC, Van der Kolk B: Reports of childhood incest and current behavior of chronically hospitalized psychotic women. Am J Psychiatry 144:1474–1476, 1987

Blom JD, Mangoenkarso E: Sexual hallucinations in schizophrenia spectrum disorders and their relation with childhood trauma. Front Psychiatry 9:193, 2018 29867612

Bourgeois C, Lecomte T, McDuff P, Daigneault I: Child sexual abuse and age at onset of psychotic disorders: a matched-cohort study. Can J Psychiatry 66:569–576, 2020 33155838

Freeman D, Garety P, Fowler D, et al: The London-East Anglia randomized controlled trial of cognitive-behaviour therapy for psychosis, IV: self-esteem and persecutory delusions. Br J Clin Psychol 37(4):415–430, 1998 9856295

Glasser M, Kolvin I, Campbell D, et al: Cycle of child sexual abuse: links between being a victim and becoming a perpetrator. Br J Psychiatry 179:482–494, discussion 495–497, 2001 11731348

Hardy A, Emsley R, Freeman D, et al: Psychological mechanisms mediating effects between trauma and psychotic symptoms: the role of affect regulation, intrusive trauma memory, beliefs, and depression. Schizophr Bull 42(Suppl 1):S34–S43, 2016 27460616

Hayes SC, Strosahl KD, Wilson KG: Acceptance and Commitment Therapy: An Experiential Approach to Behavior Change. New York, Guilford, 1999

Isham L, Griffith L, Boylan AM, et al: Understanding, treating, and renaming grandiose delusions: a qualitative study. Psychol Psychother 94(1):119–140, 2021 31785077

Keen N, Hunter ECM, Peters E: Integrated trauma-focused cognitive-behavioural therapy for post-traumatic stress and psychotic symptoms: a case-series study using imaginal reprocessing strategies. Front Psychiatry 8:92, 2017 28620323

Knowles R, McCarthy-Jones S, Rowse G: Grandiose delusions: a review and theoretical integration of cognitive and affective perspectives. Clin Psychol Rev 31(4):684–696, 2011 21482326

Lecomte T, Potvin S, Samson C, et al: Predicting and preventing symptom onset and relapse in schizophrenia: a meta-review of current empirical evidence. J Abnorm Psychol 128(8):840–854, 2019 31343181

Shulman JL, Horne SG: Guilty or not? A path model of women's sexual force fantasies. J Sex Res 43(4):368–377, 2006 17599258

Smith N, Freeman D, Kuipers E: Grandiose delusions: an experimental investigation of the delusion as defense. J Nerv Ment Dis 193(7):480–487, 2005 15985843

Tai S, Turkington D: The evolution of cognitive behavior therapy for schizophrenia: current practice and recent developments. Schizophr Bull 35(5):865–873, 2009 19661198

Varese F, Smeets F, Drukker M, et al: Childhood adversities increase the risk of psychosis: a meta-analysis of patient-control, prospective- and cross-sectional cohort studies. Schizophr Bull 38(4):661–671, 2012 22461484

12

A Bizarre and Grandiose Delusion

Persecution of a Goddess Using Social Media and Microbots

Douglas Turkington, M.D.
Helen M. Spencer, B.A.

Jaspers (1913/1963) described delusions as being fixed false beliefs out of keeping with a patient's social, cultural, educational, and religious background that are not amenable to counterargument. This dichotomous definition of the boundary between delusion and the world of non-insane beliefs has been very persuasive in terms of psychiatric education and practice. Freud (1911/1958) was similarly pessimistic about working with delusions. He described the delusion as "a sticking plaster over the unconscious" (Freud 1924/1981, p. 215) that should not be worked with using classical psychoanalysis because of the risk of causing a severe psychotic deterioration. Phenomenology and psychoanalysis therefore combined to tip psychiatric practice toward an approach of not discussing the content of bizarre delusions and instead focusing on healthier aspects of dialogue. This was linked to a treatment orientation of increasing reliance on biological approaches. Surely the bizarre nature of the systematized content and linked behavior that defied social norms was driven by ultrahigh levels of limbic synaptic dopamine? Unfortunately, this turned out not to be the case, and delusional systems (along with command hallucinations and thought disorder) proved to be the positive symptoms of schizophrenia most resistant to both standard and second-generation antipsychotics such as clozapine.

However, cognitive therapists gradually began to consider whether such bizarre delusional systems could be formulated and worked with. This development was driven by the seminal work of Aaron T. Beck, who published a case report in 1952. Beck (1952) described how (using collaborative empiricism) he had begun to work with a client with a persecutory delusional system who identified more than 100 persecutors. These "persecutors" were gradually accepted as being nonthreatening, and the unexpressed emotion of guilt was seen to lie at the heart of the delusion. Beck worked with the guilt cognitively, and the delusion receded.

In 1998, we described the case of "the Mafia man," who believed he was being persecuted by the Italian Mafia but also believed he was about to be appointed the next godfather (Turkington and Siddle 1998). He had a poor response to medication, but we were able to formulate a case by building rapport, having the patient do homework on delusions of reference, and working on the pre-psychotic period and timeline. The patient expressed negative childhood affect (sadness) in relation to a mistaken belief in his specialness related to his being appointed the next godfather. We worked with him on his depression, and he achieved a degree of social recovery. The delusion was still present but was much less prominent and allowed a reasonable quality of life.

Over time, psychoanalysts gradually returned to work with delusions, and Michael Garrett showed how cognitive-behavioral therapy (CBT) could be used to strengthen the observing ego until interpretive work on underlying conflict could be done (Garrett and Turkington 2011). The process of therapy was most clearly described by Turkington et al. (2015) on three cases of delusional systems all treated with CBT, but the caveat was that in the region of 50 sessions were needed. The case of Olivia described later in the chapter demonstrates the stages of therapy and the need to persevere through difficult phases of therapy.

Doug's Personal Reflection

This reflection is not about me personally, because as far as I know I have never had a bizarre delusional system, but it is a reflection on my experience in therapy. When a delusion systematizes, the primary delusion is protected from the benefits of sensitive questioning and reality testing by the incremental development of secondary delusions. The primary delusion is usually invested with a lot of affect (euphoria, anger, and terror seem to be the most common), and the delusion is usually acted on in ways that bring the person in contact with the police and the courts. This is frequently a disaster in relation to the possibility of developing a therapeutic alliance. Periods of time spent in prison make it harder to forge a therapeutic alliance. Often patients with delusional systems are admitted to acute or rehabilitation inpatient psychiatric wards, and the necessary skilled therapeutic work is, surprisingly, rarely attempted. This is tragic because an inpatient setting is a good place in which the seed of truth can be detected in the delusional system and worked with. It is possible to identify and work with this emotional hotspot, which is linked to an Achilles heel within the schema profile, a trauma, or a goal conflict. Such patients need expert psychiatry, psychology, or nurse therapy input and not the secondary iatrogenic disability of an—at best—only partially effective polypharmacy. It is generally the rule rather than the exception that when beginning to engage a patient with a delusional system, they are so overmedicated that sedation interferes with the engagement process. I have often had to request a gradual reduction of one of the antipsychotic medications before CBT could be attempted.

Case Example

Olivia became physically unwell at age 52 years. She had worked throughout her entire career with the same firm of accountants and was a much-valued staff member. Unfortunately, she quite suddenly developed back pain and fever and started passing dark urine. She was admitted to an acute medical ward, was diagnosed with septicemia and acute pyelonephritis, needed intravenous antibiotics, and required a prolonged period of renal dialysis. Olivia and her family were informed that she might need a renal transplant and they should prepare themselves for the fact that she might not survive. Fortunately, Olivia's health began to improve, and as she started to recover she began to feel that something very important was about to happen. She subsequently described this as a feeling of "spiritual anticipation and happiness." She became well enough to receive visitors, and her husband attended the ward, only, to his astonishment, to be rejected. Olivia was apparently waiting for somebody else.

Toward the end of the visiting period a work colleague entered the ward carrying flowers for Olivia. The flowers had been bought by her friends at the office and were an impressive bouquet. When she saw the flowers, Olivia reported, she realized that she was the Goddess and that the colleague from work had come to worship her. She told her colleague that the flowers (red carnations) were the symbol of the new religion. She angrily told nursing staff that her husband was "a wimp" and that no men would be allowed to join the new religion. Men were to have a role only in working and in procreation. This grandiose delusion, even at this very early stage, had a persecutory component. Olivia demanded to know why this particular colleague had been asked to bring the flowers, and she asked her whether people at work had been laughing at her husband and talking about her sexuality. The work colleague was ejected from the visit to join Olivia's baffled husband in the waiting area attached to the ward.

On her return home, Olivia engaged in daily confrontational arguments with her neighbors, who she said were talking about her and trying to flirt with her. Repeated denials by all concerned led to the emergence of more delusions. Olivia indicated that microbots (tiny transmitting robots) in her bloodstream were keeping people informed of everything she said and did on a day-to-day basis via social media. She next started to promote the Goddess religion. Olivia would stand on the corner of busy city-center streets, preaching about the Goddess religion and offering red flowers to people while verbally abusing any male passersby who made comments. She attracted some converts, but there was always a persecutory edge to her sermons. Her husband, afraid that she would be assaulted, tried to stop her from preaching but without success.

Olivia came to the attention of the police following an episode of public disorder in which a group of young men took offense at the anti-male rhetoric and there was a scuffle. Bottles were thrown, and people in the area feared for their safety. Referral to psychiatry followed, and Olivia exhibited very poor adherence to oral antipsychotic medication. A monthly depot was commenced, but neither the delusional system nor the linked behavior showed any sign of significant improvement. Olivia regularly received her depot from a community psychiatric nurse after being placed on a community treatment order and was referred against her wishes for CBT. She was not offered clozapine.

Phases of Therapy

Therapeutic Alliance

The first phase of CBT is to form a therapeutic alliance. The alliance is often fragile in the early stages, and missed appointments are frequent. The three key elements are engaging, reducing risk, and hanging in there as a therapist. Olivia was very reluctant to see any mental health professional (male or female) but did agree to her husband bringing her to the appointments as long as no extra medications would be added. The crucial elements of forming the therapeutic alliance were to spend a lot of time *listening and absorbing the psychotic material* and asking questions (which were *not perceived to be collusive or confrontational*). Sessions were *variable in length*; some were very brief (no more than 10 minutes), whereas on other occasions sessions up to 30 minutes were possible. The classic, more formal structure of a CBT session was impossible during this early phase. Having formed a basic alliance, we needed to achieve a joint understanding of Olivia's beliefs and make the situation safer. *Peripheral questioning* was used in relation to her belief in her identity and the Goddess religion. I (D.T.) asked her to tell me the key elements of the Goddess religion. She stated the tenets of her belief as follows: "All male-dominated institutions have been a total failure; male-oriented religion is uncaring and discriminatory; men should not be the heads of the families they live in. Males caused all wars, climate change, and disease." When working with delusions, it is very important to introduce relevant information for consideration. I asked her how her ideas related to feminist theology.

> Olivia said that she had never heard of feminist theology and declined to do any homework reading. I offered to read a bit about it (the therapist often does the homework in the early sessions) and bring my findings back to our next session for discussion. Olivia was, for the first time, mildly interested in what I would discover about this subject. I read excerpts from Simone de Beauvoir (1949) about feminist philosophy and from Carol P. Christ (1997), who had written an influential book titled *Rebirth of the Goddess* and had been fundamental in launching the Goddess movement across the United States. Discussing this material did not make the delusion worse or systematize it further. Instead, it allowed Olivia to realize that some of her beliefs were partially held by others and were at least in part true. I learned a number of things that I did not know, so I was able to show interest and enthusiasm about some of the ideas in feminist theology.
>
> Having achieved a degree of engagement, I felt it was time to attempt to make the situation safer. Could Olivia promote her beliefs without preaching on the streets? This was the first bit of homework that Olivia became involved in. We considered how other religions promoted their ideas in the current day. YouTube, blogs, and leaflets seemed most common. Olivia decided to write a blog once a week and post it. There is an apparent contradiction here because Olivia believed microbots (small transmitters in her blood) were already transmitting her thoughts to others via social media. Interestingly, Olivia did not know anything about social media, did not have an account, and did not know how to post a blog. The blog was written and posted online, and it was agreed that Olivia would wait for responses and would not preach on the streets for a week. We had successfully engaged over the first 10 sessions of CBT (3 were not attended), the risk had been reduced, and toward the end of the 10 sessions the discussion was much less controlled by Olivia and was more collaborative.

Scaffolding

The second phase includes developing scaffolding activities and coping strategies and (if appropriate) using metacognitive approaches. The concept of developing scaffolding activities relates to the fact that delusional systems are inherently weak belief structures and are prone to collapse if the appropriate trajectory is followed. Therefore the therapist scaffolds by asking the patient to consider their previous interests, skills, and hobbies and whether any of these might be reactivated.

One of Olivia's hobbies was baking high-quality cakes for others, and she had been involved in a running club before the pyelonephritis and the emergency admission. She said that she would not run again at present because others would victimize her, but she would bake a special cake for her colleagues at work. Becoming involved in buying the ingredients, baking the cake, and sending it to her work showed Olivia that she had skills, and her colleagues were very positive about what she had done. Being involved in this activity allowed her to spend a period of time when she was not entirely focused on the delusion.

Olivia agreed that her husband could listen to a recording of one of her CBT sessions, and he responded positively. He bought Olivia a treadmill and installed it out of the view of any neighbors, and she began to exercise at home by jogging for brief periods (10 minutes twice a day). This allowed a degree of structure to return to her day.

Olivia was concerned that people she met outside the home were tuning in to social media to taunt her with things she had previously said. For example, a hairdresser said to her, "Where are you going on holidays this year?" She said that she was enraged by this comment because she had spoken about holidays the day before. Olivia angrily remarked, "She obviously got this information from social media." Olivia needed a strategy for coping with her distress around the perceived persecution by others, and it was agreed that she would continue with her running and consider joining an online yoga class. She learned a yogic breathing exercise that she would use when distressed.

We decided to set a behavioral experiment—a test phrase—to see whether it was said back to her by anyone the following week. We agreed that if anyone said the phrase "trout and antique" to her in any sentence she would report it in the next session. The words "trout and antique," fortunately, were not said by anyone, and this puzzled her. Olivia concluded that not everything she thought about (or spoke about) was appearing on social media. Reduction of rumination about perceived persecution was attempted with rumination postponement and the prescription of rumination periods with the help of the image of a feather floating from the ceiling to the floor, but this approach did not help in Olivia's case. The reason for this appeared to be that Olivia was not motivated to think about any other subjects at that point in time. She completed a further eight sessions of more collaborative CBT, with only one missed session.

Examples of coping strategies and metacognitive approaches are shown in Videos 11 and 14, respectively. (For descriptions, see Chapter 20, "Decoding Delusions.")

Video 11: Coping

Video 14: Metacognitive Techniques

Exploration of the Pre-psychotic Period

Exploring the pre-psychotic period is the next and crucial therapeutic phase. How was Olivia thinking and what was she feeling in the hospital before her husband and then her friend arrived? This was explored with *inductive questioning*. Inductive questioning is a stepwise questioning approach to exploration of a particular time period. The sequence of events is discussed, as are linked behaviors, emotions, and automatic thoughts. Particular stressors are identified that may be pertinent to the emergence of the delusion.

> Olivia reported that her mood was "spiritual and excited" and that she was anticipating something—obviously not her husband's visit, as he was sent out of the ward very quickly. She said that she was "expecting someone special to arrive" and that there would be "a special gift." She said that when she saw her husband she thought, "He's a wimp," and when she saw her work colleague she thought, "Why did they send *her* in particular?" Olivia said that on seeing them both, her emotions changed from anticipation to anger. She said that when she saw the beautiful bouquet of red carnations, "everything made sense." This is an example of *delusional perception*. She said that in her opinion red carnations symbolized undying love, admiration, and affection and that at that moment she realized that she was the embodiment of a female goodness—"the Goddess"—and was to promote female rights and leadership via a new religion. She had come to believe in that instant that she was "the" long-awaited Goddess. These were four interesting sessions during which I understood much more about how the systematizing delusion had emerged.

Timeline Review

A timeline review is the next phase. This activity may require the help of family and friends to validate and develop key memories and perspectives about the past. To ensure balance, it is important to look for positive memories and achievements as well as negative memories. Olivia's timeline review took place over the next six sessions.

> Olivia noted that her work and family lives were unexceptional, describing them as "run-of-the-mill" prior to her developing a life-threatening illness. She said that her husband was a carpenter and "good at putting up shelves" but "lacking in spark, creativity, and fun." She said that she did not know why she had married him but that he had been reliable and safe. She said that her work was monotonous and that she had been overlooked for promotion. She noted that during her school years she was "middle of the class" and had not had any durable close relationships. She indicated that she lived with her mother and sister after her father left home when she was 4 years old. She said that her sister had heard her parents having a big argument and her father saying that he "would always come back to see his girls." Ol-

ivia became very tearful at this point and said that he had never come back and that she must have done something wrong. She said that he did not even send birthday or Christmas cards or presents. Olivia said that she had inquired about his situation over the years and knew that he lived nearby but had never heard any other gossip or information about how he was. It was clear that Olivia blamed herself and felt guilty and saddened by these childhood events.

Olivia agreed for her mother to be contacted for a collateral history, and her mother said that the relationship between her and Olivia's father had broken down because of her husband's excessive alcohol use; because of this, she had taken out a court order to prevent him from coming to the house to see the girls. Olivia's mother said that she had destroyed the cards and presents the girls' father had sent "to prevent them from becoming upset." Olivia's mother said that her ex-husband was still alive and living nearby and frequently asked a joint acquaintance how his daughters were doing.

Emotional Processing

The fifth phase is emotional processing, in which the patient works with the emotions that have been expressed on the timeline, including sadness, anxiety, shame, and guilt. This took place over four sessions with Olivia.

The first session was a very emotional session attended by Olivia, her elderly mother, and her sister, during which they all reevaluated their understanding of what had happened in the past. Olivia said that it had never been spoken about before but that she had always believed that she had done something very badly wrong and that was why her father had never been in touch. Her sister said that she felt the same way, and their mother said that she was only trying to protect them from more emotional pain. Old photographs were viewed, and memories were exchanged of the good and the bad times before and after their father left.

As this work was being done, much less was said about the Goddess delusion, microbots, or persecution via social media. The first signs of some normalization of social functioning appeared. Rational responses were generated for the automatic thoughts, and it was agreed that Olivia would practice these. Automatic thoughts reported while Olivia was viewing the old photographs included "It was my fault" and "He didn't love me." Rational responses included "A 4-year-old girl shouldn't be blamed for her parents splitting up," "It was nobody's fault," and "It was just one of those things" and "At least he was trying to get in contact."

Following work on guilt came a couple of sessions in which Olivia became extremely tearful, and the sadness was explained to her as her grieving over all the lost years when she felt abandoned by her father and was repeatedly searching for news of his well-being. Olivia said that she felt better after these sessions and that the tears were "healing tears." During these sessions the grandiose and persecutory delusions were rarely mentioned, and Olivia was a much more active collaborator in her CBT.

Schema Work

The key core belief (schema) and linked emotion can also be detected by asking a series of questions about the personal implication of each statement about the delusion were it to turn out to be true (downward arrow). This questioning style can be distressing if used too early in therapy. Working with the continuum of beliefs can be an effective intervention to modify a distressing core belief (schema) linked to the delusion. Key core beliefs linked to the delusion can also be identified using the Brief Core Schema Scales (Fowler et al. 2006). This scale measures the extreme negative evaluations of self and others which are commonly present in psychosis. Schema-level work includes work on goal conflict. Questioning both sides of an identified goal conflict is a technique that has been described for a full range of mental health problems patients that present with in primary care. This approach allows the patient to focus on a conflict that has never previously been verbalized for spontaneous resolution between sessions. This therapeutic approach has been called the *method of levels* and was described by Carey (2008). The techniques of method of levels therapy can be used to address goal conflicts linked to delusional systems (Tai 2016). The basic approach is to use an unstructured questioning style and to look out for disruptions in communication. The basic principle of perceptual control theory when applied to CBT is that the therapist should ask, "What went through your mind just there, when you [stopped speaking, looked away, laughed]?" The theory is that by going to that thought, the therapist and patient go "up a level" to the goal conflict, which can then be explored by asking questions about both sides of the conflict. In Olivia's case, she began to feel more comfortable about the idea of contacting her father again.

> During schema work over the next four sessions, Olivia came to believe that she was not an unloved person, had not been abandoned, and was not to blame. This shift in belief structure was achieved with rational responding and role-play. A role-play was done of Olivia speaking to her father, with me playing her father. This was done by Olivia as a 4-year-old child and then again as her adult self. This was followed by a role reversal, with Olivia playing the role of her father. Following these role-plays it became apparent that Olivia had a goal conflict in relation to her father. She stated that she was desperate to meet her father again but also wanted to avoid punishment for not visiting him sooner. This conflict was talked through during the later sessions of therapy, and Olivia was able to explore both sides of the conflict and come to a resolution.

Examples of downward arrow questioning and schema-level work are shown in Videos 6 and 12 (see Chapter 20).

Video 6: Downward Arrow

 Video 12: Schema Intervention

Reorientation

At the end of therapy, as sessions are gradually spaced out, reorientation to a more balanced social life can occur. The degree to which this can be done varies.

> Olivia continued with her Goddess blog, but it became more mainstream. She came to believe that when others said something she had said (or thought), it was usually just a coincidence. Interestingly, she decided to accept redundancy from work and set up her own business making specialty cakes for events and celebrations. Olivia stayed with her husband, and the couple worked to improve their marriage. She visited her father once and then stayed in touch by phone and social media.

Discussion

This case is fairly typical of the delusional systems we see in clinical practice. The more time that is spent in CBT listening to the patient, the more the emergence of the delusion and its various components starts to make sense. The biggest problem is engaging, and many mental health professionals do not have the time to devote to the engaging process. Acting on the counter-transference and avoiding engagement altogether or discharging the patient following a couple of missed appointments is very common. It is a patient and flexible clinician who can persevere and make therapeutic gains. In particular, the delusion is defended not only by systematization but also by a tendency for the patient to overcontrol the session. The patient will often speak all the time or not at all. They might display hostility, repeatedly interrupting the therapist or disattending. The therapist might be accused of being part of the persecutory network. The difficulties encountered in these engaging sessions are emotionally demanding for the therapist, and when one is working with patients with delusional systems, supervision is especially important.

Recovery from a delusional system normally involves the belief still being held but less extremely so, in order that social function can proceed without the need for external intervention from psychiatric services in the form of inpatient care or the use of mental health legislation to force hospitalization. It is unclear exactly which of the phases and techniques described here were the key therapeutic elements in Olivia's recovery. A case can be made for any or all of them. The therapeutic alliance is certainly key; peripheral questioning allows the delusion to be worked with while minimizing systematization, because peripheral questioning is nonconfrontational. Although the emotional processing and schema-level work seemed crucial from my perspective as the therapist, Olivia did not recognize it as such, and she never made any link between those matters, the delusional system, and her gradual social recovery.

The approach described is classical CBT but with modification. In the early sessions of working with distress linked to a circumscribed delusion or voice-hearing, it is much easier to set an agenda and construct a collaborative problem list. Goals can be set for each session, and it can be expected that an attempt will be made to complete homework that is collaboratively generated. The situation with a bizarre and grandiose delusion is different in that the emergence of structure takes slightly longer, and early sessions are more flexible in content and length. As is the case in classical CBT, we are working to develop joint understanding in a formulation, but, again, it takes longer. We work with stressors in the pre-psychotic period rather than current ones and work with cognitive restructuring and eventually schema-focused approaches linked to the delusion itself. Thus, this is CBT, but with techniques applied at a different pace and within a more flexible session structure.

Questions for Discussion

1. Can you think of cases like this in your practice where there has been a seed of truth at the heart of the delusion?

2. Might Olivia have responded to clozapine? (She would not accept medication voluntarily, so only a depot could be given.)

3. Where do patients with bizarre delusional systems end up in the long term? Are they in prison, in acute or rehabilitation psychiatric wards, or in the community?

4. Do massive delusions eventually burn out?

5. Who is best placed to deliver CBT: psychologists, nurse therapists, or psychiatrists?

KEY POINTS

- No matter how bizarre delusional content may appear, it will make much more sense once the pre-psychotic period and timeline have been explored.

- The engaging phase can be very difficult, with missed sessions and marked variability in session duration and degree of collaboration.

- Close attention should be paid to the episode of delusional perception that immediately predated the emergence of the delusional system.

- Homework will initially need to be done by the therapist and thereafter can be completed jointly.

- The seed of truth at the heart of the delusion can be worked with, but complete insight is usually not achieved.

- Negative affect (unprocessed), trauma, or goal conflict can be gradually identified and worked with.

- A degree of gradual but incremental social recovery is expected as the strength of the delusion begins to recede.

- Forty to fifty sessions of expert therapy are needed.

References

Beck AT: Successful outpatient psychotherapy of a chronic schizophrenic with a delusion based on borrowed guilt. Psychiatry 15(3):305–312, 1952 12983446

Carey TA: Hold That Thought! Two Steps to Effective Counseling and Psychotherapy With The Method of Levels. St. Louis, MO, New View, 2008

Christ CP: Rebirth of the Goddess: Finding Meaning in Feminist Spirituality. New York, Routledge, 1997

de Beauvoir S: The Second Sex. Translated by Parshley HM. London, Vintage Books, 1949

Fowler D, Freeman D, Smith B, et al: The Brief Core Schema Scales (BCSS): psychometric properties and associations with paranoia and grandiosity in non-clinical and psychosis samples. Psychol Med 36(6):749–759, 2006 16563204

Freud S: Psycho-analytic notes on an autobiographical account of a case of paranoia (1911), in The Standard Edition of the Complete Psychological Works of Sigmund Freud, Vol 12. Translated and edited by Strachey J. London, Hogarth, 1958, pp 3–82

Freud S: On Psychopathology. Harmondsworth, UK, Penguin, 1924/1981

Garrett M, Turkington D: CBT for psychosis in a psychoanalytic frame. Psychosis 3:2–13, 2011

Jaspers K: General Psychopathology (1913). Translated by Hoenig J, Hamilton MW. Manchester, UK, Manchester University Press, 1963

Tai SJ: An introduction to using the method of levels (MOL) therapy to work with people experiencing psychosis. Am J Psychother 70(1):125–148, 2016 27052610

Turkington D, Siddle R: Cognitive therapy for delusions. Adv Psychiatr Treat 4:235–242, 1998

Turkington D, Spencer H, Jassal I, Cummings A: Cognitive behavioural therapy for the treatment of delusional systems. Psychosis 7(1):48–59, 2015

13

Who Are You?

Capgras Syndrome and Other Delusions of Misidentification

Michael Garrett, M.D.

The term *delusions of misidentification* (DMI) refers to a variety of beliefs in which a person attributes a mistaken identity to the self, another person, a place, or inanimate objects. In the *Capgras delusion* (Capgras and Reboul-Lachaux 1923), an individual believes that a familiar person (often a close family member) has been replaced by a double or impostor. In the *Fregoli delusion*, a person believes that individuals who outwardly appear to be different people are the same person in disguise. *Intermetamorphosis* is the belief that a person has physically and psychically changed into someone else. In the *delusion of subjective doubles*, someone else is transformed into a physical copy of oneself (Christodoulou 1978). In *mirrored-self misidentification*, one's reflection in the mirror is believed to be another person. In *reduplicative paramnesia*, time and place as well as persons and body parts may be duplicated. DMI are grouped together because they often co-occur and interchange around the theme of the substitution of people and things. Some writers include the *Cotard delusion*, the belief that one is dead or physically atrophied internally, in the DMI group. As many as 12 DMI variants have been named.

Despite the common theme of misidentification, the clinical phenomenology of DMI is extremely varied, which has led to a proliferation of definitions, classifications, and theories. The prevalence of DMI in samples of inpatient admissions has been estimated at roughly 4%. Pandis et al. (2019) provided a recent review of 255 cases of Capgras delusion. An organic etiology was attributed to 43%; 56% were considered functional disease, mostly diagnosed as schizophrenia or schizoaffective psychosis. The median age was 37 in the functional group and 64 in the organic group; 58% were female and 42% male, and 65% showed a response to treatment, typically neuroleptics or electroconvulsive therapy, often with full resolution of DMI symptoms. The person identified as an impostor varied: 38% spouse, 27% parent, 16% child, 10% sibling, 4% second-degree relative, 10% stranger. In addition, 39% reported multiple impostors, 17% reported the doubling of inanimate objects, and 6% had committed homicide. In this chapter I concentrate on the Capgras delusion because it is the most common and best known of the DMI and because it is an exemplar of cognitive neuropsychiatric (CNP) research. I construe Capgras syndrome not as a discrete psychiatric diagnosis but rather as one variant of a wide variety of DMI phenomena and other psychotic symptoms.

Biological and Psychological Explanations of Capgras Syndrome

Maher (1988) considered delusions to be explanations for anomalous perceptions arrived at via ordinary theory-building processes—that is, the authority of the anomalous experience, not a deficit in reasoning, results in a delusion. This idea has been called the one-factor model of delusion formation. In keeping with this model, Capgras syndrome is considered to be the patient's attempt to explain an anomalous perception of a familiar face. Usually, a ventral neural track running in the inferior longitudinal fasciculus *recognizes* aspects of a face as familiar, and a dorsal track in the inferior frontal-occipital fasciculus *identifies* the face as a particular person linked to emotionally significant memories and a name. In a CNP model of Capgras syndrome, damage to the dorsal emotional track while the ventral recognition track remains intact results in the anomalous experience of seeing a familiar face that elicits no emotional response, which the patient explains by surmising the familiar has been replaced by a double (Ellis and Lewis 2001; Ellis and Young 1990). Current consensus suggests that a two-factor CNP model is required to explain the persistence of delusions. Some writers have implicated right hemisphere damage and other brain lesions. A favored psychodynamic explanation regards the Capgras delusion as a psychological defense against ambivalent feelings for a close family member. To deal with conflicted sentiments, the patient splits the image of a relative into a vilified double that the patient is free to hate and an idealized image of the original, or the reverse (Berson 1983).

Phenomenology of Delusions of Misidentification

Disturbances in face recognition and defenses against ambivalent feelings may play a role in some cases, but these mechanisms fail to account for the wide range of phenomena in DMI. In fact, the 53-year-old woman who inspired the Capgras diagnostic category appears to have had chronic paranoid schizophrenia in which the belief that family members were impostors was only one of many delusional beliefs; for example, she believed that thousands of people had been substituted, including herself, and that a host of children were imprisoned in the basement of her home. A general theory of Capgras syndrome needs to account for at least the following observations:

- Schizophrenia or schizoaffective psychosis is a comorbidity in more than half of cases of Capgras syndrome. If one places a range of delusional ideas about identity in the DMI group, the incidence of Capgras delusion and Capgras-related symptoms increases significantly. For example, ideas of reference that lead people to believe that strangers are not who they appear to be are extremely common, such as when a patient believes that a stranger is a government agent in disguise.
- Capgras delusions and schizophrenia both respond to dopamine-blocking neuroleptic medications. Although improvement in Capgras delusions may lag behind improvement in other symptoms, in general resolution of Capgras syndrome follows the course and response to treatment of the underlying psychosis. However, the observation of Kapur (2003) tends to hold true: when the medication is discontinued, the Capgras delusion reemerges unless it has been processed psychologically (by cognitive-behavioral therapy [CBT] or structured psychodynamic therapy). Cases of acute onset of Capgras syndrome in response to dopamine agonists (L-dopa) are reported, with rapid resolution following treatment with dopamine blockers.
- Capgras syndrome waxes and wanes in some patients. It is likely that this cycle of change represents the disturbance and resolution of a diffuse metabolic process rather than a cycle of organic structural brain damage and repair.
- Rapid onset of Capgras syndrome in patients with acute delirium who have no underlying premorbid psychiatric condition is reported in which Capgras delusions resolve when the delirium clears: for example,

one patient experienced transient Capgras delusions in a delirium following a myelogram.

- As is true for schizophrenia, the majority of patients with Capgras syndrome do not show evidence of focal brain lesions on CT or functional MRI. Although some investigators suggest that right hemisphere damage plays a role in Capgras syndrome, even when brain damage is demonstrable, the identified lesions are not invariably in the right hemisphere.

- The classification of Capgras syndrome into a younger functional primary group lacking demonstrable brain damage with onset, on average, 30 years earlier than secondary Capgras syndrome with dementia and other organic brain disease suggests that Capgras syndrome is a final common phenotypic expression of different diffuse disease processes.

- Some patients with bilateral ventromedial frontal damage can recognize the identity of familiar faces yet fail to generate a discriminatory skin conductance response indicating emotional identification (Tranel et al. 1995). The fact that this deficit does not result in Capgras in these patients suggests that the anomalous experience of a lack of covert emotional response is insufficient to produce the Capgras delusion.

It is impossible to explain the varied presentations of Capgras delusions and other DMI as a disturbance of face recognition or any known modular brain deficit. In DMI, not just faces but all manner of people, places, things, and body parts may be subject to duplication. Thompson et al. (1980) described a patient who claimed there were at least eight duplicates of his wife and children, each living in a separate duplicate city with a separate duplicate of himself. Other examples include the following:

- Capgras syndrome has been reported in a blind patient. Some patients claim that doubles of themselves and other people exist that they have never seen. Accordingly, an error in face recognition cannot be a necessary and sufficient condition for Capgras syndrome.

- Capgras, Fregoli, intermetamorphosis, subjective doubles, and Cotard syndromes can occur in the same patient, which suggests a single disorder with multiple expressions rather than five separate diagnostic entities. To the extent that Capgras syndrome constitutes a failure of emotional recognition, and Fregoli syndrome is considered the phenomenological opposite of Capgras syndrome (i.e., hypertrophic recognition), it is difficult to explain these polar opposites with the same modular visual processing deficit.

- How could disruptions of face recognition explain the belief that one's own identity is being physically cloned in the body of an unseen other

(Christodoulou 1978) or that one's self is an impostor (Fialkov and Robins 1978)?

- If the doubling in Capgras syndrome is a defense against ambivalent feelings, how could a typewriter ribbon or a tube of glue to which the patient has no emotional attachment be identified by the patient as a substituted object that functions as a defense against ambivalent feelings for a close family member or be the result of impaired face recognition?

- As is true for people in general, Capgras patients would not have had occasion to see their internal organs, yet on occasion patients believe that one or more of their internal organs have been replaced by duplicates. Such individuals are reporting *mental representations* of their internal organs rather than misperceptions of them—that is, they are reporting *fantasies*. The same can be said of many Capgras claims, such as one patient's claim that the sky itself and the entirety of the country of Japan had been duplicated.

- In cases of reverse subjective doubles, patients believe that they are the double of someone else who has an authentic identity; in reverse Fregoli delusions, patients believe they are capable of cloaking themselves in a variety of appearances.

- A woman wondered whether the other woman her husband had substituted as his wife was the real wife and she the impostor or if it was the other way around. She required her driver's license for assurance that she was the real wife.

- A 29-year-old man with chronic schizophrenia claimed that every time his mother put her glasses on, she changed into a local woman he disliked intensely and that this woman sometimes changed into his mother, which particularly enraged him. This patient appeared to be describing alternating mental representations of his mother and another woman, as though he were flipping through a card file of images and substituting one image for another.

These clinical observations suggest that a modular deficit in face recognition cannot explain the varied phenomenology of Capgras syndrome and that Capgras is more likely the expression of a diffuse aberration of mental functioning consistent with prevailing biological theories of schizophrenia that attribute positive psychotic symptoms to excess dopaminergic transmission. Whatever its biology, the primary disorder in DMI would appear to interfere with the ability of people to form stable, differentiated mental representations of people and things that remain associated with a subjective feeling of authenticity. Instead, mental representations multiply, dissolve, merge, and are infiltrated by primordial fantasies. This view is in keeping with Sinkman's (2008) conclusion that DMI should be regarded not

as separate diagnostic entities but rather as varying expressions of a single underlying disturbance of mental representations, in the majority of cases, one
symptom of schizophrenia among others. Capgras syndrome aside, delusions
regarding the identity of the self and others are quite common in schizophrenia. For example, patients with ideas of reference may believe that strangers are
government agents concealing their real identities. If DMI are one symptom
of schizophrenia among many that falsify mental representations of people,
what pathological process might account for such delusions?

Biological and Psychological Factors

Rather than focusing narrowly on facial recognition, Margariti and Kontaxakis (2006) suggested that Capgras patients experience a disorder of a sense
of the *uniqueness* of people and things. Young (2010) spoke of a disturbance
of *familiarity of being*. These formulations reference that property of mind
that imparts a subjective quality of stability and individual uniqueness to
mental representations of persons, places, and things. Looking at the me-
nagerie of different manifestations of Capgras syndrome, one imagines a
pathological process that erodes the felt uniqueness of a wide variety of mental representations of the perceived world, as if a psychological duplicating
ray were trained on mental images of people and things, fractionating them
into doubles, or as if images were reverberating in an echo chamber. The
nervous system is organized hierarchically from lower-level sensors such as
the retina and the cochlea, which receive stimuli from the environment and
function in relatively constrained, automatic ways, to less constrained
higher-level cortical networks shaped by the individual experience of the
organism that construct complex matrices of memories and associations
among multimodal sensory inputs. As is true of schizophrenia, the neurological disturbance that underlies Capgras delusions likely resides in the
malfunction of connections in high-level association networks.

Aberrant Biology

What clinical conditions are already known to cause a generalized disturbance of feelings of uniqueness and familiarity? Depersonalization and derealization are prime candidates, in particular *jamais vu* ("never seen") and/
or *jamais vécu* (persistent jamais vu), in which individuals feel that something they know they have seen before appears oddly unfamiliar, as if being
seen for the first time; and *déjà vu* ("already seen") and *déjà vécu ("already
lived")*, in which they feel an uncanny sense of familiarity that suggests an
experience is being repeated (replicated). There is an obvious parallel between the feeling of unfamiliarity in jamais vécu and the Capgras delusion,

in which a relative appears unfamiliar. Déjà vécu is reminiscent of the hyperfamiliarity seen in Fregoli delusions. Capgras patients frequently report jamais vu and déjà vu (Christodoulou 1986). Temporal lobe epilepsy also results in déjà vu and jamais vu. Repeated negative fearful experiences of jamais vu may predispose a person to epileptic psychoses (Sengoku et al. 1997). I am not suggesting that temporal lobe epilepsy causes Capgras syndrome. I am suggesting, as have others, that like temporal lobe epilepsy, Capgras syndrome arises from a disruption in higher-level associative networks that cannot always be visualized as focal brain damage on CT or functional MRI scans (Christodoulou et al. 2009). Consistent with there being a disturbance of varying intensity of network function that attaches a feeling of familiarity and stability to mental representations, both Vie (1930) and Sno (1994) considered DMI to have one underlying cause, ranging in expression from hypo-identification in Capgras syndrome to hyper-identification in Fregoli syndrome, with transient experiences of déjà vu and jamais vu in ordinary mental life lying along a continuum between these extremes. In a two-factor CNP model of DMI, the anomalous experience that prompts DMI would be a jamais vécu–like and/or déjà vécu–like alteration of the experience of familiarity.

Psychoanalytic Object Relations Theory

Although little is known about the neurobiology of identity, psychoanalytic object relations theory has much to say about the psychology of how individuals form mental images of people and things. The iconic computer chip that some patients claim has been embedded in their brains to monitor and control them, voices that speak to the patient, delusional mental representations of the self and others (as in the belief that one is God or the Devil), and the impostor perceived by patients with Capgras syndrome are examples of psychological objects. Object relations theory describes the development and interplay of mental representations of the self and others, including how such images are shaped by past experience, fantasy, emotions, and the need for psychological defense (Kernberg 1976). Psychological objects are not physical objects, even though they may correspond to actual people and things. They are mental representations that are *objects* of internal psychological interest. According to object relations theory, the human mind is composed of an array of self-representations and object representations, with each dyad linked via an affective valence, pairings that coalesce into fantasies that can be rendered as stories in which the self is doing something to a psychological object or an object is doing something to the self. In classic Capgras, the double is a psychological object perpetrating an imposture on the patient for a variety of reasons.

When very young children are in emotional distress, they split their mental representations of themselves and others into a "good" self and a "bad" psychological object who is imagined to be the cause of their unhappiness. The human tendency to attribute unhappiness to persecutors, first described by Melanie Klein (1935), can be seen not only in the external attribution bias that paranoid people have toward negative events (Bentall et al. 1994) but also in the ordinary penchant that many people have to blame others for their own limitations. What psychoanalysts call *projection* overlaps with what cognitive-behavioral researchers call an *externalizing bias*. In the primordial split between the self and a persecutor, people regard their suffering as having been intended by a maleficent agent rather than seeing it as a consequence of the unavoidable exigencies of reality. The persecutor is one of the oldest object-related archetypes in the human psyche.

According to psychoanalytic object relations theory, human beings retain memories of early interactions with caregivers that endure in unconscious form as mental representations of the self and others that influence how individuals behave and how others are mentalized later in life. Memories of experiences in childhood, including recollections of childhood abuse, are retained not as historically accurate analogue copies of events but rather as amalgams of fantasy and reality that are retained as mental representations of one's personal history. What cognitive-behavioral clinicians call *core beliefs* and *schemata* resemble what psychoanalysts call *unconscious object-related fantasies*. In ordinary mental life, as well as in psychosis, individuals interact with people and things not as cognitively authenticated reproductions of the external world but rather as psychic images of past experience tailored to meet their ongoing psychological needs.

Psychoanalytic theory assumes that people inevitably transfer mental representations of relationships in childhood into current interactions. *Transference* is ubiquitous in ordinary mental life. For example, although an employee's coworkers may consider their boss fair-minded, the employee who envisions his boss as constantly undermining him may have formed a mental representation of the boss that merges with his image of his hypercritical father. When the intrusion of the father imago remains unconscious, the patient experiences a neurotic conflict. If the father transference were to intrude and become conscious in psychosis, he might say that his father was secretly in cahoots with the boss, that his boss is his father in disguise (Fregoli delusion), or that the impostor who claims to be his father began sabotaging his life after kidnapping and killing his real father (Capgras delusion). The psychological operations that create the distortions of mental representations that occur in DMI borrow from the transference operations of everyday life. Implicit in this object-related dyad is a story: sadistic father bars his son from pleasures in life to which the son is entitled.

Affectively charged mental representations become characters in delusional narratives. From an object relations view, delusions are stories played out between psychological objects that are mental representations of the self and others and that express and regulate the delusional person's emotional life (Garrett 2019). The content of DMI is constructed in the internal representational world of the patient.

Relationship Between the Capgras Delusion and Ordinary Mental Life

Patients do not create the idea of doubles de novo. Rather, the patient's attempt to explain the anomalous experience of unfamiliarity in Capgras syndrome recruits a duplicative *fantasy* with deep roots in myth, religion, and culture that the patient then confuses with reality (Currie 2000). Many examples of doubles can be found in mythology and the arts. For example, the Greek sea god Proteus, thought to embody the ever-changing moods of the sea in his ability to transform himself, is an example of imposture and intermetamorphosis in Greek mythology that survives in everyday English in the word *protean*, which means "versatile," "changeable," "adaptable." The goddess Athena is forever shape-shifting in Homer's *Odyssey*. In Robert Louis Stevenson's story, Mr. Hyde is the evil twin of the good Dr. Jekyll. In Fyodor Dostoyevsky's *The Possessed*, Nikolai Stavrogin is secretly married to Marya Lebyadkina, but at a public social gathering he avoids recognizing her as his wife. He draws her aside and counsels her to think of him in that setting as merely a friend rather than her husband. When Stavrogin visits her some days later, she refuses to recognize him, insisting he is an impostor who only resembles her husband and further charging that he has murdered her real husband. In the popular cable series *Game of Thrones*, Arya becomes a shape-shifter. In the Grimm Brothers' *Iron Henry*, a frog changes back and forth into a prince. Mark Twain played with doubles in *The Prince and the Pauper*. Some readers may recall Bizarro, a flawed double of Superman, who appeared periodically in Marvel comic books. The duplicating ray that created Bizarro also created other Bizarro clones and a Bizarro world on the planet Htrae ("Earth" spelled backward). And recall Bruce Banner, who morphs into the Incredible Hulk when he is enraged.

The double idea, once pressed into service to explain an anomalous experience, leads to a delusional narrative that features the self, the impostor, and the original in a story that captures the patient's imagination. The condensation of the double idea into a demarcated story helps to explain why the delusion typically selects one or only several family members rather than all family or all people, as one might expect in an indiscriminate biological disturbance. As is true for any story, delusional narratives work best with a protagonist and a limited number of characters. Nourished by its communal roots, the double idea settles into a delusional narrative.

Fantasies and stories about doubles, impostors, doppelgangers, or identical twins serve a variety of psychological purposes in nonpsychotic persons and Capgras patients. Doubles provide a means to escape death; many people believe that their existence will continue in an afterlife that, although not an exact duplicate of their current life, is a close-enough replica for them to enjoy the company of departed loved ones much as they once did. The fantasy of a double provides an alter ego that can express forbidden sexual and violent impulses prohibited to the self. The power to transform others into different forms can be used to redeem or punish them. Because of its deep psychological roots, the double idea readily occurs to the Capgras patient to explain an anomalous perception of unfamiliarity; it endures partly because it resonates with one or more of these themes. If one believes, as I do, that Capgras syndrome is a consequence of a disturbance in mental representations, and if we ask, this being the case, why Capgras and other DMI attract more attention than other delusions that are more common, we might conclude that just as the imagination of Capgras patients is captured by fantasies of doubles, so too the imagination of mental health professionals is captured by Capgras syndrome because it resonates with fantasies of doubles, twins, and doppelgangers latent in their psyches.

A Case of Animal Intermetamorphosis

Courbon and Tusques (1932) described a female with intermetamorphosis who experienced a progression of delusional beliefs culminating in Capgras syndrome. She believed first that two of her young hens had been switched for older ones and later that the man she had once regarded as her husband was the reincarnation of a neighbor. In this case, animal doubling preceded the Capgras delusion. Like most clinicians, my personal experience treating classic examples of Capgras imposture is limited: a young man who thought that his mother and all other people except himself were robots with simulated blood, not including a group of authentic women who had left Earth to colonize another planet and who remained in voice contact with him; and an adolescent who claimed his parents were impostors and ran away from home to pursue vagabond travels, as had his father when he was the same age.

Assuming that DMI lie along a continuum, I now describe a patient who did not experience classical Capgras delusions but who described what might be called the psychological intermetamorphosis of her cat. This case summary is intended to illustrate how disturbed patterns of childhood attachment and intense emotions in the present can combine to sculpt delusional mental representations of the self and others.

Case Example: Metamorphosis of a Pet Cat Into a Would-Be Murderer

Alicia believed that her once-beloved pet had transformed into a murderer. On the surface, her delusion appeared to be a truth claim about the world, but in psychotherapy the cat was revealed to be a persecutory object, a character in an allegorical story expressive of a terrible life crisis she was facing. Alicia had been physically and sexually abused as a child, but despite her consequent mistrust of most people, she had established a secure relationship with Valerie, her partner of 15 years. Alicia was referred to me by her prescribing psychiatrist for psychotherapy after she spiraled into a suicidal depression unresponsive to medication. Alicia reported that she felt suicidal because her cat was planning to murder her in order to have Valerie all to herself. The cat would do this, she thought, by biting her in the jugular one night as she lay asleep, as a lion might bring down a gazelle on the Serengeti.

The following backstory emerged in our first several sessions. Several weeks before the onset of the cat delusion, Valerie had taken a new job. Still insecure in her attachments, Alicia was accustomed to calling Valerie at work to "check in" several times a day, a routine they had both enjoyed for years. Alicia now sensed a hesitancy in Valerie's voice. Phone conversations felt rushed, as if Valerie wanted to get off the phone quickly. Alicia began to wonder whether she was tiring of their relationship. When she shared her concerns, Valerie explained that unlike her previous job, where her desk had been in a relatively private area, she now worked in an open space where her new boss discouraged private phone calls. She reassured Alicia that her brusqueness on the phone did not indicate any change in her feelings. These reassurances only made matters worse. Valerie's change of heart seemed so self-evident to Alicia that she could draw no other conclusion than that Valerie was lying. Her apparent withdrawal of love and her deceit terrified and infuriated Alicia. It was then that she came up with the cat idea.

When exactly had Alicia come to this belief? One night, as she and Valerie were about to go to sleep, she took special note of her cat lying down *between* the two of them. She had seen her cat do precisely this hundreds of times before, but in the context of Alicia's extreme emotional distress, this mundane event was perceived in an anomalous way with new personal meaning. The cat's *physical* coming between symbolized an *emotional* coming between that signaled the cat's intent to steal her partner. Just as patients with Capgras delusions draw on doubling stories available in their culture, Alicia drew on personal experiences of childhood abuse to compose a narrative of her partner, herself, and the cat. In CNP parlance, her altered experience of phone conversations and her altered perception of the cat were anomalous experiences of familiars that demanded an explanation. The seeming oddness of Valerie's phone conversations and the seemingly portentous gesture of the cat parallel the seeming oddness that Capgras patients perceive in a relative. Alicia's terror and anger, incited by the prospect of losing her partner's love, had transformed her mental representation of the cat into a persecutor and altered her perceptual experience of the world to correspond with her story.

The reader may wonder why Alicia did not just get rid of the cat. It was not because of a *deficit in belief evaluation* regarding the mental capacities of real cats. Alicia desperately needed to keep the cat in her delusional narrative for two reasons. First, she much preferred to believe that the cat had come between her and her partner rather than that Valerie had fallen out of love with her for some inexplicable reason she could do nothing about. If the cat was responsible, rather than Valerie, in Alicia's fantasy Valerie's love might still remain potentially intact and could possibly be reinstated. Alicia preferred to blame the other woman (the cat) rather than a philandering spouse. Second, in her delusional narrative, only one character was capable of murder—the cat. Alicia's rage at Valerie for betraying her went missing from her own mind and appeared in her mental representation of her pet. In this way, the cat was a projected disavowed aspect of herself.

Multifactor Models of Delusions of Misidentification

Having briefly outlined object relations theory and the case of Alicia, I now frame psychoanalytic object relations theory within a multifactor CNP model of delusion formation (Corlett et al. 2010; Garety et al. 2001; Langdon and Coltheart 2000). In their recent review of CNP, Connors and Halligan (2020) suggested that something may be missing from CNP theories and concluded that limitations encountered in CNP explanations of delusions may be due, "in part, to some of the inherent assumptions of cognitive neuropsychology and the failure to adopt methods for potentially non-modular processes." Unlike CNP, psychoanalytic models do not envision modular neurological deficits and do not expect that psychological disturbances are transparently expressed. Rather, they expect psychopathology to be articulated obliquely and symbolically, in the form of thoughts, feelings, and behavior whose less than fully conscious meaning must be inferred. I suggest that the absence of psychodynamic psychology in CNP models of delusions may in part account for the limitations in CNP models to which Connors and Halligan alluded.

Attention

A person's attention is drawn to an anomalous perception. A seemingly mundane event is given special attention because 1) its significance is promoted by a generalized biological process that enhances its salience, as with ideas of reference linked to excess dopamine; 2) as in Capgras delusions, a biological disturbance in the mental representation of the uniqueness of people and things confers a patina of peculiarity to otherwise familiar perceptions; or

3) the event symbolically resonates with an affectively charged unconscious object-related fantasy, which then infiltrates perception, leading to a subjective experience that feels odd because it is a hybrid of emotion and perception (Marcus 2017) that carries strong personal meaning for the patient. In such moments meaning is not experienced as a cognition about a perception, but rather the meaning of the event is fused with and seemingly self-evident in the perceptual experience itself. CBT for psychosis offers a powerful tool for separating cognitions from perceptions in psychotherapy.

In Capgras delusions, biology creates an anomalous state of familiarity that psychology secondarily elaborates with the impostor delusion. In the case of an event that resonates with a powerful object-related fantasy, psychology is primary and biology is secondary because the intrusion of an unconscious fantasy creates an anomalous experience of the real world that the patient elaborates in a delusional explanation. Alicia did not experience a biologically determined generalized disturbance of salience or familiarity. Rather, the resonance of the symbol of the cat's coming between her and her partner, driven by her terror and rage, transformed the mundane into the anomalous extraordinary.

Explanation

The anomalous experience invites an explanation. When the anomalous experience follows the intrusion of an unconscious fantasy, the explanation sought has in effect already been formulated in the unconscious object-related dyad that is expressed in a delusion in which a psychological object is doing something to the self or the self is doing something to an object. In Alicia's case, her mental representation of her cat as intent on stealing her partner's love was shaped by mental representations of caregivers who had neglected her in childhood. In cases of Capgras delusions traceable to disturbances in face recognition or another biological cause, the anomalous experience of a familiar face resonates with a fantasy of doubles that suffuses the human imagination and that the individual patient embellishes and elaborates with specific personal meanings.

Privileged Hypothesis

Hypotheses are privileged according to individual personal biases (e.g., jumping to conclusions, first-person sensory information, externalizing biases). Regardless of whether biology or psychology is primary in the genesis of the anomalous perceptual experience, as it resonates with an activated fantasy, the delusional belief becomes the privileged hypothesis. Invested with significant affect, as was true in Alicia's case, the delusion *feels* real, and this *feeling of reality* is mistaken for reality proper. The fantasy-based hypothesis is privileged because the patient *feels* that something they have long unconsciously imagined has come true. To the extent that a biologically based alteration of the conscious experience of uniqueness and familiarity persists, a bias in favor of first-person, observationally adequate current experience would be expected to inevitably overwhelm past beliefs about reality. Jamais vécu–like self-states that last for months and even years eventually are seen as incontrovertible evidence in support of the delusion.

Reevaluation

The prioritized list is subject to a rational unbiased reconsideration that does not automatically advance one hypothesis over others. This is a crucial—if not *the* crucial—step in CNP two-factor models, which posit a *deficit in belief reevaluation* that fails to question delusional hypotheses that defy common sense. From a psychoanalytic perspective, it is not only, or even primarily, the absence of cognitive belief reevaluation but rather the presence of psychological processes essential to the maintenance of the delusion that are not, in their essence, rational. The phrase *reality testing* has a scientific ring implying that knowledge of what is real is based on a data-driven cognitive testing process that discriminates fantasy from reality. This is not entirely true. Nonpsychotic persons have little trouble distinguishing perceptions of the real world from wishful thinking, daydreams, and other instances of imagination without submitting these states of mind to a reality test. In areas of experience not caught up in a delusion, persons with psychosis are generally able to do the same. They know very well how to move around their apartment without trying to walk through a wall. They may say of their conviction that their neighbor is a government agent or that their spouse is an impostor, "I know what it feels like to imagine things, like flying to the moon. When I am thinking about my neighbor, I don't feel at all like how I feel when I am imagining something." Consensual reality requires that a person maintain differentiated subjective boundaries between thoughts, feelings, fantasies, perceptions, and memories. Because these boundaries blur in psychosis, a delusion explaining an anomalous event that is a hybrid of emotion and perception endures because it is *felt* to be true.

A delusion is a story that is in some way meaningfully (symbolically) expressive of a person's mental life. One would not expect a symbol or metaphor to dissolve in response to a cognitive challenge. For example, if someone were to tell you, "She is a breath of fresh air!" you might say, "I know her; that is so true." You would not say, "That's ridiculous. A person isn't a breeze. You are delusional. You suffer from a deficit in belief reevaluation." To the extent that a delusion is a symbolic expression framed in an allegorical story, one would not expect it to yield to a logical argument. Failure to recognize an utterance as having a metaphorical dimension creates the impression of a *deficit in belief reevaluation*. In an integrated approach to the treatment of psychosis, psychopharmacology aims to dissipate the biological base of anomalous experiences, and in psychotherapy, cognitive-behavioral techniques provide a superior method for helping a patient see the *literal falsity* of delusions and a psychodynamic approach helps the patient to explore the *figurative truth* of the delusion.

CNP models postulate deficits in belief reevaluation in comparison with Aristotelian logic, a rule set in which A cannot be simultaneously B or partially B. Yet in psychosis, A and B are readily assumed to be the same on the basis of what is known as *predicate logic*, in which if the subjects of two statements share the same predicate, they are considered the same: for example, "The president lives in a white house. I live in a white house. Therefore, I am the president." The thinking of persons with psychosis follows definable rules, but the rules are not Aristotelian. In *Interpretation of Schizophrenia*, an important book rarely cited in CNP models, Silvano Arieti (1974) detailed this conception of cognition in psychosis.

Circumscribed Delusion

Instead of rejecting the delusional hypothesis as inconsistent with prior experience or suspending judgment ("I don't know"), the patient not only embraces the delusional belief but also looks for confirmatory evidence that supports it. From a psychoanalytic point of view, although the delusional belief is literally false, it is in some way figuratively true. The delusion survives in a mental space cordoned off from consensual reality similar to the psychic arena where daydreams are entertained, but with an essential difference. In ordinary daydreaming, the daydreamer can multitask, attending to reality and fantasy at the same time, ready to snap back into reality as need be. Delusional people are like daydreamers who are too desperately invested in their imaginings to muster much interest in consensual reality. Rarely do patients act as one would expect were the delusion essentially a truth claim about the real world. Instead, the delusion becomes a circumscribed expression and central regulator of emotional life.

Finally, I would like to say something more about the mental duplicating process in DMI. Alterations of self-experience are common in, even pathognomonic of, psychosis, including feelings of *diminished ipseity* (the vital three-dimensional self normally at the center of experience fades) and *hyperreflexive self-awareness* (people become observers of their thoughts rather than fluent thinkers of their thoughts, and their thoughts take on the quality of perceived objects) (Sass and Parnas 2003). In my opinion, the curious doubling effect reported in DMI may occur when persons with psychosis call to mind the mental representations of themselves and doubles featured in their DMI stories, when, in a state of diminished ipseity and hyperreflexive self-awareness, they observe their mental representations of the characters in their delusional narratives as if they were perceiving objects and people. In a cognitive sequence that approaches a regression of mirrors, an image comes to mind that has the quality of a perceived object, and in the process of continuing to think about that image, in a state of hyperreflexive self-awareness, these persons observe themselves observing, which results in a seeming second perception of the image, which is experienced as a double of the initial mental representation, a sequence of thinking about thinking that can be multiplied to a third or beyond in DMI. To coin a word, the *perceivedness* of the mental representation creates the illusion of duplicated objects. The duplicating process in DMI may function like a kind of echo chamber for thoughts. I was led to this idea by a patient who heard the voice of an entity he called MindGirl, who repeated his thoughts to him verbatim as they emerged in his stream of consciousness. In a state of hyperreflexive self-awareness, his monitoring of his own thoughts resulted in a hallucinated echo of his thoughts—that is, his thoughts were doubled.

In conclusion, I have characterized Capgras delusions and other DMI as likely issuing from a generalized disturbance of the subjective experience of familiarity, which constitutes an anomalous experience that, in keeping with CNP two-factor models, invites an explanation that leads to a delusion. The anomalous experience of altered familiarity may result from biological distortions of perception or from the intrusion of intense object-related fantasies that distort perceptions of reality. The DMI delusion condenses around an object-related fantasy that is expressed in a delusional narrative. Construing DMI as disturbances in internal object relations rather than as disorders of perceptual stimuli helps the therapist to understand the varying phenomenology and the persistence of DMI delusions, as in the following case example of treatment provided by Douglas Turkington, with commentary by the chapter author (M.G.). See also Video 13 and Chapter 20, "Decoding Delusions."

 Video 13: Capgras Intervention

Case Example: A Case of Capgras Delusion ("Her Upstairs")

Robert had been given a diagnosis of schizophrenia and was maintained on a depot antipsychotic. His core delusion was that his mother, whom he lived with and who looked after him, was not his real mother but an impostor who looked like his mother and dressed similarly. He also had a delusion that he had won the lottery and his prize was being withheld. Despite his symptoms, Robert was working in a supported placement. His attitude toward his mother was dismissive and at times argumentative. His mother tended to occupy the upstairs rooms in the house, and he referred to her as "her upstairs." Interestingly, Robert was dismissive and hostile to female mental health professionals and social workers but polite and respectful to male staff, which in psychodynamic terms likely reflected a negative maternal transference.

Engagement in CBT was attempted by a male therapist under supervision. Peripheral and Socratic questioning about the Capgras delusion were unhelpful, and Robert did not entertain any alternative hypotheses. He learned a coping strategy of mindful walking, which he used as a form of distraction when becoming stressed by his delusions. A therapeutic alliance was partly formed, but little progress was made until Robert was working on the timeline and remembering the period of time prior to the emergence of the Capgras delusion. Helping a patient to construct a timeline grounded in a linear narrative frame helps some patients gain access to painful recollections otherwise repressed. Robert vividly recalled an incident under a bridge. It related to a real episode when he was 7 years old and his parents were separated. He was living with his father, who took him to visit his mother at a meeting under a bridge. By his report, his mother did not behave in the way expected. He thought that his mother would have been very affectionate toward him but perceived her as being angry, being distressed and rejecting of him, and focusing her attentions on his father. He was upset at his mother's behavior and remembered being puzzled on the drive back home and wondering if the woman they had met really was his real mother.

All episodic memory is to some degree shaped by fantasy. As a child, Robert had been unable to experience the encounter under the bridge in any way other than a child's self-referential way ("She doesn't love me" vs. "Adult relationships are complicated. She was preoccupied trying to reconcile with my father, so she didn't pay attention to me"). Fifteen years later, he developed delusional mood following a difficult work situation and one day realized that his real mother had been murdered. He remembered seeing an item of what he believed to be her clothing on the *Crimewatch* television program. At that moment, many years after the incident under the bridge, the crime show provided a bridge into consciousness for what had been a childhood memory that the woman under the bridge could not have been his mother. The crime show was a nidus in the present around which a traumatic memory could crystalize as the Capgras delusion.

Why 15 years after the bridge? It is likely that some mounting grievance against "her upstairs" led him to perceive the clothing on the crime show as belonging to his real mother, who must have been murdered. In his fantasy, if his real mother had been taking care of him rather than the impostor upstairs, he surely would have fared better in life. From that point on, his behavior toward his mother changed dramatically. CBT focused on a role-play of the scene under the bridge, with Robert and the therapist playing the different roles of father, mother, and son. This processing of the emotions from the time and reframing of the meaning of the event facilitated a change in his behavior toward his mother and female mental health staff. He was less dismissive and less hostile. The Capgras delusion had not disappeared but seemed to be less troublesome and probably less dangerous.

Personal Reflection

Consider a moment in everyday life when you may feel confused about the identify of another person, an occasion that provides an opportunity to explore connections between belief formation in everyday life and DMI. For example: While walking on a sidewalk, you see a person halfway down the block who looks like a female colleague and friend. As you approach each other, you prepare to say hello, but shee abruptly turns and crosses the street, appearing not to have noticed you. You wonder, is the person who just now crossed the street really your friend, or is she a stranger who resembles her? You wonder, if the person is your friend, is she pretending not to see you to avoid you—a distressing thought—or was she absorbed in her thoughts and truly didn't notice you? Perplexed and taken aback that your colleague might be avoiding you, a dark thought crosses your mind that in your imagination rescues your friendship but creates new anxieties: "Maybe it was someone pretending to be my colleague? That would explain the resemblance and the avoidance. Whatever her motive, she didn't want me to get close enough to uncover her disguise." Noticing moments like this one in your mental life can support connection to and understanding of individuals who present with DMI.

Questions for Discussion

1. Looking back at the personal reflection, can you think of times that this has happened for you? How would you think this situation through? Was it your mistake in identifying a stranger as a friend, a distracted or avoidant friend, or a person in disguise? All these explanations are a conceivably true. How would you entertain a range of alternative beliefs in a situation like this one in which certainty about reality is not immediately self-evident?

2. In addition to the examples in the chapter, can you think of any other examples of the fantasy of duplicates in popular culture, in films, television programs, books, or other art forms?

KEY POINTS

- Capgras syndrome is best considered not as a distinct disorder with a distinct etiology but rather one example among many of delusions of misidentification (DMI) that occur frequently in people given a diagnosis of schizophrenia and in patients otherwise diagnosed.

• Because DMI may include a belief that things a person has never seen are fraudulent or duplicated, as in the belief that one's inner organs have been falsified, DMI are perhaps best thought of as disturbances of representations of internal psychological objects rather than disturbances of perception.

• Brain lesions are found in some but not all patients with DMI, which suggests that the organic pathology associated with DMI may reside in disturbances of connectivity rather than localized brain injury.

• In keeping with the two-factor neuropsychiatric model of delusion formation, DMI patients use fantasies of doppelgangers and other such fantasies of cloning and duplication that occur in ordinary mental life to explain their anomalous experience of recognizing but not emotionally connecting with an otherwise familiar person.

• DMI may respond to neuroleptics, psychotherapy, or a combination of both.

References

Arieti S: Interpretation of Schizophrenia, 2nd Edition. New York, Basic Books, 1974

Bentall RP, Kinderman P, Kaney S: The self, attributional processes and abnormal beliefs: towards a model of persecutory delusions. Behav Res Ther 32(3):331–341, 1994 8192633

Berson RJ: Capgras' syndrome. Am J Psychiatry 140(8):969–978, 1983 6869616

Capgras J, Reboul-Lachaux J: L'illision des socies dans un deliere systematise chronique. Bull Soc Clin Med Ment 11:6–16, 1923

Christodoulou GN: Syndrome of subjective doubles. Am J Psychiatry 135(2):249–251, 1978 623347

Christodoulou GN: Role of depersonalization-derealization phenomena in the delusional misidentification syndromes. Bibl Psychiatr (164):99–104, 1986 3718466

Christodoulou GN, Margariti M, Kontaxakis VP, Christodoulou NG: The delusional misidentification syndromes: strange, fascinating, and instructive. Curr Psychiatry Rep 11(3):185–189, 2009 19470279

Connors MH, Halligan PW: Delusions and theories of belief. Conscious Cogn 81:102935, 2020 32334355

Corlett PR, Taylor JR, Wang XJ, et al: Toward a neurobiology of delusions. Prog Neurobiol 92(3):345–369, 2010 20558235

Courbon P, Tusques J: L'illusion d'intermetamorphose et de charmes. Ann Med Psychol (Paris) 90:401, 1932

Currie G: Imagination, delusion and hallucinations, in Pathologies of Belief. Edited by Coltheart M, Davies M. Oxford, UK, Blackwell, 2000, pp 167–182

Ellis HD, Lewis MB: Capgras delusion: a window on face recognition. Trends Cogn Sci 5(4):149–156, 2001 11287268

Ellis HD, Young AW: Accounting for delusional misidentifications. Br J Psychiatry 157:239–248, 1990 2224375

Fialkov MJ, Robins AH: An unusual case of the Capgras syndrome. Br J Psychiatry 132(4):403–404, 1978 638395

Garety PA, Kuipers E, Fowler D, et al: A cognitive model of the positive symptoms of psychosis. Psychol Med 31(2):189–195, 2001 11232907

Garrett M: Psychotherapy for Psychosis: Integrating Cognitive-Behavioral and Psychodynamic Treatment. New York, Guilford, 2019

Kapur S: Psychosis as a state of aberrant salience: a framework linking biology, phenomenology, and pharmacology in schizophrenia. Am J Psychiatry 160(1):13–23, 2003 12505794

Kernberg O: Object-Relations Theory and Clinical Psychoanalysis. New York, Jason Aronson, 1976

Klein M: A contribution to the psychogenesis of manic-depressive states. Int J Psychoanal 16:145–174, 1935

Langdon R, Coltheart M: The cognitive neuropsychology of delusions, in Pathologies of Belief. Edited by Coltheart M, Davies M. Oxford, UK, Blackwell, 2000, pp 183–216

Maher B: Anomalous experience and delusional thinking: the logic of explanations, in Delusional Beliefs. Edited by Oltmanns TF, Maher BA. New York, Wiley, 1988, pp 15–33

Marcus ER: Psychosis and Near Psychosis: Ego Function, Symbol Structure, Treatment, 3rd Edition. New York, Routledge, 2017

Margariti MM, Kontaxakis VP: Approaching delusional misidentification syndromes as a disorder of the sense of uniqueness. Psychopathology 39(6):261–268, 2006 16960464

Pandis C, Agrawal N, Poole NA: Capgras' delusion: a systematic review of 255 published cases. Psychopathology 52(3):161–173, 2019 31326968

Sass LA, Parnas J: Schizophrenia, consciousness, and the self. Schizophr Bull 29(3):427–444, 2003 14609238

Sengoku A, Toichi M, Murai T: Dreamy states and psychoses in temporal lobe epilepsy: mediating role of affect. Psychiatry Clin Neurosci 51(1):23–26, 1997 9076856

Sinkman A: The syndrome of Capgras. Psychiatry 71(4):371–378, 2008 19152286

Sno HN: A continuum of misidentification symptoms. Psychopathology 27(3–5):144–147, 1994 7846229

Thompson MI, Silk KR, Hover GL: Misidentification of a city: delimiting criteria for Capgras syndrome. Am J Psychiatry 137(10):1270–1272, 1980 7416284

Tranel D, Damasio H, Damasio AR: Double dissociation between overt and covert face recognition. J Cogn Neurosci 7(4):425–432, 1995 23961902

Vie J: Un trouble d l'idenfication des personnes: l'illusion des sosies. Ann Med Psychol (Paris) 88:214–237, 1930

Young G: Delusional Misidentification. New York, Nova Science, 2010

14

Thought Disorder or a Problem With Communication?

David Kingdon, M.D., FRCPsych
Kate V. Hardy, Clin.Psych.D.
Kenneth Sandoval Jr., M.S., M.S.W., LCSW

Thought disorder is a broad term that can cover both the form and the content of thoughts. When thought disorder concerns the *content* of thoughts, it is referred to as a *delusion*, an *overvalued idea*, or an *obsession*. However, thought disorder is more commonly used as shorthand for disordered speech, and in this chapter we focus on such abnormality of form and process and how this relates to any linked delusion. When the term thought disorder is used to refer to the form and process of speech, the focus is specifically on the articulation or communication of thoughts, and thus this is also typically referred to as *disorganized speech* or *formal thought disorder*. DSM-5 (American Psychiatric Association 2022) includes formal thought disorder as a key symptom in the diagnosis of schizophrenia and other psychotic disorders (Roche et al. 2015), and this disorder has been shown to have a negative impact on social functioning, which indicates the potential for significant disability. In addition, clinicians may find it challenging to engage and understand patients who are presenting with thought disorder in therapy, and there is a risk that these individuals may slip through the cracks if treatment providers are potentially overwhelmed by the presence of disordered speech or pessimistic about the potential for therapeutic change because of communication difficulties. Thus, it is essential to consider key intervention techniques to support individuals with disorganized speech when working with false beliefs.

A fundamental question is whether the process of thought disorder, or its form, is actually a disorder of production or communication. Is it a disorder of *thoughts* (i.e., the production and flow of thoughts), or is it a disorder of *communication* (i.e., the individual has difficulty articulating and communicating their thoughts to others)? Therapeutically speaking, cognitive therapists have focused on the latter (Kingdon and Turkington 1994, 2005; Turkington and Kingdon 1991). The intention has been to understand what the individual is trying to convey—and it has been presumed that this is possible—rather than assuming that the thoughts are unintelligible, nonsensical, and essentially beyond comprehension. The individual may be very difficult to understand, and their experiences and beliefs difficult to convey, but taking the time and effort to work with different forms of thought disorder can be highly effective and can improve communication in a way that in turn results in a rich and informative formulation. Such a formulation will often make sense of the delusional content as well. Subsequently, this is very engaging for the individual, who begins to feel that they are being understood or at least that the practitioner is making every effort to comprehend that person's experience. However, this is not always an easy process, and, as we demonstrate in this chapter, different techniques may be used to support interventions when working with thought disorder. It may be that family, friends, community members, or practitioners who are familiar with the person and their culture can be enlisted to aid this communication process when progress is initially proving difficult. Ultimately, taking the stance that thought disorder is a disorder of communication and is fundamentally understandable aligns with the normalizing and recovery-oriented philosophy of many psychotherapeutic approaches for working with psychosis, including cognitive-behavioral therapy for psychosis (CBTp).

Key Features of Thought Disorder

Thought disorder is somewhat disregarded in diagnoses in which positive symptoms (delusions and hallucinations) and, variably, negative symptoms are more prominent but usually features in broader descriptions of psychosis. In contrast, Bleuler (1951) described a loosening in the association of ideas as one of the primary and fundamental disturbances in "the group of schizophrenias." Overinclusiveness in thinking, described by Cameron (cited by Mayer-Gross et al. 1969), has also been regarded as an important feature involving the "inclusion of irrelevant ideas and confusion of thought" (p. 265). Schilder (also cited by Mayer-Gross et al. 1969) conceptualized conscious thinking as guided by a "determinative idea"—a goal toward which clear and relevant thoughts progress—and therefore formal thought disorder as an interference in this process.

Detecting Thought Disorder

Thought disorder can be detected through an examination of writing, art, music, or the spoken word. The latter is most common, but disruption in written communication also occurs frequently and sometimes displays thought disorder more clearly with confusing sentence structures. When an individual is writing lengthy descriptions, the descriptions can be used to assess thought disorder and may also provide an insight into traumatic events or issues pertinent to the individual. Art can also be abstract but meaningful, although explanations may be essential to understand its significance.

Disorder of the stream of thinking is quite common. This includes *thought blocking*, which may be described as going blank or an abrupt and complete emptying of mind. The flow of speech may reduce considerably, resulting in *poverty of speech* and *poverty of content*, in which what is said is limited and lacks variety and spontaneity. It is important to note that this is different from experiencing a distraction or intrusion of a different line of thinking. When an individual is distracted by internal or external stimuli or is experiencing intrusion of a different line of thinking, there can appear to be a *loosening of associations*, which makes it difficult to follow the train of thought as spoken aloud. Examples of this include *knight's move thinking*, in which the individual switches to a different line of thought that is linked but tenuously so; *derailment*, when thinking goes off in a direction without completion of the initial expression; *circumstantial thinking*, in which thinking progresses along a line of thought and covers a number of seemingly unrelated topics before returning to the initial subject area; and *tangential thinking*, in which the conversation progresses abruptly to a completely different subject area without ever returning to the initial subject. *Flight of ideas*, which is said to be more common in mania as seen in bipolar disorder, can also occur in psychosis, and here speech jumps between different topics that are somewhat tenuously linked either by subject, puns, or the sounds of the words (clanging). When the stream of thought becomes particularly distorted, the words may lose grammatical structure and manifest as a word salad. *Pressured speech* may also be present, whereby the individual produces rapid speech without pause that is difficult for the interviewer to interrupt. In addition, speech can be *perseverative*, whereby a single word or topic is repeated, or can echo the speech of the interviewer, as is the case in *echolalia*.

Sometimes speech can appear, and be, witty, facetious, or jocular—words used outside of their context but in an original way that can be quite illuminating and creative—or it can be garrulous and actually off-putting to the listener, thus affecting personal relationships and potentially the ability to form a therapeutic relationship. Philosophical and mystical or technological content may fill the conversation, and the person may write copiously but with a high degree of idiosyncrasy, including books, epistles, plays, and poetry. However, it is essential to consider whether the deficit in understanding lies in the presentation by the individual or in the reception by the listener. For example, the clinician may erroneously assess the individual as creating neologisms (new words) or new ideas if the person repeatedly uses a concept, word, or phrase with which the clinician is unfamiliar.

The person's awareness of problems in communicating thoughts may be explained as perplexity, bewilderment, poor concentration, or emptiness. A "woolly" vagueness may be present. The content of speech may involve alliterations, analogies, symbolic meanings, or the condensation of topics or words into neologisms or hybrids, such as the use of "unillegal" to mean totally illegal.

Speech can become highly idiosyncratic, for example, using private meanings, or writings can use punctuation and grammar in eccentric or simply incorrect ways. Words similarly may not just be made up but may also include known words that have private individual meanings attached that can sometimes be very difficult to elicit. For example, "exactment" might be used to convey something about precision but with a powerful but unclear additional meaning of considerable importance to the individual. The challenge, therefore, is to detect thought disorder, achieve improved communication, and then work toward an exploration of the delusional content and impact and toward recovery.

Case Example

Kelly was hospitalized for physically assaulting her boyfriend. She believed that he was working for her enemies and trying to take her children. She also believed that she was being imprisoned at the hospital against her will, leaving her children vulnerable to harm. Kelly was referred for CBTp because of ongoing refractory symptoms of psychosis, specifically, profound symptoms of thought disorder and fixed systematized delusional beliefs. Kelly's symptoms prevented effective communication with others, which had adverse impacts on her ability to benefit from treatment on the unit. CBTp was initiated with the aim of increasing Kelly's ability to communicate effectively with others in an effort to improve her engagement in treatment and thereby improve her overall prognosis.

At the onset of treatment, Kelly presented with unique strongly held beliefs, rapid speech, interweaving delusional themes, neologisms, words with private meanings, and tangential thought processes. Kelly believed that she was the queen of an alien race engaged in a civil war for control of her planet. Kelly further believed that she and her children were hiding on Earth to avoid being harmed or captured by her enemies. Kelly used idiosyncratic forms of communication, such as neologisms and clanging. She refused to use traditional words and phrases, fearing that if she did, her enemies would learn that she was hiding on Earth with her children and would find them. These idiosyncratic forms of communication made it extremely difficult for others to understand her. In addition, her rapid speech and her jumping from one bizarre topic to the next made conversations difficult to follow.

Psychological and Social Causes of Thought Disorder

Communication is a social process shaped through reciprocal exchanges. A key contributor to formal thought disorder is considered to be a lack of communication practice, such that communication is often replaced by an internal dialogue. In other words, being isolated or living in an environment where communication is fraught and confusing can lead to a lack of opportunities to interact meaningfully with others. This has particularly been an issue in large psychiatric hospitals, where patients may have very limited opportunities for social interaction and rewarding communication exchanges. However, it can also occur at home or in community dwellings where communication opportunities are limited. Over years this can lead to a withering away of communication skills and the development of idiosyncratic ways of communicating. Thoughts still flow in the person's mind but may evolve in a nonconstructive way, which makes it increasingly difficult for them to be understood by others when they do finally start to speak. Attempts to communicate may then be met with confusion, dismissal, or colluding and unintentionally patronizing responses, resulting in the individual further limiting their communication and an increase in isolation. As seen in the case example, social isolation was a causative factor in Kelly's thought disorder.

There is some evidence that community-based services, in which living arrangements for people with persistent psychosis are in small-scale community settings instead of large psychiatric hospitals, lead to an increase in social networks. Leff and Trieman (2000) followed up with a large cohort of patients who left mental hospitals in London as they closed and concluded, "There was no change in the patients' clinical state or in their problems of social behaviour. However, they gained domestic and community living skills. They also acquired friends and confidants" (p. 217).

Anxiety needs to be considered an important cause of thought disorder, and this can lead to rambling, speaking too quickly, losing the flow of thought, interrupting, difficulty in interacting, and an increase in unintelligibility. Thought blocking is often confused with not speaking or being overly talkative, particularly when an individual is experiencing stress. Struggling to convey meaning may lead to the formation of new words that, if not questioned, can become entrenched. Without feedback from people in their environment, individuals may not recognize that they are not being understood, and thus communication challenges persist and become reinforced. The anxiety related to the delusion about harm to her children would have been a powerful factor in exacerbating Kelly's thought disorder.

Thought disorder can also be affected by more general learning disabilities and by physical health problems, such as deafness and speech impairment. These should be considered during assessment in order to have a fuller understanding of the contributory factors. It is also important to assess for the presence of delusional thinking that may contribute to disorganized communication. For example, an individual could hold the belief that they are the leader of an alien nation committed to a vow of silence who will communicate via hieroglyphs representative of an ancient alien language. Thought disorder may become linked to or even lead to delusions. Blocking can be interpreted as thought withdrawal, in which the person thinks that their thoughts are being removed by someone, an organization (e.g., the government), or something (e.g., aliens or satellites), or similarly, they may believe that their ability to think is being interfered with, as part of paranoid beliefs. Thought insertion may similarly have a delusional interpretation. For example, the individual may believe that thoughts are being put into their mind by others, especially if these thoughts are unpleasant, violent, or sexual in content.

It may also be necessary to consider the potential for a defensive function to the thought disorder. For example, communication may become more disorganized when the person is recounting traumatic experiences or current stressors and thus may serve as a way to avoid discussion of these topics. Conversely, speech may become more organized when the person is recounting past events (including traumatic ones) that preceded the onset of psychosis or describing neutral, non-psychosis-based topics. Being aware of this in the interview and monitoring for changes in speech and the severity of thought disorder throughout the exchange can provide valuable insights into the influence of topics on the presence of disordered speech.

Personal Reflection

Psychotic experiences are considered on a continuum, and the same paradigm can be applied to thought disorder. Imagine being in an important job interview and being asked a question. It is quite feasible that you feel anxious in this situation, and as you start to answer you become an observer of your communication and possibly aware of thoughts that you are having while answering the question. These thoughts might include "Am I making sense?" "Do they like this answer?" "Oh goodness, I can't believe I just said that; they are going to think I am stupid," or "Shut up, shut up, shut up." However, you continue to answer the question, and you notice that the response is becoming slightly garbled: you started talking about your experience pertinent to the position, but now you are telling a story about a chicken and you are not quite sure how you got there. As you check in on the interview panel, you notice their eyes have glazed over, people are starting to shift uncomfortably, one interviewer has a fixed smile on her face, and there is one person who is nodding encouragingly and willing you to finish the sentence. With that, you trail off into a series of mumbles and "I hope I answered your question" before bolting for the door. Although this does not portray the full extent of experiencing thought disorder, it does highlight the role anxiety can play in disordered speech production and the influence of observers engaged in the exchange.

Prognosis and Cultural Aspects of Thought Disorder

Thought disorder may follow a worsening trajectory over time, and early intervention for individuals with psychosis offers the opportunity to directly intervene to prevent this (Roche et al. 2015). There does seem to be an overall reduction in the severity, frequency, and presentation of thought disorder in clinical practice observable over the past 40–50 years, which suggests that increased awareness of the importance of intervening early and the shift toward community-based and recovery-oriented care that engages individuals with psychosis in meaningful social role functioning may be having a positive impact.

Cultural issues always need to be taken into account in the context of whether an unusual belief is culturally syntonic or a delusion and whether thought disorder is or is not present. Consultation with natural supports who are familiar with the individual can aid in this process by highlighting changes in speech from baseline and also identifying speech structure that may be consistent with the cultural background of the individual. For example, some cultures may use more metaphors and abstract ideas to describe difficulties and emotional or physical pain. Communication difficulties may be due to misunderstanding by the practitioner or therapist. When either the therapist or the individual is communicating in a non-native language, strong accents and colloquialisms may make communication more challenging even without the presence of thought disorder. When such difficulties are present, there are more opportunities for language to be misunderstood, and these challenges may become more extreme if the individual is agitated or anxious. When the individual has limited social contact beyond their family, there may be a type of shorthand communication that has developed among family members that is learned and reinforced within the family system. Thus, family members may be able to act as translators, but it is important that they are used only as a bridge, with the intent of supporting the individual in communicating effectively with people outside the family as well.

Case Example (*continued*): Progress With Cognitive-Behavioral Therapy for Psychosis

Kelly's history of bizarre beliefs and disorganized behaviors secondary to command hallucinations caused multiple problems in her life. She began to experience interpersonal difficulties, increased stress at work, social isolation, and a worsening of psychosis over time. These problems also led to her physically assaulting her boyfriend, which had resulted in her current hospitalization. Prior to Kelly's hospitalization, her family had become increasingly concerned about her welfare and the welfare of her children. In the weeks prior to Kelly's physical assault on her boyfriend, she was experiencing a multitude of stressors. Kelly was working two jobs, and she was the primary support system for her two young children. Her delusional fear of being discovered by her enemies led to increased isolation, and eventually to Kelly losing her job, and her kids stopped attending school. Kelly was engaged in an unhealthy intimate relationship fraught with arguments and physical fighting, which made it difficult for her to learn how to communicate with others in a healthy and constructive manner and contributed to the development of her idiosyncratic communication style. Kelly's fixed delusional system also contributed to the ongoing development of her thought disorder. Specifically, her belief that she was from another planet and needed to communicate through neologisms and clanging made communicating with Kelly difficult and confusing for others. Prior to Kelly being hospitalized, her beliefs and behaviors had led to her causing serious harm to others. The assault on her boyfriend caused her significant ongoing emotional pain and distress. Thus, many of her beliefs served to protect her from this intense emotional pain (guilt).

Historically, Kelly's delusional system reinforced her safety behavior of isolating, which led to a worsening of her psychosis, a decreased need for sleep, and criminal behaviors and strengthened the fear of losing her children. This fear in turn contributed to the development of her thought disorder.

Addressing Thought Disorder

As already highlighted, clinicians may find thought disorder intimidating and overwhelming, so they feel unable to work therapeutically. Sitting with someone who is producing incomprehensible speech can certainly be challenging, and clinicians may feign understanding of what someone is trying to communicate for fear of appearing ignorant or impolite. The practitioner may feel able to deal only with basic practical issues, such as medication management, or may simply give up altogether and not try to pursue conversation. However, as demonstrated earlier, ignoring or passively listening to the disorganized speech and not attempting to clarify, provide feedback, or intervene is potentially counterproductive, and by taking this approach we as clinicians are doing patients a huge disservice. It can also lead to frustration on both sides. In contrast, using skills to explore thought disorder can lead to a rich narrative that can aid formulation over time, support the individual in learning more adaptive communication strategies, and, most important—even when communication remains difficult—improve the therapeutic relationship, which ultimately may aid social recovery.

Working with thought disorder is primarily a communication task in understanding what the person is trying to convey. It requires patience, perseverance, and sometimes imagination on both sides. Working from a strong therapeutic relationship is essential, but time spent supporting effective communication will also enhance this relationship (see Chapter 7, "Collaboration, Not Collusion"). The content of what is articulated, and how it influences communication, will need to be addressed, but this is not the focus of this chapter.

Establishing a Goal for Addressing Thought Disorder

Establishing a goal for addressing thought disorder allows the clinician to name challenges in understanding the patient's communication style. As mentioned previously, this can feel uncomfortable for many clinicians. However, it is important to remember that the clinician is coming from a position of genuinely wanting to understand the experience of the patient, and the current communication style is making this challenging. Presenting this goal as a genuine desire to understand the patient's perspective and being willing to put in extra effort to structure the session to ensure the goal is met can help address any discomfort the patient or clinician may feel.

Assessing Thought Disorder

Assessing thought disorder is part of the overall process of gathering information and developing a therapeutic relationship. Recognizing different examples and causes of thought disorder (as described previously) can help to disentangle the presentation. When thought disorder is present and in what context need to be monitored. When a patient presents with thought disorder in the acute phases of illness, they are likely to improve quickly with other treatments, such as stress management and medication. Nevertheless, working to develop communication and the relationship is critically important to future progress and collaboration so that valuable time and understanding are not lost while waiting until the patient is better.

Understanding the circumstances that lead to the psychosis and being able to prompt if necessary or recognize that unusual references are related to recent or past experiences or a delusional belief can help form a better understanding of this experience. Looking for associations with unpleasant, unhappy, or traumatic events can provide clues to obscure connections or neologisms generally. Curious exploration of the meanings of words or connections through gentle Socratic questioning can demonstrate a genuine interest in the internal experience of the individual and can support collaborative exploration and express a commitment to developing a shared understanding. Family, friends, and cultural supports can decipher comments that may seem unintelligible to the uninitiated and may be helpful in supporting communication initially. Examining the thought disorder can provide valuable clues to underlying processes related to belief formation and history because the disorder can become more pronounced and interfere with communication when troubling events, thoughts, or periods in the person's life are recounted.

Thought-disordered speech can be challenging to follow, and the clinician may find that at the end of the session they are unable to repeat content verbatim. They may be fully aware that a lot of speech occurred but be unable to recount exactly what was discussed or the topics covered. This is because the idiosyncratic nature of the speech does not fit into a generally accepted rubric of reciprocal speech and speech comprehension. Assessment of thought disorder can be greatly helped if the clinician is able to write down verbatim key phrases and concepts that can be reviewed at a later date. If possible, recording the session can also be helpful for assessment and, as will be seen later, may aid intervention. Simply slowing the pace of speech and taking one phrase or sentence at a time can do much to help elucidate meaning.

Formulating Thought Disorder and Delusions

Formulation of thought disorder sits within the broader case conceptualization, but its links to thoughts, feelings, behaviors, and events can be worth pulling out in its own right, especially when thought disorder is impeding management, constructive interaction, and recovery (Palmier-

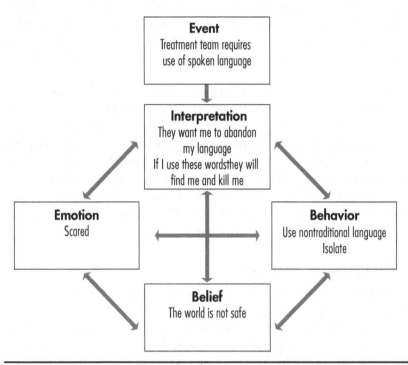

FIGURE 14–1. Cognitive-behavioral therapy for psychosis case formulation for Kelly. .

Claus et al. 2017). Case formulation helps the therapist understand the patient and their symptoms in cognitive terms; this process is dynamic and guides intervention. Kelly's delusional system involved a fear for the safety of her family and adversely impacted how she communicated with others. Therefore, a primary goal of treatment was to help Kelly increase her effective communication with others while helping her to feel safe (Figure 14–1).

Intervening With Thought Disorder

Structuring Sessions

Patients with thought disorder can benefit from setting a simple agreed-on agenda in order to structure the session. This might include a conversational review of the previous week and session, discussion of the current situation, and possible issues to address. This helps to provide structure in conversation and allows the clinician to have something to refocus the patient toward if the patient frequently goes off topic. Pausing frequently to provide and elicit mini-summaries, with as much contribution from the individual as they can manage and tolerate, helps to ensure shared understanding of the exchange. Conversation may flow freely, but in the event that it becomes circular or unproductive, the clinician can refocus the patient on the agenda.

Structure can also be enhanced by having the patient write down topics or write out narratives for the clinician to then review and potentially identify themes to work with. Developing a timeline and asking the patient to add important life events to this timeline is another way of structuring and organizing conversation. This timeline can also allow the clinician to begin to form links between life experiences and the onset of mental health symptoms. Diagrams linking events, behavior, thoughts, and feelings can be particularly helpful but may need to be simplified and sometimes used just to link two or three issues or clarify a single concept.

Providing Feedback

Checking on a regular basis that content has been correctly understood or that at least the gist of the conversation is understood helps to improve collaboration and shape communication. Noting when agitation, distress, or enjoyment occurs in the conversation provides clues for the clinician as to the emotions elicited by different topics. This can then be highlighted for the patient and explored if they agree. Topics that elicit positive emotions may be used to enhance the sessions further, such as starting and ending with a topic that the patient enjoys discussing; humor can be a natural, warm, and relaxing part of the interaction and can come from both participants. The aim is to support conversational flow, sometimes with deviations or interruptions from the clinician to reinforce understanding of structure. The clinician should be aware that the patient may experience this as frustrating or quite exhausting if it is too frequent and repetitive. Thus, it is important to strike a balance between retaining a positive relationship and improving communication, with the former generally trumping the latter. It can be helpful here to choose a section of the session or a specific topic to apply structure around. The clinician should remember to provide reinforcement for any positive change in communication style, highlighting for the patient how much they have enjoyed the conversation that day, how much better they understand their patient's experiences, or how appreciative they are of the patient's efforts to help the clinician understand their perspective through clearer communication.

Role-play can be used as a form of feedback, with the patient providing comments on the clinician's communication style in different scenarios and then switching roles as the patient is coached in this interaction. When possible this can be audio recorded and played back to the patient to aid in learning and feedback, and indeed recordings of full sessions can be very helpful for some patients.

Remaining Curious

It is essential that the clinician remain curious throughout and treat the exchange as an opportunity to learn more about, and from, the patient. Discussion can be like a game or a quiz and can be presented in a manner that is quite entertaining for both the patient and the clinician, whereby both parties engage in guessing what is meant and are open to sometimes being right and sometimes being wrong. The process can be therapeutic, even when the thought disorder is quite profound, and the grounds for a positive working relationship set. Teasing or joking is not unusual, as long as it comes from a place of genuine positive regard and curiosity. It is often signaled by nonverbal means and can be reciprocated when needed with a gentle request for clarification. When the clinician comes from this curious position of seeking knowledge about the individual's world, the patient is usually forthcoming; as the individual becomes more relaxed, their thought disorder can improve and their ability to respond increase. Thought disorder may be concealing important issues, and as trust and the relationship improve, its function becomes less relevant and important material emerges.

Anxiety and Stress Management Skills

Teaching stress inoculation skills can help to reduce stress and hyperarousal secondary to internal stimuli or distressing or traumatic thoughts and events. Reducing hyperarousal helps to improve the effectiveness of other intervention strategies.

Case Example (*continued*): Kelly's Progress With Cognitive-Behavioral Therapy for Psychosis

Intervening with thought disorder takes time, patience, and a strong therapeutic alliance. Initially, Kelly was reluctant to engage in treatment. She believed that her treatment team did not understand her and that doing what they asked would threaten her family, causing her significant distress. Kelly was engaged in treatment. However, her difficulty communicating effectively with others had a negative impact on her progress. Kelly's desires to be understood, connect with others, and ultimately reunite with her children were her primary motivations for therapy. Once Kelly realized that her treatment team was trying to help her communicate so that she could be reunited with her children, she became increasingly more open and engaged in treatment.

Therapy often involved engaging in active listening, inquiring curiously, reframing and reflecting thought content, and helping Kelly learn to communicate in a mutually agreed-on manner. This involved spending considerable time building trust and rapport and inquiring curiously about her beliefs and experiences. This was done not for the purpose of changing her beliefs (at least not initially) but rather for the purpose of understanding them. Inquiring curiously while reflecting and reframing thought content helped Kelly and the team to begin discussing and ultimately challenging unhelpful thoughts and beliefs and develop mutually agreed-on ways of communicating. These alternative forms of communication were presented in a tentative, nonthreatening manner and were subject to collaborative change. Reminding Kelly that the treatment team was only going to focus on thoughts and beliefs that were causing problems for effectively communicating with others was helpful.

Setting an agenda with Kelly was essential. This helped structure sessions and guide communication, helping Kelly recognize when she was going off topic and when her thought process was difficult to follow. Exploring significant life events and constructing a timeline with Kelly helped her and the clinician to understand how her history informed the development of her thoughts and beliefs and was the foundation for case conceptualization. Providing feedback helped to clarify communication and provided opportunities for the therapist to reflect and reframe Kelly's thought content, shaping and reinforcing a more adaptive and collaborative communication style. This adaptive communication style ultimately led to improvements in communication. Once this was achieved, Kelly and the clinician collaboratively explored thoughts and beliefs to better understand the context in which her beliefs were developed and maintained over time. Socratic questioning was used to ultimately explore and change unhelpful thinking patterns. Remaining curious and seeking to understand Kelly's experience was essential throughout the process of therapy. Kelly also engaged in weekly group CBTp to help reinforce many of these concepts.

Over time (2–3 years), although Kelly continued to experience delusions related to her planet of origin, her delusional system became more flexible and amenable to change. She was able to reduce the intensity of her emotional arousal, which allowed her to become increasingly more open to alternative ways of thinking and ultimately challenge unhelpful thinking patterns. In time, Kelly also developed shared ways of communicating with others. She was able to recognize when her thoughts were becoming tangential and was able to get back on track with minimal prompting from staff. These gains improved her overall prognosis in treatment and ultimately led to her discharge from the hospital into community outpatient treatment.

Conclusion

Thought disorder is a common symptom alongside delusions and has varying degrees of severity. Clinicians may perceive it as overwhelming to address, and individuals presenting with thought disorder, especially in its more extreme forms, may be excluded from treatment. However, working from a position of genuine curiosity and desire to understand the individual can support assessment and formulation, which can lead to effective interventions to aid more accessible speech and ultimately to the potential for increased social interaction and engagement.

Questions for Discussion

1. How do you feel when working with someone with thought disorder? Do you notice any reluctance to engage around the thought disorder and address it directly? If so, what might that reluctance be about, and how can you address it?

2. Consider a reflective practice and identify what thoughts and feelings you might have if you were struggling to communicate with people around you. How might you then act?

3. What kinds of resources can you use to support increased structure in the session? How might you support your patient in moving toward more effective communication?

KEY POINTS

- Patients with formal thought disorder commonly present with delusions of varying degrees of severity. Thought disorder tends to be more severe when emotional expression is heightened, such as when delusions or trauma are being discussed.

- The clinician should identify different types of thought disorder presentations and understand the interplay among culture, thought content, and process.

- When addressing formal thought disorder clinically, the goal is to increase and improve effective communication with the therapist and others.

- Clinicians can engage in a number of strategies, including inquiring curiously, clarifying the meanings of words and statements, and modeling effective communication.

- Working from a strong therapeutic relationship allows the patient and clinician to collaboratively develop an agreed-on form of communication to aid formulation, intervention, and recovery. Working with the thought disorder allows an effective cognitive-behavioral therapy intervention for the delusion.

References

American Psychiatric Association: Diagnostic and Statistical Manual of Mental Disorders, 5th Edition, Text Revision. Washington, DC, American Psychiatric Association, 2022

Bleuler E: Textbook of Psychiatry. Translated by Brill AA. New York, Dover, 1951

Kingdon DG, Turkington D: Cognitive-Behavioral Therapy of Schizophrenia. Guilford, 1994

Kingdon DG, Turkington D: Cognitive Therapy of Schizophrenia (Guides to Individualized Evidence-Based Treatment; Persons JB, series ed). New York, Guilford, 2005

Leff J, Trieman N: Long-stay patients discharged from psychiatric hospitals: social and clinical outcomes after five years in the community: the TAPS Project 46. Br J Psychiatry 176:217–223, 2000 10755067

Mayer-Gross W, Slater E, Roth M: Clinical Psychiatry, 3rd Edition. Baltimore, MD, Williams & Wilkins, 1969

Palmier-Claus J, Griffiths R, Murphy E, et al: Cognitive behavioural therapy for thought disorder in psychosis. Psychosis 9(4):347–357, 2017

Roche E, Creed L, MacMahon D, et al: The epidemiology and associated phenomenology of formal thought disorder: a systematic review. Schizophr Bull 41(4):951–962, 2015 25180313

Turkington D, Kingdon DG: Ordering thoughts in thought disorder. Br J Psychiatry 159(1):160–161, 1991 1888967

15

Cognitive-Behavioral Therapy for Delusions Within Japanese Culture

Akiko Kikuchi, Ph.D.
Douglas Turkington, M.D.

Cognitive-behavioral therapy for psychosis (CBTp) has been shown to reduce delusions when added to standard care (Bighelli et al. 2018; van der Gaag et al. 2014). Culture influences delusional content. The subject matter of delusions reflects the values of a culture and changes with time (Rathod et al. 2015). Therefore, CBTp targeting delusions benefits from cultural considerations and adjustments according to patients' ethnic and cultural backgrounds. Indeed, a growing body of research suggests that the effectiveness of CBTp can be improved by adapting the delivery method to the culture of the patient (Habib et al. 2015; Naeem et al. 2015; Rathod et al. 2013).

Previous studies discussed the adaptation of CBTp in Asian cultures such as Hong Kong (Ng et al. 2003), Pakistan (Husain et al. 2017; Naeem et al. 2015), and China (Li et al. 2015). However, the literature on the cultural adaptations for CBTp in Japanese culture remains lacking. Thus, in this chapter we focus on individual CBTp for delusions in the context of Japanese culture.

Cognitive-Behavioral Therapy in Japan

CBT in Japan began in the late 1950s with applied research on learning theory for abnormal behavior. In the 1980s, interest in cognitive therapy increased, particularly in psychiatry. The World Congress of Behavioral and Cognitive Therapy, held in Kobe in 2004, greatly increased awareness of CBT's effectiveness among a wide range of helping professionals (Ishikawa et al. 2020). From 2004 to 2007, a national project funded by the Ministry of Health, Labor and Welfare conducted a 16-week manualized CBT program for major depressive disorder that showed promising results (Fujisawa et al. 2010). Following this, CBT for mood disorders was added to the National Health Insurance Scheme in April 2010. Subsequently, in 2016, CBT for obsessive-compulsive disorder, social anxiety disorder, panic disorder, and PTSD was also covered by the National Health Insurance. Although CBT training systems subsidized by the Ministry of Health and Labor exist, dissemination in routine clinical settings remains a challenge. Training opportunities and cultural adaptation have been advocated as being critically important for promoting the widespread use of CBT (Ono et al. 2011).

Features of Japanese Culture in Relation to Cognitive-Behavioral Therapy for Psychosis

Causal Attribution, Stigma, and Help-Seeking

According to previous studies, in Japan, mental disorders tend to be seen as caused by a weakness in an individual's personality or the result of nervousness (Nakane et al. 2005). Such causal attributions are likely to have an impact on reducing help-seeking (Mirza et al. 2019). Japanese people are known for their low utilization of mental health services (Nishi et al. 2019; Substance Abuse and Mental Health Services Administration 2015). They are reluctant to talk about mental disorders, except with family members (Jorm et al. 2005). Stigma is a contributing factor to this low utilization of mental health services (Naganuma et al. 2006). In an effort to address stigma, the name *seishin-bun-retsu-byo* (schizophrenia or split-mind disease) was changed at the national level to *togo-shiccho-sho* (integration disorder) in 2002. This renaming is said to have helped improve mental health literacy (Koike et al. 2016).

Delusional Content and Conformism

Tateyama et al. (1998) compared the schizophrenic delusions of 324 inpatients in Tokyo, 101 inpatients in Vienna, and 150 inpatients in Tübingen, Germany. Specific and direct themes such as persecutory delusions (poisoning) and religious guilt were prominent in Europe, whereas atypical reference delusions such as being slandered were more common in Japan. The authors considered that this difference stemmed from the type of self in the two cultures: the individual-oriented self in Europe and the group-oriented self in the "culture of shame" of Japan. *Taijin kyofusho* (interpersonal fear disorder) is a "syndrome found in Japanese cultural contexts characterized by anxiety about and avoidance of interpersonal situations due to the thought, feeling, or conviction that the individual's appearance and actions in social interactions are inadequate or offensive to others" (American Psychiatric Association 2022, p. 879). Although social anxiety disorder and *taijin kyofusho* have similar symptoms, the origin of the fear differs. The primary fear in social anxiety disorder is characterized by a self-centered fear of being evaluated negatively by others. In contrast, the primary fear in *taijin kyofusho* is the fear that one may have a negative influence on others (Nakamura et al. 2002). *Taijin kyofusho* is considered a broader concept than social anxiety disorder and in clinical practice is often comorbid with schizophrenia.

A common theme frequently found in Japanese delusions and *taijin kyofusho* is an emphasis on not being disliked by one's group. For the Japanese, the well-being of the group tends to take precedence over the comfort of the individual. The conformism of trying not to be disliked by one's group was reinforced during the Edo period (1603–1868). Failure to follow in-group norms was punishable by ostracism from all situations except firefighting and funerals. This social ostracism was the most significant punishment next to the death penalty.

Cognitive-Behavioral Therapy for Psychosis for Japanese Patients: A Culturally Relevant Note

The components of treatment in CBTp for delusions among the Japanese are not different from what has been proposed for Western cultures: 1) developing a therapeutic alliance and including the patient's perspective, 2) developing alternative explanations for psychotic symptoms, 3) reducing the impact of positive and negative symptoms, and 4) offering alternatives to traditional medical approaches to address adherence (Turkington et al. 2006). However, there are cultural influences that merit attention when one is providing CBTp in Japan. Table 15–1 presents the points to be considered in this regard. These points were extracted from my (A.K.) experience practicing CBTp in Japan after learning it in the Western context. Each point is discussed after the two case examples.

TABLE 15–1. Cultural considerations for the practice of cognitive-behavioral therapy for psychosis in Japan

1. A hierarchical relationship is assumed in supportive relationships.

2. People may refrain from expressing their real thoughts to show respect.

3. People tend to avoid definitive or straightforward expressions.

4. The family exerts a major impact on the therapy process of the individual.

5. The influences of culture differ across individuals.

Case Example 1

Phase 1: Engagement

Ken was a man in his mid-30s. He was admitted to a medium-security unit after attacking his colleague with a hammer. When a psychiatrist asked why he was in a secure unit, he replied, "It's because I have schizophrenia and I need treatment." However, at the first session with the psychologist, he ranted that his hospitalization was unjustified. His colleague was the one to blame, and the root cause of the attack was his mother, who was not his real mother. He said he had been kidnapped as a child, and the colleague he had attacked was the abductor. The therapist confessed that she was confused by the complicated background of the attack and requested that Ken slowly tell his side of the story. Ken agreed.

Phase 2: Sowing the Seeds of Doubt

For several sessions, Ken discussed incidents he considered important. Several of them were about the kidnapping or about how he knew his mother was not his real mother. Ken talked about seeing a dead body in the room and hearing the radio talking about him. He described how he had hid on an island for weeks because he was afraid to be mistaken for a murderer. The therapist frequently responded with "That's unbelievable," and Ken said, "I know, but it's true." The therapist asked him to write a life chart to enable her to follow the numerous incidents.

In the next session, Ken drew a life chart (Figure 15–1), and the therapist took notes as he explained. His life contained periods of being physically abused by his father, being abandoned by his mother, running away from home, being chased by debt collectors, being admitted to a psychiatric hospital, and attacking his colleague for constantly nagging him for money but never paying back. Happy periods were observed as well. He especially looked back on the days when he had had a stable job as a delivery person. The therapist expressed how impressed she was that he had survived many hardships and had been relatively well for a while before his first admission to the psychiatric hospital. Ken said he wanted to lead a proper life. Thus, recovering a proper life was agreed on as the long-term goal for therapy.

The therapist then asked Ken whether he had forgotten to mention the kidnapping in the life chart. Ken froze for a moment with a puzzled look on

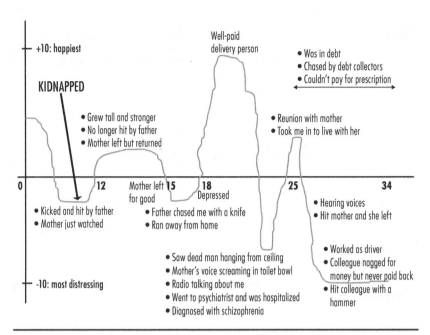

FIGURE 15–1. Life chart of Ken.

his face but then quickly and determinedly pointed to a time in his childhood. The therapist added "KIDNAPPED" to the life chart.

Phase 3: Exploring the Evidence for the Delusion

Ken's mother was scared of him because of the violence he had inflicted on her in the past. Ken became unstable when his mother visited him at the hospital or spoke with him on the phone. He told the therapist about his ambivalence. If she was not his real mother, then why would she visit him? The therapist recommended looking into evidence for and against the fake mother and introduced a worksheet for "evaluating thoughts" (Morrison et al. 2008, p. 39). Ken sounded as if he completely believed his mother was fake. However, he noted the conviction as 40%–50%. He cited past abandonments and his mother's words "You're just a kid I found under a bridge," an expression used by parents in Japan to admonish bad behavior. Ken took those words literally. He could only come up with evidence supporting his mother to be a fake. The therapist advised him to take the time and fill in the worksheet whenever he found anything else to write.

One day, Ken excitedly told the therapist he had come up with the absolute solution to determine whether his mother was fake. Contrary to the therapist's expectation, he did not propose genetic testing. Ken said he would reveal the secret adoption if he could access the family registry stored in the city government. With the support of the therapist, he looked up the procedure to obtain a copy of the complete family registry and made a formal request.

Thought: My mother is not my real mother.	Conviction: 40%~50% Feeling: Fear 80%
Evidence supporting the thought	Evidence **not** supporting the thought
Her face looks different from what I remember as a child. She is pale and looks like a dead person.	She looks very different when she wears makeup.
When I was with her, it didn't feel like I was with a family member.	Sometimes it does feel like I'm with family. She visits me.
She once said, "Why are you here?" She meant I wasn't her son.	Maybe she meant, "Why are you here? Isn't it time for work?"
She abandoned me as a child.	She came back several times.
She abandoned me as an adult.	I questioned her and hit her, nagged her for money. She couldn't take it.
My mother once told me I was just a kid found under a bridge.	<u>The family registry says I'm Mom's child</u>.

How much do you believe in the thought now?
2%~3%
What emotions do you feel now?
Relief 65% Anxiety 20% (She might disappear again..She is getting old.)
Do you think this was a fact or just a thought?
It was a thought. Delusion?
Is there another possible explanation for this experience?
I was probably sick. I thought she was cruel to me because I wasn't her real child.

FIGURE 15–2. Evaluating thoughts, 1.
Source. Worksheet adapted from Morrison et al. 2008, p. 39.

A week later, Ken received a document from the city government. He wanted the entire multidisciplinary team to be with him when he opened it. His name and the word *child* were written clearly in the family registry. He was not an adopted child. He was silent for a long time. Ken completed the worksheet (Figure 15–2) in the next therapy session. He now found counterevidence and concluded that his mother was real. The result was not surprising to the treatment team because Ken and his mother looked very much alike.

A cascade of questions followed. If the mother was Ken's birth mother, it meant that the root cause of the attack did not exist. The story of the kidnapping and the secret adoption to enslave him did not stand anymore. However, Ken did have a memory of an abduction. Had he been saved from the kidnapping? He did not have any memory of a rescue. Ken was confused. He willingly decided to work on the second worksheet to weigh the evidence of the kidnapping. This process was difficult for him, and it lasted over several sessions. One day, as part of peripheral questioning, the therapist asked Ken the approximate age of the abductor in the kidnapping. He

Thought: I was kidnapped as a child by X.	Conviction: 100% Feeling: Anger 120%
Evidence supporting the thought	Evidence **not** supporting the thought
I have a clear memory of X abducting me.	X does not look younger in the memory. He looks the same as today.
I was kidnapped and strapped into the passenger seat of a truck. I remember looking out the window.	The view from the truck window was the same as the view I had when I worked as a driver. Memory mix-up?
I remember lighting a petroleum tank on the abductor's truck and causing an explosion.	It may have been a dream. I asked my friend if he had seen the news about the explosion, but he said he had no idea what I was talking about.

How much do you believe in the thought now?
4%

What emotions do you feel now?
Confusion 20%–30%

Do you think this was a fact or just a thought?
I remembered it vividly and frequently, so I believed it.

Is there another possible explanation for this experience?
It was a memory mix-up.

FIGURE 15–3.   Evaluating thoughts, 2.

Source.   Worksheet adapted from Morrison et al. 2008, p. 39.

closed his eyes to remember the abductor and looked shocked when he opened them. "He looked just like how he looks today.... Impossible! He should look at least 20 years younger!" Ken and the therapist agreed to take time to think about how such a thing could happen.

In the next session, Ken said, "I know what happened. Memories got mixed up. I had a memory of being strapped to the passenger seat of a truck and looking out. I thought that was my memory of being kidnapped. But then I realized it was the same view I had seen when I worked as a truck driver. I used to drive a truck to make deliveries." Ken completed the rest of the worksheet (Figure 15–3).

Phase 4: Working on Current Issues

Ken was unhappy. Now that he knew his mother was real, the abandonment felt worse. He felt stupid for believing his mixed-up memories. The therapist attempted to shift gears and discuss the future. However, her efforts were in vain. Ken remained preoccupied with his relationship with his mother. In fact, he did not know what a normal relationship between an adult son and a mother looked like. The therapist suggested a survey. Ken was tasked with interviewing 10 unmarried male staff and asking them how frequently they met with their mother. The therapist informed the entire staff about the survey plan beforehand. Ken was surprised by the results. The majority of the interviewees met with their mothers only once or twice a year. He asked additional questions and found that several interviewees had worked to pay their tuition to become nurses. All of them made a living and were independent. As a result of the survey, Ken's resentment that his mother had abandoned him and had not even cared to pay for his schooling decreased. He decided to visit his mother once a month or every other month after discharge. Ken's definition of a proper life was changed to securing a job, getting a girlfriend, and visiting his mother.

Ken developed a liking for CBT. During an overnight leave from the hospital, he heard two men on the street talking about his attack. Ken became anxious but decided to listen closely. In fact, the men were only talking about their destination. Ken proudly reported, "I told myself '*stop and think*,' just like how we practiced, and tried not to jump to conclusions." During the rest of his stay at the secure unit, Ken consulted a lawyer to help him clear his debts, practiced keeping track of finances with the nurses, and developed a staying-well plan with the therapist. He was finally discharged.

Case Example 2

Shin became agitated when he was convinced that colleagues in a job center were slandering him and attempting to hinder future opportunities. He panicked. After failing to jump off a building, he tried to burn his hair using a cigarette lighter. He was admitted to an acute psychiatric ward. After 1 month, his psychiatrist referred him for CBT. The referral note explained that he no longer heard voices but still strongly believed his colleagues were after him.

Phase 1: Engagement

In the first phase of treatment, Shin did not believe that he needed "CBT, whatever that is." He said he used to experience auditory hallucinations but now heard only the voices of the spirits residing within him. He was extremely cautious when discussing the spirits to gauge whether the therapist would take it as a sign of deterioration. Shin explained that auditory hallucinations "can be drowned out by medication"; however, the spirits remained untouched because they were not symptoms. He seemed to relax after finding out that the therapist would not advise the psychiatrist to increase his medication just because he talked about spirits. The therapist explained the Activating event, Belief, Consequence (ABC) model and said that CBT addresses stress through the person "changing the thinking" and trying new behaviors. Shin showed interest in CBT as a form of a new psychological technique. In particular, he became fond of the phrase "Haste makes waste," which the therapist happened to use in the session.

Phase 2: Exploring the Delusion

Over a few sessions, Shin gradually revealed the entire delusional system of the spirits inside him (Figure 15–4). The system excluded his self-categorized auditory hallucinations. Several of the spirits were actual people in his life.

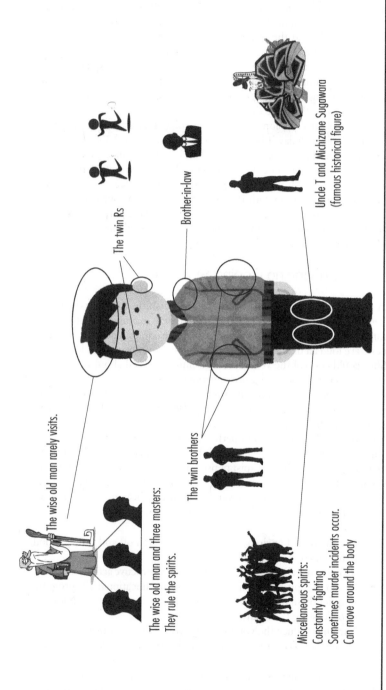

FIGURE 15–4. Locations and names of spirits residing within Shin.

He said that spirits had begun to live within him when he was 20 years old. Shin believed in their presence because of the bodily sensations and voices. Shin had tried to burn his hair because the wise old man had commanded him to do so. He said the intention was to release the accumulating evil power from his brain. The wise old man had left after the incident; nowadays, the three masters were suppressing the voices of other spirits to support Shin. According to Shin, all the spirits intended to support him despite saying harsh things. He wanted them to keep him company but was distressed by them at the same time.

Two consecutive sessions of reviewing voice diaries revealed that Shin was hearing voices all day. The content was 70% advice and 30% harshness. When distressed by the voices, he would seek advice from the masters and engage in conversation. The therapist shared her concern about the lack of balance between his human and spirit relationships when seeking advice. He agreed. Shin came up with the idea of seeing a job counselor because getting a job was one of his goals. Moreover, it served the purpose of seeking advice from a human being. In this manner, he could balance out the types of advice he was receiving.

Phase 3: Enhancing Coping Strategies

Shin started consulting a job counselor. Cherishing the phrase "Haste makes waste," he decided not to jump immediately to employment but first to complete a course on becoming a nursing care equipment specialist. The voices were loud all day. The masters were saying they wanted to leave soon so Shin could control the voices himself. Shin panicked about the masters leaving; however, he became more motivated to learn how to cope with the voices. The therapist gave him an information sheet called "Understanding Voices" (Kingdon and Turkington 2005, p. 190). When asked about coping strategies, Shin hesitantly talked about a "mind switch" that he used to turn off the voices. The effect was imperfect but functional for the majority of the time. In addition, he regularly used the "Haste makes waste" mantra to curb his impatience. The therapist praised him for his creativity. Ken asked, "Do you really think this is good?" He seemed suspicious and happy at the same time. Over the course of several sessions, he became more creative with his coping strategies, which included the following:

- When you get anxious, turn the mind switch off and do two good behaviors (e.g., chores).
- To prevent feeling useless, schedule two constructive activities per day.
- When the spirits are noisy, show them an educational TV program to quiet them down. The spirits like the programs on the National Broadcasting Company.
- Earplugs reduce the volume of the voices by one-third.
- When the voices are loud, taking meals alone and in silence is helpful.

As Shin became increasingly confident in controlling the voices, he even asked his doctor to prescribe him as-needed medications. Although he continued to believe that the spirits' voices were not hallucinations, he found medication helpful in calming his nerves to deal better with the spirits. At this point, the masters were telling him the date of their departure. Shin was no longer scared. He felt that he could manage the spirits better. In one session, Shin described the farewell party that was held the day before the departure of the masters. He said they went to a Chinese restaurant, ordered dumplings, and drank beer as they reflected on the days they had spent together. The therapist asked whether the other customers saw the masters. Shin looked at the therapist with disbelief and said, "Of course not. They are in a different parallel world. I didn't say anything out loud because that would have scared the people around me." The masters left the next day and did not return.

Phase 4: Developing a Staying-Well Plan

Shin finished his training course and was certified as a nursing equipment specialist. He continued to invent creative coping strategies, and sharing them became a major part of the sessions. The most effective strategy was called the "lava bath." When the voices began making nasty remarks, Shin would find a place to lie down, relax, and imagine a volcanic eruption taking place in his brain. When the imaginary lava trickled down his body, he would actually feel the heat. To his surprise, several of the spirits melted in the lava and vanished. He did not know how to interpret this but said that perhaps their time had come. When he got up, he noticed the ashes of the spirits on the floor, and he vacuumed them up. By the end of the 18th session, only two spirits remained. One was a spirit of a 10-year-old boy, and the other was a former wise old man who had now become a kind and wise old woman. Shin did not mind their company. Collaboratively, the therapist and Shin developed a staying-well plan. Shin reflected on his suicide attempt and said that bullying was not the only stressor. His mother's arthritis had worsened, and he was worried about her and his future. He also felt guilty about being unemployed, and the voices were loud and hostile. His early warning signs were worries about money, insomnia, anxiety, agitation, negative thinking, external blaming, and voices. The plan was full of his creative coping strategies.

Phase 5: Ending the Therapy

Shin's mother was invited to the last session. Shin was initially anxious as he shared the staying-well plan with his mother. The mother stated that she was interested in what her son was doing in therapy because he was more emotionally stable and active. Without a doubt, she was proud of his progress. Shin calmed down and became increasingly talkative when he saw that his mother was happy with his achievements in therapy.

Discussion

The two cases in this chapter feature several cultural aspects that merit consideration when using CBTp with Japanese patients with delusions. The issues presented have much in common with counseling with Japanese patients in general, and some have been pointed out as sometimes puzzling for therapists with Western backgrounds.

A Hierarchical Relationship Is Assumed in Supportive Relationships

In Japan, patients typically perceive psychiatrists and psychologists as people to respect and learn from (Rathod et al. 2015, p. 205). In a culture in which therapists are perceived as authorities who can solve problems or directly give instructions on what to do (Nippoda 2012), patients can be confused when a therapist takes a collaborative approach. In both Ken's and Shin's cases, a hierarchical relationship was assumed between the patient and the CBT therapist. The therapist acted as a teacher-like figure, taught patients thinking skills, and gradually transformed the relationship into a more collaborative one. In the first case, Ken underwent therapy with a psychologist for the first time. In the beginning, he seemed to wonder where to locate her in the hierarchy but continued to use honorific speech. In the second case, Shin was able to explore different coping strategies only when the therapist, the figure of authority, acknowledged them as effective.

People May Refrain From Expressing Their Real Thoughts to Show Respect

When attempting to implement cognitive restructuring, it is essential for therapists to avoid pushing patients to select the most adaptive interpretation. When pressed, patients may try to guess and say what they assume the therapist wants them to say or may respond with "I don't know." This scenario frequently occurs out of respect for the therapist. Patients will attempt to avoid speaking against a figure of authority; inwardly, however, they may firmly keep their original delusional interpretation.

For the Japanese, separating the private self (real intentions) from the public self (pretense or facade) is routine (Ohnishi and Ibrahim 1999). Westerners also display true feelings and pretense. However, they try to match these versions of the self, whereas the Japanese are comfortable separating them. In CBT with Japanese patients, building a relationship that enables patients to talk about their true feelings and not just the public self is important.

In the case of Ken, although he was frustrated about the hospitalization, he did not express his frustration to the psychiatrist, whom he saw as the top-ranking figure of authority. In Shin's case, the trigger for his self-harming behavior was revealed only at the very end of the therapy. Often patients show respect by minimizing conversation with the therapist. Similarly, many patients take antipsychotic medication out of politeness to the psychiatrist; however, they may not necessarily believe that they have psychosis. Such tendencies are part of this crucial cultural issue of separating the private and public selves.

People Tend to Avoid Definitive or Straightforward Expressions

One aspect to consider when identifying thoughts is that the Japanese tend to avoid the use of definitive expressions. Even when their thoughts are full of black-and-white ideas, typically they automatically soften the thoughts when expressing them by adding filler words, such as *maybe* and *perhaps*. Such ambiguous expressions render the determination of counterevidence difficult. When the level of belief conviction is high, the therapist should verify whether the identified thoughts are being expressed as extreme. For example, if the patient says, "There is a possibility the phone is bugged," ask if they actually feel that the phone is bugged. Moreover, direct denial of an idea should be avoided in conversations (Ohnishi and Ibrahim 1999). Therefore, denying a thought for its irrationality is not preferable. A well-accepted approach would be to seek a more balanced view. In Shin's case, the concept of balancing the types of advice he received (i.e., from spirits and human beings) was well accepted because of this premise.

The Japanese tend to emphasize reading the context and guessing the meaning of ambiguous expressions. For example, the word *sumimasen* can mean "I'm sorry" or "thank you," "anybody here?" or "excuse me," according to context. In the same manner, the statement "I will consider it" requires reading the context to verify whether it means "no." Thus, one should read between the lines to grasp the meaning. An example of this tendency is a patient who is distressed by derogative voices that frequently call him a "loser." When the therapist asks whether calling another person a "pink giraffe" for a sufficient number of times would transform him into one, the patient replies "maybe" when in fact he means "no," only to avoid saying "no" to the therapist. This high-context communication can become the seed for delusions. In Ken's case, his mother's statement "You're just a kid I found under a bridge" was understood as evidence of her being a fake birth mother, when the mother only stated it to reprove his behavior.

The Family Exerts a Major Impact on the Therapy Process of the Individual

Ken's delusion evolved around his relationship with his mother, and so did his recovery process. Shin seemed to need his mother's validation to feel confident about his change process. From Western perspectives, these cases may be understood as people in need of individuation to achieve recovery. However, such cases, in which the family is crucial to recovery, are common in Japan. In Japanese culture, the family exerts a significant impact on the decision-making of the patient. Thus, the influence of the family should always be considered when one is providing psychotherapy to Japanese patients.

The Influences of Culture Differ Across Individuals

Different cultures exhibit distinct features. However, stereotyping should be avoided. In today's highly globalized world, cultural adaptation is one form of the individualization of treatment because the influence of culture can be manifested in many forms. The following example can help to illustrate this concept. An inpatient believed that an earthbound ghost possessed him. He feared that anyone who became close to him would die. To prevent this from happening, he performed rituals, such as chanting Buddhist scriptures for hours; arranging talismans; and simulating waterfall ascetic practice by taking long, cold showers. During a session, when he was discussing the appearance of the earthbound ghost, it became clear that the ghost had legs; traditional Japanese ghosts do not have legs. In addition, the ghost had a pointed tail. The patient became upset because he might have mistaken the devil for a Japanese ghost. If this were the case, then the effect of the Buddhist rituals may have been questionable. The therapist suggested that the patient consult with a priest to discuss the devil's appearance and behavior. The patient was unaware of Christian rituals used to ward off devils, so he was anxious in the days before meeting the priest. During this waiting period, no one close to him died. When the patient returned from the meeting with the priest, he excitedly reported to the therapist that he understood that trying to live as a good person was more effective than performing rituals in keeping him free from demonic influence. Thus, the amulets, scriptures, and water practices were no longer necessary.

The CBT model is generic and can be used across cultures. However, cultural adaptations should be made to enhance its effectiveness. We hope that this chapter provides helpful ideas for therapists implementing CBTp in the context of Japanese culture.

Personal Reflection

The first author (A.K.) is Japanese. She lived in New York from age 2 to age 7 and spent time with children from many countries from kindergarten to the first grade of primary school. She returned to Japan and started school, where a teacher said, "Raise your hand if you have a question." A.K. raised her hand a few times. No other student did. After the third class, the teacher told her, "Come and ask me after class if you have a question because you are interfering with the progress." A.K. did not know why the teacher was angry.

Strange communications happened at home, too. When A.K.'s mother gave gifts to people, she would say, "It is just a trifle" even though the item was a beautiful gift she had chosen with great effort. As a child, A.K. thought, "In Japan, the words we say and the meaning we convey are different." It took her years to be able to read between the lines of Japanese culture, even though she rapidly forgot how to speak English. It was a valuable experience for her to realize that speaking the language does not necessarily mean understanding the culture.

A.K. went on to graduate school to become a psychologist. In Japan, psychologists were trained not to listen to delusions because listening to the delusions would worsen them. When patients start to talk about their delusions, the therapist should return to talking about everyday life as soon as possible. During her hospital placement, A.K. met a patient who was desperate to talk about the conspiracy of a secret organization. She listened to his story with a vague smile and asked, "What did you eat for lunch today?" The patient looked angry and sad but then answered what he had for lunch. Perhaps he was being polite to the psychologist because she was the professional in a white coat. At the time, A.K. ignored her regret of being rude and told herself that this was the professional response.

Time passed. The above two experiences have become a resource for A.K. when listening to the delusions of Japanese people while using the framework of cognitive behavior therapy, which was born in the West.

Questions for Discussion

1. How do you tell whether a Japanese patient is speaking from a public-self viewpoint?

2. If a Japanese patient does not ask questions in therapy, does this mean that they clearly understand the content?

3. When the parents of adult Japanese patients want to observe the therapy session, is this a sign of overinvolvement?

KEY POINTS

- In Japan, a hierarchical relationship is typically assumed in supportive relationships. A collaborative approach can be established only gradually.

- Japanese people may refrain from expressing their real thoughts to show respect. Separating the public and private selves is routine practice in Japan.

- Japanese people tend to avoid definitive or straightforward expressions. They commonly use indirect expressions instead of directly saying "no."

- The family exerts a major impact on the therapy process of the individual.

- The influences of culture differ across individuals and can manifest in many forms.

References

American Psychiatric Association: Diagnostic and Statistical Manual of Mental Disorders, 5th Edition, Text Revision. Washington, DC, American Psychiatric Association, 2022

Bighelli I, Salanti G, Huhn M, et al: Psychological interventions to reduce positive symptoms in schizophrenia: sytematic review network meta-analysis. World Psychiatry 17(3):316–329, 2018 30192101

Fujisawa D, Nakagawa A, Tajima M, et al: Cognitive behavioral therapy for depression among adults in Japanese clinical settings: a single-group study. BMC Res Notes 3:160, 2010 20529252

Habib N, Dawood S, Kingdon D, Naeem F: Preliminary evaluation of culturally adapted CBT for psychosis (CA-CBTp): findings from Developing Culturally Sensitive CBT Project (DCCP). Behav Cogn Psychother 43(2):200–208, 2015 24382109

Husain MO, Chaudhry IB, Mehmood N, et al: Pilot randomised controlled trial of culturally adapted cognitive behavior therapy for psychosis (CaCBTp) in Pakistan. BMC Health Serv Res 17(1):808, 2017 29207980

Ishikawa S, Chen J, Fujisawa D, Tanaka T: The development, progress, and current status of cognitive behaviour therapy in Japan. Aust Psychol 55(6):598–605, 2020

Jorm AF, Nakane Y, Christensen H, et al: Public beliefs about treatment and outcome of mental disorders: a comparison of Australia and Japan. BMC Med 3:12, 2005 16004615

Kingdon DG, Turkington D: Cognitive Therapy of Schizophrenia (Guides to Individualized Evidence-Based Treatment; Persons JB, series ed). New York, Guilford, 2005

Koike S, Yamaguchi S, Ojio Y, et al: Effect of name change of schizophrenia on mass media between 1985 and 2013 in Japan: a text data mining analysis. Schizophr Bull 42(3):552–559, 2016 26614786

Li Z-J, Guo Z-H, Wang N, et al: Cognitive-behavioural therapy for patients with schizophrenia: a multicentre randomized controlled trial in Beijing, China. Psychol Med 45(9):1893–1905, 2015 25532460

Mirza A, Birtel MD, Pyle M, Morrison AP: Cultural differences in psychosis: the role of causal beliefs and stigma in white British and South Asians. J Cross Cult Psychol 50:441–459, 2019

Morrison AP, Renton JC, French P, Bentall RP: Think You're Crazy? Think Again: A Resource Book for Cognitive Therapy for Psychosis. New York, Routledge, 2008

Naeem F, Saeed S, Irfan M, et al: Brief culturally adapted CBT for psychosis (CaCBTp): a randomized controlled trial from a low income country. Schizophr Res 164(1–3):143–148, 2015 25757714

Naganuma Y, Tachimori H, Kawakami N, et al: Twelve-month use of mental health services in four areas in Japan: findings from the World Mental Health Japan Survey 2002–2003. Psychiatry Clin Neurosci 60(2):240–248, 2006 16594950

Nakamura K, Kitanishi K, Miyake Y, et al: The neurotic versus delusional subtype of taijin-kyofu-sho: their DSM diagnoses. Psychiatry Clin Neurosci 56(6):595–601, 2002 12485300

Nakane Y, Jorm AF, Yoshioka K, et al: Public beliefs about causes and risk factors for mental disorders: a comparison of Japan and Australia. BMC Psychiatry 5:33, 2005 16174303

Ng RMK, Cheung M, Suen L: Cognitive-behavioural therapy of psychosis: An overview and 3 case studies from Hong Kong. Hong Kong J Psychiatry 13(1):23–30, 2003

Nippoda Y: Japanese culture and therapeutic relationship. Online Readings in Psychology and Culture 10(3): 2012

Nishi D, Ishikawa H, Kawakami N: Prevalence of mental disorders and mental health service use in Japan. Psychiatry Clin Neurosci 73(8):458–465, 2019 31141260

Ohnishi H, Ibrahim FA: Culture-specific counselling strategies for Japanese nationals in the United States of America. Int J Adv Couns 21:189–206, 1999

Ono Y, Furukawa TA, Shimizu E, et al: Current status of research on cognitive therapy/cognitive behavior therapy in Japan. Psychiatry Clin Neurosci 65(2):121–129, 2011 21414087

Rathod S, Phiri P, Harris S, et al: Cognitive behaviour therapy for psychosis can be adapted for minority ethnic groups: a randomised controlled trial. Schizophr Res 143(2–3):319–326, 2013 23231878

Rathod S, Kingdon D, Pinninti N, et al: Cultural Adaptation of CBT for Serious Mental Illness: A Guide for Training and Practice. Hoboken, NJ, Blackwell, 2015

Substance Abuse and Mental Health Services Administration: Racial/Ethnic Differences in Mental Health Service Use Among Adults (HHS Publ No SMA15-4906). Rockville, MD, Substance Abuse and Mental Health Services Administration, 2015

Tateyama M, Asai M, Hashimoto M, et al: Transcultural study of schizophrenic delusions: Tokyo versus Vienna and Tübingen (Germany). Psychopathology 31(2):59–68, 1998 9561549

Turkington D, Kingdon D, Weiden PJ: Cognitive behavior therapy for schizophrenia. Am J Psychiatry 163(3):365–373, 2006 16513854

van der Gaag M, Valmaggia LR, Smit F: The effects of individually tailored formulation-based cognitive behavioural therapy in auditory hallucinations and delusions: a meta-analysis. Schizophr Res 156(1):30–37, 2014 24731619

16

Trauma and Delusions

Charles Heriot-Maitland, Ph.D., D.Clin.Psy., M.A., B.Sc.

Types and Dimensions of Delusions

The most common type of delusions is paranoid or persecutory delusions, in which a person perceives themselves to be under a threat of some kind, usually believing that other people intend to harm them. Other common types include delusions of being controlled (beliefs that one's own thoughts, feelings, or behaviors are being externally controlled), delusions of grandeur (beliefs of one's own power or importance), and delusions of reference (beliefs that events in the environment have personal significance). Psychological approaches have typically regarded delusional beliefs as occurring on a continuum with "normal" beliefs (van Os et al. 2009), which suggests that what distinguishes a delusion from any other belief is no single feature but an interaction of multiple different dimensions (e.g., the dimensions of belief conviction, incorrigibility, interference with functioning, distress, and preoccupation) (Freeman 2007; Heriot-Maitland and Peters 2015).

Trauma Pathways to Delusions

The evidence for a causal link between trauma and psychosis is substantial and, as Bentall et al. (2014) pointed out, is comparable to the causal evidence linking smoking to lung cancer. Childhood trauma increases the odds of psychosis by 2.8 (Varese et al. 2012), and there is evidence for a cumulative relationship such that the more trauma experienced, the greater the odds of psychosis (Shevlin et al. 2008). There are suggestions that different types of trauma may lead to different symptoms of psychosis; for example, Bentall et al. (2014) argued that childhood sexual abuse may be more linked to voice-hearing and that attachment-disrupting events may be more linked to paranoia. However, this specificity case is not so clear because although there is evidence in support of it (Bentall et al. 2012), there is also evidence to the contrary, such as that linking sexual abuse to paranoia (Murphy et al. 2012), attachment disruption to voice-hearing (Pilton et al. 2016), and childhood adversities to global effects on different symptoms (Longden et al. 2016).

In this chapter, there is no assumption of a specific trauma type in the pathway to delusions, but there is a focus on *interpersonal* traumas more generally. This includes adverse experiences that occur between people, which could be related to attachment or sexual abuse and equally could be related to other interpersonal threats, such as bullying, violence, or neglect, as well as experiences of marginalization, discrimination, and oppression. In other words, it is the interpersonal (social) domain of a threat, harm, or injury that is the focus here.

There is evidence for direct links between interpersonal trauma and delusions. For example, Johns et al. (2004) showed that paranoid thoughts were significantly associated with victimization experiences. There is also evidence for indirect pathways from trauma to delusions via social mechanisms such as social defeat (Seo and Choi 2018) and shame (Carden et al. 2020). In reviewing the neurocognitive research, Green and Phillips (2004) also drew attention to social mechanisms, presenting evidence that delusional processing is linked to processing of social threat. Interestingly, they found a vigilance-avoidance pattern with delusions, whereby there is an initial vigilance to social threat and a subsequent avoidance of threat at a later stage of information processing. This led the authors to conclude that delusional processes may be linked to evolutionary processes developed to help people detect and respond to social threats (Green and Phillips 2004). A similar argument has been proposed in the literature on compassion-focused therapy (CFT) approaches to psychosis, in which delusions are linked to evolved social mentalities for threat protection, in particular in the context of dominant-subordinate social interactions (Heriot-Maitland 2022).

Trauma-Focused Understandings and Interventions for People With Delusions

De-shaming Psychoeducation

It is important for a trauma-focused intervention for people with delusions to be built on solid psychoeducation and formulation. Psychoeducation about how minds and brains operate, especially under conditions of extreme threat, is crucial to help counteract the high levels of shame experienced by survivors of trauma; by people with psychosis-related diagnoses; and, even more pertinent for this chapter, by patients who have both traumatic experiences *and* a psychosis-related diagnosis.

One of the key aims of psychoeducation for these patients is to develop a de-shaming—"It's not your fault"—understanding about what is happening in their minds. However, the "It's not your fault" message alone is not sufficient because this could leave a patient feeling disempowered and hopeless in the belief that the delusions are out of their control. For example, in the medical model of delusions (i.e., delusions are manifestations of medical illnesses, such as schizophrenia), there is a clear "It's not your fault" message (i.e., "It's not your fault because the delusions are caused by your illness"). This can be helpful from the perspective of de-blaming and de-shaming; however, attributing cause to a disease process (which is out of one's control) can leave a patient disempowered and reliant on *external* solutions, namely, mental health professionals and psychiatric drugs. The problem with this is that it can create out-of-control patterns linked to anxiety (e.g., anxiety about psychosis or relapse) as well as submission/defeat patterns linked to depression (e.g., submitting to an illness identity and to professionals with superior insight into and solutions for one's condition). Interestingly, a review found that disease-based models of understanding psychosis can actually *increase* stigma for people in this patient group (Carter et al. 2017). This chapter argues for an "It's not your fault, but it is your responsibility" message, one that is not only de-shaming but empowering. As illustrated in the following case example, this psychoeducation is rooted in an evolution-informed understanding of brain patterns and functions, with the possibility of continuous reshaping, transformation, and growth of these patterns.

Case Example 1

Dean is a 24-year-old man who finds it hard to leave the house because when he goes out, he believes that people are looking at him and laughing at him. He finds this very distressing. He has been told by his mental health team that this is not real and is "just part of his illness." They tell him that he has to take antipsychotics to treat the chemical imbalance caused by schizophrenia, which is making him believe things that are not real. Dean has recently started worrying that maybe people are laughing at him because they know about his schizophrenia and think he is "crazy" or "a weirdo." Dean has very low social confidence and has also lost a lot of confidence in his own mind and judgments. He questions his ability to make good decisions. It feels much safer to stay at home. The antipsychotics do help him to feel calmer and get more sleep, but he fears he will not be able to cope without them and might have to take them forever.

At school, Dean was bullied by a group of three boys. They bullied him over a 5-year period with constant name-calling and rumor-spreading, which led to Dean feeling excluded from the wider peer group as well. He had no idea who had or had not heard these rumors about him. Maybe everyone knew and was laughing at him? On two occasions, Dean was also physically assaulted by the boys, but he does not remember all the details; it is a bit of a blur. He did not tell his parents about the bullying and assaults because he was too embarrassed.

Key Psychoeducation Messages

This case example demonstrates how psychoeducation can be both de-shaming and empowering, each of which is crucial in a trauma recovery process, in particular with interpersonal trauma, in which a patient has been in a threatening, subordinated position in relation to powerful other(s). The therapist conveyed the following key messages to Dean:

1. Our brains have a built-in threat system that has an important evolutionary function. Its job or function is very simple: to detect danger and respond to it. The threat system does not function for our happiness or mental health; it functions for our survival, which means it has a natural bias toward threat detection and protection, using the principle of better safe than sorry. That is its job.
2. The more the threat system gets activated, the more sensitized it becomes. Similar to training a muscle in the gym, the more we exercise it, the stronger it becomes. If someone has had to use their threat system a lot in their life, such as through prolonged experiences of trauma, bullying, or conflict, then the threat system has been exercised more, has become stronger and more dominant, and is more readily activated.
3. Your brain is not broken. It has been doing its job of threat protection very well, under extremely difficult circumstances. Scanning for real and potential threats is *highly functional* under the circumstances of being bullied and excluded socially at school. There is nothing to fix in your brain; it is more a question of reorganizing and growing.
4. It is *not your fault* that our brains have evolved in this way, with built-in better-safe-than-sorry algorithms, and it is *not your fault* that your early social experiences have shaped how your threat system has become exercised and attuned over time. But now we can see and understand what patterns are being activated in your brain. You now have choices and opportunities to *intentionally* create new patterns and to reorganize and transform the patterns that your mind creates.

Considering the evolutionary context in psychoeducation can help to create a *common humanity* experience, in which a patient can feel more connected and "normal" rather than isolated and abnormal. The idea of re-shaping and repatterning our brains (e.g., through neuroplasticity, which is a lifelong process; Lillard and Erisir 2011) also helps to elicit hope for the future and a path that patients can direct and implement themselves (with the support of others) rather than being wholly dependent on others and on treatment.

Additional psychoeducation that is relevant for people with trauma and delusions is around dissociative processes and how the mind has automatic responses to deal with distressing situations. It can be helpful for patients to have a general understanding of how our minds are capable of adapting to what is going on in our environments; that minds will do what is necessary to survive, which might even include dissociating, hallucinating, or creating alternative realities. As we will see, such strategies could be crucial to surviving and continuing to function in extreme situations. Another important area of psychoeducation is the normalizing of delusional thinking and how this occurs on a continuum in the general population; for example, 10%–15% of the general population have fairly regular delusional ideation (Freeman 2006). In a poll of American adults, 42% were found to believe in haunted houses, and 33% believed that the Earth has been visited by extraterrestrial beings (Newport and Strausberg 2001). The continuum of delusions may further contribute to normalizing, destigmatizing, and de-shaming processes.

Formulating Delusions, and Their Possible Functions, in the Context of Trauma

The evolution-informed psychoeducation outlined earlier is centered on principles of understanding our evolved minds and brains and how they function. The general direction has been away from themes of "abnormal brains" and toward a theme of "normal brains operating under difficult circumstances." This theme continues in this subsection on formulating delusions. Here delusional beliefs are conceived as strategies rather than symptoms—strategies that our "normal brains" might adopt under situations of extreme adversity and trauma.

There are a number of ways in which delusions could be operating as (functional) strategies for people in the context of trauma. A threat belief, for example, may help to sustain an *oriented* and *mobilized* threat system (Heriot-Maitland 2022), which can protect a person from external or internal threats. If the threats are more enduring and culturally ingrained—for example, the experience of systemic racism in communities and institutions—the requirement for threat protective patterns may be more enduring, with (belief) strategies that are more entrenched. In the following subsections, I elaborate on ideas about the function of delusions as 1) an oriented and mobilized threat system, 2) managing overwhelming emotion and defeat states, and 3) providing meaning and control. A case example on how a delusion-as-strategy formulation might look in practice then follows.

An Oriented and Mobilized Threat System

Delusions may be functional posttrauma in protecting people from external threats, such as fear of further harm, humiliation, or injury from others. To prevent further harm, it is protective to have one's threat detection and responses switched on (mobilized). A delusional belief may, for example, elicit responses such as "stay on guard," "keep a distance from others," or "lock your doors and windows." It does not necessarily matter what the actual *content* of the delusion is; the important thing, as far as threat protection and survival are concerned, is the mental, physical, and behavioral *response* elicited by the delusion.

Consider the example of someone who has been sexually abused in childhood and then as an adult develops delusions of alien abduction. The content of the delusion does not actually match the content of the trauma in that there is a different source of threat. However, the protective response elicited by an alien abduction belief is still likely to be highly relevant and functional in protecting against sexual abuse (e.g., being highly vigilant to sounds and movements at nighttime and being ready to defend oneself). In the book *How to Defend Yourself Against Alien Abduction* (Druffel 2010), the following techniques are suggested: block their mind control, fight back, summon your inviolate rights, guard your loved ones, seek strength in numbers, sense them coming, and create a personal shield. The point is, as outlined in the psychoeducation described earlier, the job of the threat system is to survive (better safe than sorry), so the mind will do what is necessary for protection, even if that involves creating a delusional framework to mobilize the threat system.

Managing Overwhelming Emotion and Defeat States

The function of delusions to protect against threats may apply not only to potential external threats (from others) but also to *internal* threats (from one's own feared emotions, memories, and mental states). An example of an internal threat that is relevant to trauma survivors is the fear of one's own feelings of helplessness and powerlessness. In this case, it may be functional to hold a delusion that keeps the mind oriented toward a current threat in the external world when the alternative (of encountering one's own internal states and memories of helplessness and powerlessness) may be far harder. Here the delusion is keeping the individual in fight-or-flight mode, which is preferable to and more mobilizing than being in freeze or submit modes (i.e., defeat states), which are demobilizing. Again, the important aspect is not necessarily the *content* of the delusion but more the process of what this delusion is doing for the person.

Providing Meaning and Control

Another function that a delusion may serve is to provide meaning (when there is no meaning, direction, or purpose) and control (when one is feeling lost and out of control). In a qualitative study, my colleagues and I asked people to talk about the immediate situational context in which their initial psychotic-like experience had arisen. We found that "eleven of 12 participants were experiencing an intense emotional experience, accompanied by deep existential questioning in eight participants," and that the "cognitive shift" accompanying the psychotic experience for many seemed to provide an adaptive solution to this emotional or existential crisis (Heriot-Maitland et al. 2012, p. 45). One participant, Clive, who felt he had reached a dead end in life, reported that with the arrival of his psychotic-like experience, "There's more meaning, there's more purpose, and there's more direction" (p. 42). It may be that attributing meaning *in itself* is protective against vulnerable states. In the context of trauma-related helplessness and out-of-control feelings and memories, the process of meaning-making can provide orientation and control (Westermann et al. 2018), can provide emotion regulation, and can offer an immediate choice of protective responses. Again, under the brain's better-safe-than-sorry algorithm, these may be far more important priorities for survival than arriving at an *accurate* explanation. If we keep in mind the fact that our brains have evolved over many millions of years, it is easier for us to understand why, when under threat, our brains might favor survival over rational accuracy. It is better to be safe (with rapid processing and responding) than sorry (with slow rational thinking).

The following case vignette and Figure 16–1 show an example of formulation. Some patients, when formulating, may experience their delusions as a threat, and others might experience them as a strategy (to manage a threat). The case of Kim has been chosen because her delusions were formulated as both a threat and a strategy. On the one hand, they were a strategy for Kim to use to manage the threat of intense feelings (traumatic loss and grieving), and on the other, they were experienced as a current threat to her (spiritual attacks), which elicited other strategies (e.g., withdrawal, shame, self-criticism). It is important to note here that psychotic experiences themselves can often be traumatic, and post-psychotic trauma is an important process in itself, especially when combined with shame (Turner et al. 2013). Aspects of psychosis treatment (e.g., hospitalization, restraint, enforced medication) can themselves elicit a trauma reaction, so it is important to consider the bidirectional nature of trauma-delusion relationships.

Case Example 2

Kim is a 52-year-old woman who for many years believed that she had a special ability to communicate with spirits. This gave her useful insights and intuitive knowledge about people's *real* intentions; however, the gift also made her a target for evil spirits who wanted to take it away from her. These beliefs started shortly after Kim lost her baby daughter, which was also around the same time that her relationship with her partner broke down. Kim grew up with a mother who had been diagnosed with schizophrenia and who often talked about experiences of demonic possession. Her father was a gentle man but was very depressed and was unable to cope with his wife's condition. He ended up retreating into himself, drinking heavily, and neglecting Kim.

Kim's spiritual beliefs may have initially had the function of providing a sense of connection and companionship, as well as direction and purpose after her trauma (and perhaps a sense of specialness and self-worth as well). She never grieved the loss of her daughter because she did not feel safe with strong emotions. As a child, and through her experiences with her mother and father, she had learned that emotions were bad, destructive, and scary.

Interventions for Patients With Trauma and Delusions

It is not within the scope of this chapter to describe how to deliver a trauma-focused intervention. Trauma work from different psychotherapy traditions, such as trauma-focused cognitive-behavioral therapy and eye movement desensitization and reprocessing, has been described widely in the literature. These evidence-based techniques for trauma exposure and processing have been successfully and safely applied in populations with psychosis and would therefore apply here. The concern here is not so much how to work with trauma but rather how to formulate and identify the targets of trauma work for patients with delusions. The central argument is for an approach that regards brains as *normal* (not abnormal) and regards delusions as *strategies* (not symptoms).

Personal Reflection

It should come as no surprise that our brains are capable of creating stories, metaphors, and alternative realities to help us process sensory-emotional information. Our brains do this every night when we go to sleep. Have you ever had a dream that takes an emotional concern of yours and creates a whole new scene or story around it? I remember very clearly waking up one morning from a dream in which my brain had created a whole visual story around the sound of my alarm clock going off. My dream had contextual-

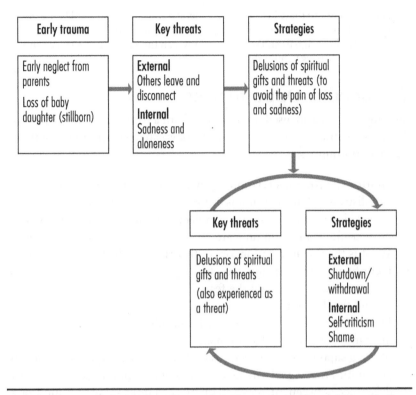

FIGURE 16–1. Delusions formulated as strategies of threats (or both).

ized a sensory experience (hearing the alarm sound) with an elaborate story (about a fire engine rushing to a burning building). This made me wonder: If my brain could do this for one type of sensory stimulus (a sound), could it do the same for another, such as a smell or a change of temperature in the room? Would my brain create a story, narrative, or metaphor around these sensory experiences too? What if the sensory stimulus were internal rather than external—for example, an emotion (anxiety), a physical sensation or pain, or maybe a memory? What if the memory were a trauma memory?

Sleep researchers have suggested that during rapid eye movement sleep, our brains may be engaged in a form of emotional processing, in that our brains extract the gist of an emotional concern and then form abstract links from this theme to disparate memories and clusters of information (Walker 2017). Walker (2017) referred to this as *overnight therapy*, which implies that this is functional and helpful to us. Given that our brains do this naturally to help us with our emotional concerns, why are we so averse to it when someone is awake? Why are our treatments and services (and research outcome measures) so targeted at shutting this process down? What if we took a different approach of listening to and exploring these beliefs, stories, and metaphors? What if we looked beyond the surface-level content and more into the symbolic or emotional meaning? What is going on here for this person? Why are these beliefs being generated for this person and being re-sponded to in a defensive manner? What (emotional) function is being served by these signals and responses? How can therapy help to alleviate the emotional distress behind this?

Therapeutic Opportunities

Building a trauma-focused intervention from a formulation that considers delusions as strategies rather than symptoms can open up a range of thera-peutic opportunities:

- Shifting the patient's relationship with a delusion from one of conflict and distress ("This delusion is a threat to me") to one of curiosity and exploration ("This delusion may reflect something my mind is trying to protect me from, communicate, or resolve. What is that something? What is the threat, emotion, or conflict that may be behind this?")
- Identifying the therapeutic targets (e.g., threat experiences and memo-ries) for trauma work and the feared or avoided emotions that may be behind the delusions
- Identifying the interpersonal, social, and cultural contexts (e.g., abusive, discriminatory, racist) that are maintaining social threat activation and offering support and resources, as well as new social experiences and op-portunities that signal safeness and acceptance (for a discussion of the difference between safeness and safety, see Heriot-Maitland and Long-den 2022)
- Preparing the patient for what intense feelings and conflicts might start to surface as the delusions start to reduce or weaken
- Setting up the route for trauma work (e.g., graded exposure to the mem-ories, emotions, and conflicts so that they can be safely accessed and in-tegrated)
- Addressing the patterns of self-shaming, self-criticizing, and self-stigma-tizing (and "illness" self-identifying) that can often trap patients and hinder their progress toward therapy goals

The following case example provides an illustration of what these inter-vention steps look like in practice. This illustration uses parts work, a ther-apy technique that conceptualizes the mind as a collection of multiple parts representing different states of mind and emotion. The concept of *parts* or *multiple selves* has been adopted in a number of different therapy ap-proaches, such as ego state therapy (Watkins and Watkins 1997), internal family systems (Schwartz and Sweezy 2019), structural integration theory (van der Hart et al. 2006), gestalt therapy (Perls 1992), and CFT (Gilbert 2010). In the case of working with trauma and delusions, the parts can represent both those that have become feared, avoided, or dissociated through trauma and the (delusional) parts that are the functional strategies created to deal with the trauma-related threats carried forward in time. The case example focuses on a sad part (the sad self) and a paranoid part (the paranoid self). However, depending on the patient and their beliefs, the parts could be represented differently (e.g., "the part that strongly holds belief XXX").

Case Example 3

Femi is a 35-year-old African British man who has paranoid beliefs that people in the streets want to beat him up. He grew up in a care home after his mother gave him up for adoption. At age 22, Femi married a woman whom he adored, and they had a son together. Ten years ago, Femi got into a fight at work after a long period of being racially harassed and taunted by some colleagues. He was badly injured in the fight, but because he was blamed for starting it, he ended up losing his job. At home Femi became very depressed. His wife started to become scared of him and his temper and became very protective of their 3-year-old son. The marriage broke down, and Femi's wife took their son away to live abroad. She broke off all contact with Femi. Femi blamed himself for losing his job, his wife, his family—everything.

Mapping out parts and selves can be a helpful tool for visually representing the patient's formulation and internal conflicts (Figure 16–2, panel 4), and it can also set up the process of *being in a relationship with parts*, with the aim of resolving these conflicts. The patient can develop more calm curiosity toward the delusion-based parts, asking questions such as "When did this part come along in my life?" "When is this part most active? Is it when I'm feeling overwhelmed? Unsafe? When I need a break?" or "What does this part do for me and help me with?"

The observer position (represented by the eye in Figure 16–2) is important. Indeed, in CFT (Gilbert 2010), this self-to-self relational stance is specifically trained with compassionate motives and competencies. Referred to as the *compassionate self*, it becomes an inner helper to guide the therapy process and a self-identity and motivational stance from which to do the trauma work. In CFT, it is argued that this training up of the compassionate mind is the crucial factor in creating the conditions for trauma work (as opposed to the specific techniques per se for exposure, processing, and so on).

Intervention Steps

Femi's treatment took place over a series of six steps that follow a trauma-informed formulation (Figure 16–2):

1. Creating *internal* cues of safeness (from Femi's body) through practices with breathing, posture, and imagery
2. Creating *external* cues of safeness through (nonracist) social experiences of equality, inclusion, and acceptance
3. De-shaming psychoeducation, which helped Femi become a mindful observer of his better-safe-than-sorry patterns
4. Formulating relationships between Femi's feared parts (from trauma) and protective parts (from delusions)
5. Learning to access and engage with parts that may be *behind* a delusion (for Femi, this is sadness and shame)
6. Building resources for safe exposure to and integration and processing of his trauma memories and emotions

By the time the trauma exposure work occurs (Figure 16–2, panel 6), the patient has already developed a formulation; has built up resources (e.g., grounding skills, safety and safeness plans); and has practiced accessing and engaging with different emotions, such as sadness and anger. There are specific ways of helping patients differentiate and relate to different emotional parts. For example, in CFT (Gilbert 2010) so-called multiple selves practices guide the patient to focus in on one emotion, say, the part of them that feels angry, and then explore what their angry self might be thinking, what this self might want to do, how this feels in the body, and what kind of memories it elicits. The patient then does the same with their anxious self and sad self and then explores how these parts might work and relate *together*, such as considering "What does your anxious self think about your sad self?" and so on. This guided discovery is essential for helping patients to differentiate functions; crucially, it also prepares people with delusions to identify and tolerate (in the body) the emotions that may surface once their delusions start to shift.

Using chair work, acting, and role-play techniques in therapy can really support the patient's embodiment of their multiple selves. They can experience the postures and movements of each self, which allows them to practice being present with and validating these emotions. They can develop tools to help ground them in stronger parts of themselves and take care of the more vulnerable parts of themselves. They can practice setting up graded exposure to the emotions they struggle with the most, which feel more out of control. Essentially, the patient is preparing for whatever intense emotions and conflicts are likely to surface when the delusions start to weaken. Remember, the delusions are protective, so it is important to tread very carefully, and, arguably, the delusions should not be challenged at all, or at least not until you have an understanding of and are prepared for what is behind them. Simply taking a delusion away and exposing the

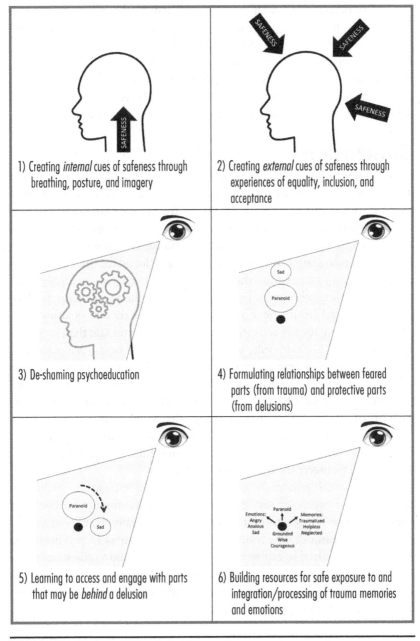

1) Creating *internal* cues of safeness through breathing, posture, and imagery

2) Creating *external* cues of safeness through experiences of equality, inclusion, and acceptance

3) De-shaming psychoeducation

4) Formulating relationships between feared parts (from trauma) and protective parts (from delusions)

5) Learning to access and engage with parts that may be *behind* a delusion

6) Building resources for safe exposure to and integration/processing of trauma memories and emotions

FIGURE 16–2. Intervention steps that follow a trauma-informed formulation.

patient to their emotional pain underneath could be risky and may lead to the patient becoming suicidal or resorting to using other strategies (e.g., alcohol, drugs) to take the place of the delusional strategy. It is a bit like pulling the rug from beneath someone's feet when they have nowhere to land. From this perspective, the aim of therapy is not so much about removing or reducing a delusion; it is about helping the patient to safely access and resolve the underlying trauma and emotional conflicts so that over time the delusional strategies become less necessary and may (naturally) subside.

Conclusion

This chapter highlights the evidence for trauma in pathways to delusions. The chapters suggests an approach to treatment that involves sharing psychoeducation about how brains are *normal* (rather than abnormal) and developing formulations about how delusions are *strategies* (rather than symptoms) in the context of trauma. Providing an evolutionary context helps patients to appreciate how brains have developed for the evolutionary tasks of survival, with natural threat protection biases that are highly functional for dealing with immediate threats but can be problematic for longer-term mental health once a threat has passed. Trauma is an extreme threat that automatically activates our protective (better safe than sorry) responses. This is not our fault; however, because our brains are constantly relearning and repatterning, we can create and learn new experiences, such as how to feel safe (both with others and with our own emotions in our bodies). We learn to switch out of threat protection patterns and switch into patterns of safeness. This chapter argues that interventions for delusions should aim not to challenge or remove delusions but rather to understand their function and to work with the trauma and conflicts underneath so that a delusional (protective) strategy is less necessary.

This approach potentially offers a different angle from the traditional approaches of psychosis services. Typically, the treatment approach has been to reduce symptoms (antipsychotics are literally "anti"—against—psychotic symptoms). The more we learn about trauma in psychosis, the more we are required to evolve our existing practices and to adapt our treatments and services. This chapter provides some illustrative examples of how it might look if we were to genuinely put a trauma focus at the heart of our support for people with psychosis.

Questions for Discussion

1. Has a belief ever served a function of helping you, or someone you know, to get through a difficult time? Maybe a religious belief?

2. If you held in mind that someone's delusional belief might be protecting them from painful trauma memories and emotions, how would you talk to that person differently?

3. Is it possible that our own psychiatric (diagnostic and treatment) frameworks are also serving some function for us as mental health workers? That is, could these institutional systems be protecting us from the trauma we would otherwise encounter in our work?

4. How can we all (as patients, as families, as workers, and as service providers) find the courage to compassionately open up to and engage with the trauma behind delusions?

KEY POINTS

- Through evolutionary processes, our brains have developed built-in better-safe-than-sorry patterns that serve the function of threat protection and survival and prime us for threat-focused attention, processing, and responding.

- A patient's delusions can be formulated as strategies with a specific function (often threat protection) in the context of adverse life experiences.

- Building on this evolution-informed psychoeducation and formulation, the therapeutic process can help patients with distressing delusions

  - Become more mindfully observant of their own threat-focused algorithms

  - Recognize that these are understandable strategies that were highly functional in the context of previous experiences, in particular trauma

  - Recognize that these strategies are not their fault, that they are evolved and automatic and that their brain was doing what was necessary to survive

  - Cultivate (biopsychosocial) states that signal safeness and groundedness

- Once patients are able to access and activate patterns of safeness, the intervention can support their exposure to, engagement with, and resolution of trauma-related memories, fears, and emotional conflicts that may be driving the delusions.

References

Bentall RP, Wickham S, Shevlin M, Varese F: Do specific early life adversities lead to specific symptoms of psychosis? A study from the 2007 the Adult Psychiatric Morbidity Survey. Schizophr Bull 38(4):734–740, 2012 22496540

Bentall RP, de Sousa P, Varese F, et al: From adversity to psychosis: pathways and mechanisms from specific adversities to specific symptoms. Soc Psychiatry Psychiatr Epidemiol 49(7):1011–1022, 2014 24919446

Carden LJ, Saini P, Seddon C, et al: Shame and the psychosis continuum: a systematic review of the literature. Psychol Psychother 93(1):160–186, 2020 30426672

Carter L, Read J, Pyle M, Morrison AP: The impact of causal explanations on outcome in people experiencing psychosis: a systematic review. Clin Psychol Psychother 24(2):332–347, 2017 26805779

Druffel A: How to Defend Yourself Against Alien Abduction. New York, Three Rivers Press, 2010

Freeman D: Delusions in the nonclinical population. Curr Psychiatry Rep 8(3):191–204, 2006 19817069

Freeman D: Suspicious minds: the psychology of persecutory delusions. Clin Psychol Rev 27(4):425–457, 2007 17258852

Gilbert P: Compassion Focused Therapy: Distinctive Features. London, Routledge, 2010

Green MJ, Phillips ML: Social threat perception and the evolution of paranoia. Neurosci Biobehav Rev 28(3):333–342, 2004 15225975

Heriot-Maitland C: Compassion focused therapy for voice-hearing and delusions in psychosis, in Compassion Focused Therapy: Clinical Practice and Applications. Edited by Gilbert P, Simos G. London, Routledge, 2022, pp 549–564

Heriot-Maitland C, Longden E: Safety and safeness, in Relating to Voices Using Compassion Focused Therapy: A Self-Help Companion. London, Routledge, 2022, pp 43–62

Heriot-Maitland C, Peters E: Dimensional approaches to delusional beliefs, in Schizotypy: New Dimensions. Edited by Mason OJ, Claridge G. London, Routledge, 2015, pp 165–179

Heriot-Maitland C, Knight M, Peters E: A qualitative comparison of psychotic-like phenomena in clinical and non-clinical populations. Br J Clin Psychol 51(1):37–53, 2012 22268540

Johns LC, Cannon M, Singleton N, et al: Prevalence and correlates of self-reported psychotic symptoms in the British population. Br J Psychiatry 185:298–305, 2004 15458989

Lillard AS, Erisir A: Old dogs learning new tricks: neuroplasticity beyond the juvenile period. Dev Rev 31(4):207–239, 2011 24648605

Longden E, Sampson M, Read J: Childhood adversity and psychosis: generalised or specific effects? Epidemiol Psychiatr Sci 25(4):349–359, 2016 26156083

Murphy J, Shevlin M, Houston J, Adamson G: Sexual abuse, paranoia, and psychosis: a population-based mediation analysis. Traumatology 18(1):37–44, 2012

Newport F, Strausberg M: Americans' belief in psychic and paranormal phenomena is up over last decade. Gallup News Service, June 8, 2001. Available at: https://news.gallup.com/poll/4483/americans-belief-psychic-paranormal-phenomena-over-last-decade.aspx. Accessed January 29, 2023.

Perls L: Concepts and misconceptions of gestalt therapy. J Humanist Psychol 32(3):50–56, 1992

Pilton M, Bucci S, McManus J, et al: Does insecure attachment mediate the relationship between trauma and voice-hearing in psychosis? Psychiatry Res 246:776–782, 2016 27817908

Schwartz RC, Sweezy M: Internal Family Systems Therapy, 2nd Edition. New York, Guilford, 2019

Seo J, Choi JY: Social defeat as a mediator of the relationship between childhood trauma and paranoid ideation. Psychiatry Res 260:48–52, 2018 29172098

Shevlin M, Houston JE, Dorahy MJ, Adamson G: Cumulative traumas and psychosis: an analysis of the National Comorbidity Survey and the British Psychiatric Morbidity Survey. Schizophr Bull 34(1):193–199, 2008 17586579

Turner MH, Bernard M, Birchwood M, et al: The contribution of shame to post-psychotic trauma. Br J Clin Psychol 52(2):162–182, 2013 24215146

van der Hart O, Nijenhuis ERS, Steele K: The Haunted Self: Structural Dissociation and the Treatment of Chronic Traumatization. New York, WW Norton, 2006

van Os J, Linscott RJ, Myin-Germeys I, et al: A systematic review and meta-analysis of the psychosis continuum: evidence for a psychosis proneness-persistence-impairment model of psychotic disorder. Psychol Med 39(2):179–195, 2009 18606047

Varese F, Smeets F, Drukker M, et al: Childhood adversities increase the risk of psychosis: a meta-analysis of patient-control, prospective- and cross-sectional cohort studies. Schizophr Bull 38(4):661–671, 2012 22461484

Walker M: Why We Sleep: Unlocking the Power of Sleep and Dreams. New York, Scribner, 2017

Watkins JG, Watkins HH: Ego States: Theory and Therapy. New York, WW Norton, 1997

Westermann S, Gantenbein V, Caspar F, Cavelti M: Maintaining delusional beliefs to satisfy and protect psychological needs. Z Psychol Z Angew Psychol 226(3):197–203, 2018

PART III
Working With Delusions in Different Settings

17

A Cognitive-Behavioral Therapy Approach to Working With Delusions in Forensic Settings

Patricia Cawthorne, D.N., M.Sc. (CBP), RMN

Personal Reflection: "Through a Glass, Darkly?"

The phrase "through a glass, darkly," attributed to the Apostle Paul (1 Corinthians 13:12), is often viewed as a metaphor for our relationship with reality or truth. The implication is that in life we only ever get to view ourselves in a distorted or imperfect way—as if represented "darkly" and as somewhat obscured, as we are in our mirror images. As a result, it is only through death and our experience of the afterlife that we ever truly get to see ourselves clearly, as we really are.

As a clinician working with patients with delusions, I often think about this. About how much of what we do involves unearthing—and perhaps painfully highlighting—with our patients a version of themselves that they either cannot or perhaps do not want to see. This is particularly true of forensic patients. And is it any wonder that they may want these aspects of themselves to remain hidden? How many of us apply our own "filters" to the reality of some of our less-desirable traits, characteristics, or even situations, and how many of us perhaps completely avoid looking at ourselves in any meaningful way at all? (As a concrete example, how often have you provided a 10-year-old image of yourself to accompany a biography for a conference flier?) And of course, although there is an element to this that is "just human nature," and perhaps vain and/or self-promoting, there is also another element that is perhaps highly anxiety-provoking and painfully, personally threatening. To look at this element, let alone share it with and reveal it to another human being, takes a great deal of courage.

How much do we think about what is truly involved in the exposure of our patient's unfiltered self when we do this work? What happens to our patients after they leave our sessions having been exposed in this way? How many of us would be prepared to allow ourselves to be truly "seen" by another person in this level of detail? This leads me to conclude that many of the patients I have worked with over the years have been some of the most courageous individuals I have ever met. I'm not sure I could do it myself.

Cognitive-Behavioral Therapy for Psychosis: Background

Early intervention for forensic patients with delusions is relatively rare. More typically, by the time these patients progress from experiencing the initial onset of delusional thinking, through to first presenting to their general practitioner (usually with multiple co-occurring psychosocial difficulties), and then moving on to secondary care services and beyond, significant periods of time—often years—will have elapsed. This may result not only in the continuous and negative reinforcement of these beliefs, many of which may involve paranoid ideation accompanied by a significant sense of threat and an inability to tolerate this so-called threat-control override (TCO; Link and Stueve 1994), but it may also have led to some individuals inflicting severe, sometimes fatal, violent attacks on others in their attempt to counter such beliefs and the distress associated with them. Bjørkly (2002) conducted a literature review that examined potential associations between delusions and violence and found that persecutory delusions, in particular those co-occurring with emotional distress, may increase the risk of violence. Within the same review, Bjørkly (2002, p. 617) also found that "there is limited but tentative support for the existence of an association between symptoms of perceived threat and internal control override and violence" (Bjørkly 2002, p. 617; Cawthorne 2019).

Prior research also suggests that cognitive-behavioral therapy for psychosis (CBTp), which encompasses the treatment of delusions, is most effective when offered at as early a stage as possible—the so-called *critical period* hypothesis. According to this hypothesis, rapid deterioration in the prognosis for untreated psychosis may occur if the duration of illness from onset to the start of treatment exceeds 5 years (Birchwood et al. 1998; Zaytseva 2011). However, notably, demographic characteristics taken from one study involving patients in a high secure hospital (HSH) in the United Kingdom indicated that the length of illness for this patient group was on average almost 14 years from onset (ranging from 1 to 50 years) and that patients had already been in the hospital for more than 4.5 years (ranging from 1 month to 30 years) by the time CBTp began (Cawthorne 2019).

Despite the apparent crucial importance of the need to intervene as early as possible with psychosis in order to optimize treatment outcomes and to address the specific delusional ideation that may be driving serious violence, very little application of CBTp in forensic services in the United Kingdom has been reported. This finding is compounded by the fact that current clinical guidelines recommend that CBTp be offered to all individuals diagnosed with schizophrenia or psychosis (including adults with complex psychosis) whose symptoms have not responded adequately to antipsychotic medication, to those experiencing persisting symptoms and/or depression, and to those who are in remission (National Institute for Health and Care Excellence 2014, 2020; Scottish Intercollegiate Guidelines Network 2013). The importance of implementing CBTp with forensic patients with delusions has been recognized by a number of national and international experts in HSH services (e.g., Benn 2002; Garrett and Lerman 2007), who have also commented on the role that this can potentially play in helping to reduce risk (Cawthorne 2019).

Some serious limitations to the implementation of CBTp in forensic services have also been identified. These include the failure to address some unique forensic and/or other contextual issues, such as the presence of co-occurring offending behaviors or comorbid personality disorder, either within the treatment protocols used or in relation to the outcomes achieved following their delivery (Bentall and Haddock 2000; Haddock et al. 2009). In recognition of these issues, and to help support the future delivery of CBTp in one UK-based HSH, Allan et al. (2002) developed a bespoke forensic CBTp intervention known as the *CBTp (f) program* (Cawthorne 2019).

CBTp (f) Program

The Garety et al. (2001) model of the positive symptoms of psychosis is central to the CBTp (f) program. However, this model has been augmented to include a focus on the role of underdeveloped and overdeveloped behavioral strategies, based on the work of Davidson (2000). This helps provide a more expansive formulation of the complex and problematic relational and behavioral aspects of personality functioning arising from core beliefs that are often found in this specific population. Furthermore, this addition

TABLE 17-1. Core beliefs and personality disorder

Typical core belief	Behavioral strategies	
	Overdeveloped	Underdeveloped
Borderline personality disorder		
I am bad.	Self-punishment	Self-nurturance
No one will ever love me.	Avoidance of closeness	Openness to relationships
I cannot cope on my own.	Overdependence	Independence
Antisocial personality disorder		
I can do what I want.	Autonomous	Sharing
Other people will get in my way.	Combative	Group identification
Don't get close to others.	Self-sufficiency	Intimacy

Source. Excerpt from CBTp (f) treatment manual (Allan et al. 2002).

of Davidson's (2000) conceptualization framework provides enhanced understanding of how these behavioral and relational patterns might be implicated in the maintenance of psychotic symptoms (e.g., delusions) and/or their appraisals in this group (Tables 17–1 and 17–2).

In the finalized version of the CBTp (f) program, Davidson's (2000) conceptualization of either underdeveloped or overdeveloped behaviors has been added into the diagrammatic representation of Garety et al.'s (2001) model as "associated behavior," as depicted in Figure 17–1.

The following case examples describe how this model has been applied in work with two forensic patients with delusions.

Case Example 1: Working With a Grandiose Delusion

Mark was an inpatient in an HSH, having been admitted following a hostage-taking situation involving the use of a firearm. He had entered a public library and "staged a protest," insisting that the people present should recognize him as Jesus and not as someone who was mentally ill. Mark asked the library reception staff to call the police and explain what was happening, saying that he looked forward to "having his day in court" so that he could expose corruption in public offices, in keeping with his responsibilities as the risen Christ.

Mark had been in the hospital for more than 18 months and was not making any progress. He was extremely distressed and frustrated at his clin-

TABLE 17–2. Core beliefs and psychosis

	Behavioral strategies	
Typical core belief	Overdeveloped	Underdeveloped
Punishment paranoia/derogatory auditory hallucinations		
I am bad/vulnerable.	Self-punishment	Self-nurturance
I am unlovable.	Avoidance of closeness	Openness to relationships
People will harm me if I displease them.	Pleasing others, compliance	Independence
Persecutory paranoia		
The world is unfair.	Autonomous	Sharing
People are dangerous.	Combative	Group identification
Don't get close to others.	Self-sufficiency	Intimacy

Source. Excerpt from CBTp (f) treatment manual (Allan et al. 2002).

ical team's lack of agreement with his delusional stance and could see no end to his incarceration as a result.

Phase 1: Engagement and rapport-building. In this phase, the therapist is demonstrating flexibility, starting by working from the patient's own perspective and shortening sessions if they become too arousing or disturbing. In Mark's case, this began with discussion about his frustration at "seeing no way out" other than "lying to you all about what I think, and I'm not prepared to do that." The therapist identified Mark's dilemma as an apparent impasse that was occurring between him and his clinical team, which might therefore be helpfully explored in an attempt to strengthen mutual understandings about each other's positions. As a result, a strong engagement was achieved, and Mark was reassured that the CBTp was not intended to "brainwash" him.

Phase 2: Clarification of context for the onset of the delusion and detailed analysis of its impact. In this phase, the therapist gradually moves from an empathic listening style to a more structured assessment interview. At this point, Mark was able to describe in detail his experience of multiple anomalous (mainly visual) experiences that had occurred when he was in prison. He also recalled and described embarking on a "search for explanations" for these experiences for some time before eventually giving them an external attribution, which had culminated in the formation of the belief that he was Jesus. However, when Mark initially told others about this, he was met with scorn and mockery. As a result, this recently formed belief extended to include the additional belief that, as Jesus, it was also his duty to prove his identity by "calling out" others' corruption, just as Jesus had done in the biblical story about when he had overthrown the tables of the money changers in the temple.

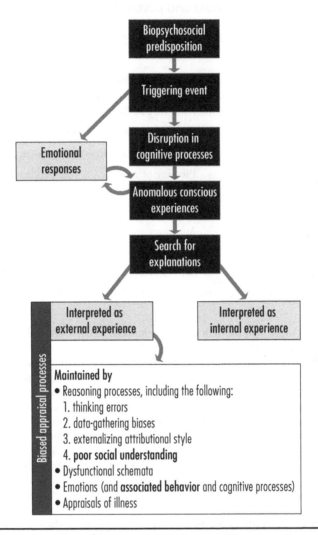

FIGURE 17–1. **Cognitive model of the positive symptoms of psychosis (after Garety et al. 2001).**

Phase 3: Formulation (including relationship to risk and identification of overdeveloped and underdeveloped behaviors). The delusion can then be formulated in accordance with a bespoke forensic CBTp intervention (Allan et al. 2002; see Figure 17–2).

Phase 4: Verbal reattributions. In this phase, the patient learns how to make links between their thoughts, feelings, and behaviors and their current delusion (and its impact on his functioning). For Mark, this phase began with him recording everyday seemingly innocuous thoughts, feelings, and behaviors about his relationships with staff and his peers on the ward. Through

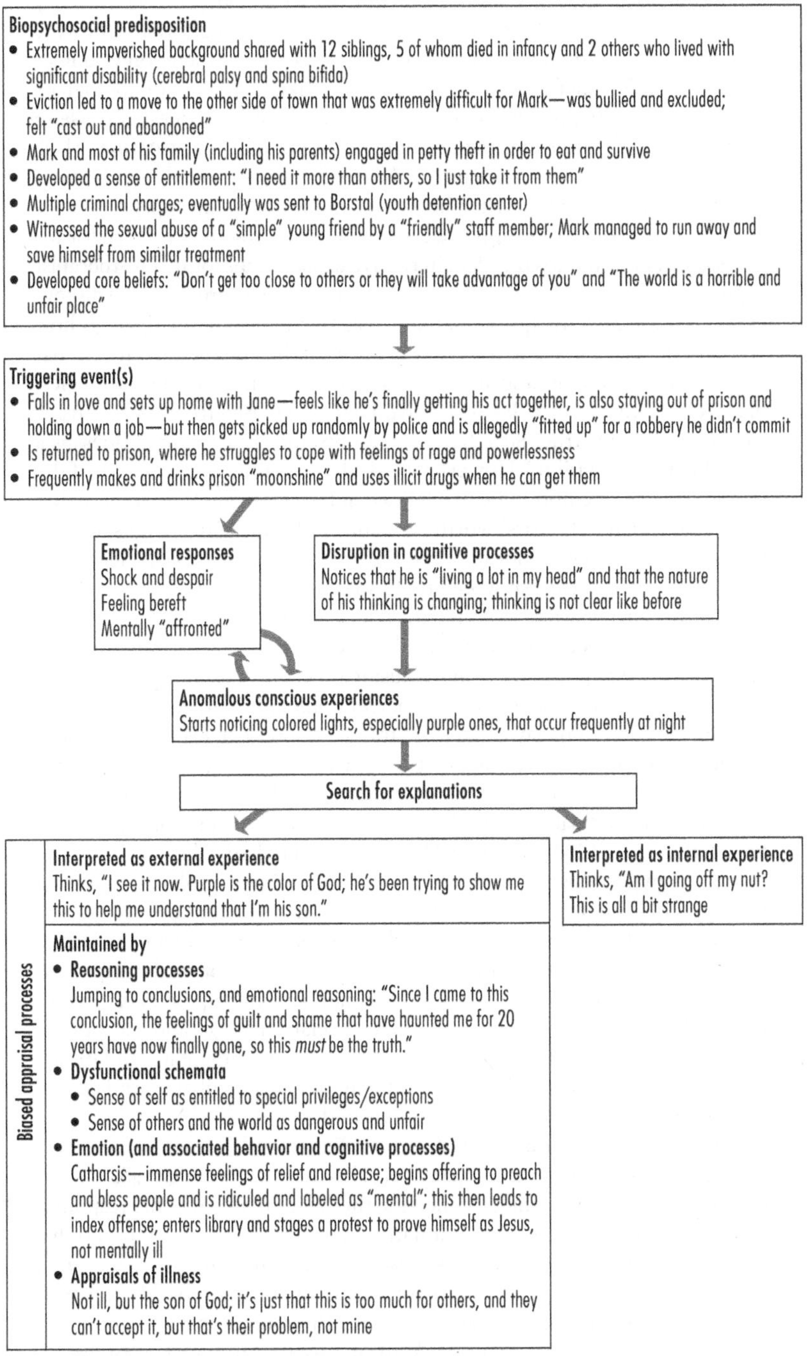

Biopsychosocial predisposition
- Extremely impverished background shared with 12 siblings, 5 of whom died in infancy and 2 others who lived with significant disability (cerebral palsy and spina bifida)
- Eviction led to a move to the other side of town that was extremely difficult for Mark—was bullied and excluded; felt "cast out and abandoned"
- Mark and most of his family (including his parents) engaged in petty theft in order to eat and survive
- Developed a sense of entitlement: "I need it more than others, so I just take it from them"
- Multiple criminal charges; eventually was sent to Borstal (youth detention center)
- Witnessed the sexual abuse of a "simple" young friend by a "friendly" staff member; Mark managed to run away and save himself from similar treatment
- Developed core beliefs: "Don't get too close to others or they will take advantage of you" and "The world is a horrible and unfair place"

Triggering event(s)
- Falls in love and sets up home with Jane—feels like he's finally getting his act together, is also staying out of prison and holding down a job—but then gets picked up randomly by police and is allegedly "fitted up" for a robbery he didn't commit
- Is returned to prison, where he struggles to cope with feelings of rage and powerlessness
- Frequently makes and drinks prison "moonshine" and uses illicit drugs when he can get them

Emotional responses
Shock and despair
Feeling bereft
Mentally "affronted"

Disruption in cognitive processes
Notices that he is "living a lot in my head" and that the nature of his thinking is changing; thinking is not clear like before

Anomalous conscious experiences
Starts noticing colored lights, especially purple ones, that occur frequently at night

Search for explanations

Interpreted as external experience
Thinks, "I see it now. Purple is the color of God; he's been trying to show me this to help me understand that I'm his son."

Interpreted as internal experience
Thinks, "Am I going off my nut? This is all a bit strange"

Biased appraisal processes

Maintained by
- **Reasoning processes**
  Jumping to conclusions, and emotional reasoning: "Since I came to this conclusion, the feelings of guilt and shame that have haunted me for 20 years have now finally gone, so this *must* be the truth."
- **Dysfunctional schemata**
  - Sense of self as entitled to special privileges/exceptions
  - Sense of others and the world as dangerous and unfair
- **Emotion (and associated behavior and cognitive processes)**
  Catharsis—immense feelings of relief and release; begins offering to preach and bless people and is ridiculed and labeled as "mental"; this then leads to index offense; enters library and stages a protest to prove himself as Jesus, not mentally ill
- **Appraisals of illness**
  Not ill, but the son of God; it's just that this is too much for others, and they can't accept it, but that's their problem, not mine

FIGURE 17–2. Mark's formulation.

keeping a thought diary, Mark began to notice that he had a distinct tendency to sometimes jump to conclusions. For example, he thought that staff were ignoring him and then felt slighted and started to avoid them, only to later reattribute this belief to his having been "mistaken" when staff apologized for having been temporarily delayed in dealing with his request because of another urgent matter that required their more immediate attention. Mark also noticed that he was more inclined to make erroneous judgments about others' intent toward him when he was feeling low and entrapped.

Gradually Mark was supported to begin examining the evidence for his delusional belief and to consider alternative explanations for it. The therapist supported this process by gently guiding his reflections (using guided discovery) and using Socratic questioning, such as "Can you talk me through how you experienced and made sense of the purple light shining in your cell that night?" Mark made significant progress with this combination of strategies; his level of conviction in his delusional belief decreased from "100% true" to "probably 20% true; 80% have my doubts and think mental illness is a more likely explanation." However, Mark also explained that because of the intense release of emotion he had felt when he eventually formed his belief (the feeling that "20 years' worth of feelings of guilt and shame suddenly left" him), he preferred not to let go of this belief in its entirety, lest these feelings recur because that would be "unbearable."

A little further work was therefore done with Mark, with the therapist working within his delusional belief. This resulted in Mark generating several alternative hypotheses for his delusional belief: 1) drinking moonshine and using drugs likely heightened his perceptions and led to distortions in his vision; 2) the delusion may have been a trauma response to his alleged wrongful incarceration; 3) the delusion may be indicative of mental illness, confirming the paranoid schizophrenia diagnosis he had been given; and 4) the content of the first part of the delusion was accurate—that is, this meant that he was the son of God. Although Mark preferred to hedge his bets and stick to an 80% hypothesis 3 and 20% hypothesis 4 combined explanation for the main part of his delusion, he was also clear that he no longer believed or felt that he needed to protest and demand that others accept his identity as Jesus. Mark was also able to recognize that the second and additional component of his delusional belief was linked to, and had been maintained by, his core beliefs about himself (as being entitled to special privileges and exceptions) and about others and the world (as being dangerous and unfair) and his associated overdeveloped behavioral strategies of being combative and autonomous when these core beliefs were activated.

Phase 5: Behavioral reattributions. Behavioral reattribution strategies can either follow or accompany verbal attribution strategies. As part of helping Mark examine the evidence for the belief that it was his responsibility, as Jesus, to call out corruption in others (i.e., the extended part of his primary delusion and the part responsible for maintaining his risk to others), the therapist designed a behavioral experiment whereby Mark had to research stories in the newspapers and on the television news about instances of exposure of corruption. Within a week, Mark had recorded almost 20 of these "outings" of corruption, none of which appeared to have required divine intervention. Mark then fed the evidence gained from this behavioral experiment back into his verbal reattribution homework and then was able to drop this part of his delusional belief entirely.

Phase 6: Reevaluation of risk. A reevaluation of the impact of Mark's now holding a significantly modified belief was then undertaken and was used to inform and update his risk assessment. His perceived level of risk was lower, and he was referred for transfer to a medium secure service shortly after the CBTp work concluded.

Case Example 2: Working With a Persecutory Delusion

James was a 28-year-old single man who was admitted to an HSH 4 years earlier following a near-fatal attack on his family physician. When he was just 18 years old, James had been involved in a serious accident on a farm. This accident almost killed him and left him with life-altering changes to his abdomen, mainly his bowel. It also took a long time for James's treating physicians to finally agree on the exact nature of his ongoing bowel difficulties. Following this, James had developed difficulties managing chronic pain and had started using cannabis on a regular basis as a means of self-medicating to cope with the pain.

Several months prior to the attack, James had presented to his physician for a pain management review while under the influence of cannabis. His physician had commented on this at the time. Shortly after this visit, James started hearing voices. Believing that his physician was the driving force behind the multiple derogatory voices that he was hearing, James stabbed him as he left the surgery one evening.

Four years after the attack, James continued to hold the delusional belief that his physician had been persecuting him, just as he had previously reported, although he conceded that his voice-hearing had improved since his admission and since he had begun taking clozapine. James also gave his reduced voice-hearing a delusional interpretation, saying he believed that it had lessened because his former physician had "clearly learned his lesson" following the attack, thus appearing to justify his actions.

Phase 1: Engagement and rapport-building. In the early stages of this phase, the therapist noted the amount of trauma that James often described when frequently reflecting on how his life had been before the farmyard accident. It was also noted that James frequently returned to describing chronic suicidal feelings that had persisted for some time following the accident. The therapist used a great deal of empathy and flexibility at this stage in the therapeutic alliance, often making time within sessions for James to tell his story and begin to develop a self-formulation of his difficulties. Like the therapist, James also paused and noted multiple "significant moments" and "significant shifts," such as in his views about himself (moving from having previously seen himself as a young man on the cusp of his physical and sexual prowess to seeing himself as a "disabled, smelly, and ugly physical wreck"). James was often tearful in these early sessions, and the therapist gently supported him to express and process feelings of loss, anger, and the pain of coming to terms with his significantly altered physical state.

Phase 2: Clarification of context for the onset of the delusion and detailed analysis of its impact. In keeping with the planned trajectory of therapy, in this phase, the therapist began to gradually move from an empathic listening style to a more structured assessment interview. To help facilitate this, the therapist worked with James to build a timeline (presented in a pictorial graph-like format) of his life experiences to date. To do this, James and the therapist focused their attention on mapping out some of the significant moments and shifts (in thinking) that James had described in earlier sessions, such as when his sense of himself had shifted, when he had begun having suicidal thoughts, when he recalled first being aware of the voices, how and when his experiences of physical and emotional pain had begun and how this pain had developed over the years, when he had begun to use cannabis and how his use had steadily increased to the point where he was using cannabis daily—sometimes several times a day—and when he had first begun having ideas about his physician persecuting him and when this had developed into a full-blown paranoid delusion that he had eventually acted on at the point of the index offense.

James took the lead in building this timeline, often adding to it as a between-session homework exercise. James reported that the use of the timeline had been a "real revelation" to him. He often commented on areas where he had "clearly got it wrong" in his recollection of how things had actually been for him, in particular in relation to his dealings with his physician. He noticed that significant points of distress in his life often correlated with those times when he was feeling most "disgusted" with himself, such as when he had had a temporary colostomy and afterward turned up "stoned" at his physician's office. James and the therapist also noted how a stark inverse relationship appeared to emerge between his chronic suicidal feelings (which decreased significantly) and the point when his delusion about the physician persecuting him had become more fully formed (and increased significantly). James commented on this, saying, "I remember it clearly. It was like, instead of being sad, I got mad—boiling mad! And I felt alive again because I had a mission. My mission was I had to make him stop punishing me!"

This appeared to suggest that James's persecutory delusion may have also been functional in that it helped to elevate his mood and improve his chronic suicidal ideation. Other authors have already commented on the potential for some beliefs to be functional (see, e.g., Chapter 8, "Cognitive-Behavioral Therapy for Paranoia"), noting that movement to another, new belief will be easier if the new belief also serves a similar function. However, this apparent increase in insight within James, although welcomed, was also handled very cautiously by the therapist, who was aware of the potential for this to perhaps have a counter-effect, possibly leading James to experience feelings of demoralization and hopelessness, thereby increasing his risk of suicidal thinking once again (Schwartz and Petersen 1999). No such feelings were noted in James.

Phase 3: Formulation (including relationship to risk and identification of overdeveloped and underdeveloped behaviors). The completion of the timeline in phase 2 significantly informed and shaped the development of James's formulation, which was completed in phase 3 (Figure 17–3).

Phase 4: Verbal reattributions. By the time therapy moved into this specific phase, James had already been engaging in using strategies such as "examining the evidence for and against" his delusional belief and "considering alternative explanations"—particularly when he and the therapist were immersed in the earlier timeline compilation and exploration. As a result, James's level of conviction in his delusional belief had decreased. He had shifted from believing that it was 100% true that his physician was the source of the voice that continued to persecute him to believing this to be only 10% true by this point. James also explained that his remaining doubt centered on his level of affect, which he noted tended to shift (and increase) at those times when he thought about his physician. He commented, "When I think of him, I just feel it so strongly. In those moments it's really hard, and I have to remind myself that these are just thoughts and feelings and that I don't have to act on them." James was also able to recognize that the previous level of his conviction in his delusional belief was linked to, and had been maintained by, his core beliefs about himself (as being flawed, yet someone who needed to be able to protect others) and about others and the world (as being cruel, hostile, and uncaring) and his associated overdeveloped behavioral strategies—of being suspicious and mistrustful—when these core beliefs were activated.

Phase 5: Behavioral reattributions. When working with James, the therapist used more indirect behavioral experiments designed to help him improve his sense of self, counter occasional thoughts of self-disgust, and help him to integrate and adapt to his bowel condition. For example, James reported that he often spent a lot of his weekly allowance buying extra toilet paper. By doing this, he was able to avoid feelings of shame and embarrassment at having to ask cleaning staff for an additional supply because of his more frequent need to go to the toilet. The therapist helped James to develop basic assertion skills and successfully request a regular increase in his toilet paper allocation because of his ongoing physical condition. James was then able to use this evidence of increased self-care and of his being "worth looking after" when challenging occasional, transient suicidal thoughts.

Phase 6: Reevaluation of risk. A reevaluation of the impact of James now holding a significantly modified belief was then undertaken and used to inform and update his risk assessment. Further work was planned with James to help him process underlying trauma related to his earlier accident.

Discussion

Both cases demonstrate that despite a number of reported limitations in implementing CBT for delusions in forensic settings, it can be done, with good effect, particularly if it is supported by a clearly structured and accessible treatment manual or program to help guide therapists who undertake this work (Cawthorne 2019). Although this approach involves a level of complexity—the underpinning model is drawn from both a cognitive model of the positive symptoms of psychosis (Garety et al. 2001) and a conceptual framework related to core beliefs in personality disorder (Davidson

Biopsychosocial predisposition
- First child in sibship of three (has a brother who is 1 year younger and a sister who is 2 years younger)
- Born via emergency cesarean section delivery (due to mother having a severe asthma attack during labor?); mother suffered postnatal depression
- Family history of psychotic illness (i.e., aunt had paranoid schizophrenia and grandmother had depression with occasional psychotic episodes)
- Father "not a great coper" and left much of James's care to his mother, despite her poor mental health at times, which (along with other things) caused marital tensions; as these tensions grew and other pressures arose, James's father began drinking to excess and developed alcoholism
- Family/home life characterized by frequent high levels of expressed emotion (mainly due to mother's ongoing emotional distress, father's poor coping, and the stress of having three young children to care for with very little social or financial support); father's alcoholism also led to unemployment
- Family was socially isolated and avoided others; inferred "rule" = "You keep your problems to yourself; it's nobody else's business"
- James was "embarrassed" to bring friends into his home because of father's drinking and mother's mental health and because the house was often dirty, smelly, and untidy
- Became vigilant and hypersensitive to father's mood; father was occasionally violent toward James, his siblings, and his mother, and James would often intervene, only to bear the brunt of the violence, which was displaced onto him
- Insecure attachment history arising from multiple factors outlined here
- Developed core schema of a sense of self as "flawed; yet someone who needs to be able to protect others" and others/the world as "cruel, hostile, and uncaring"
- Parents eventually divorced, mother recovered physically and mentally and worked hard to (successfully) build stability and financial security
- James and his siblings matured and benefited from increased stability and security at home

Triggering event(s)
- At age 18, James was involved in a farmyard accident that caused a severe abdominal injury; this eventually led to him having a chronic bowel condition
- Received multiple diagnoses and got "lost" in a series of tests/medical consultations, which led to a sense of being "sent around the houses" by "so-called experts" who "couldn't care a toss about me"
- Eventually had a total colectomy, followed by a temporary ileostomy; 4 months later the ileostomy was reversed, but he had lasting bowel difficulties
- Frequent (daily) cannabis use to self-medicate abdominal pain and to "escape the reality of the situation"
- Father died suddenly
- After the last operation, James had difficulties picking up his previous life, relationships, and career (higher education, financial services course), which had only just started
- Went to a general physician for pain management consultation but was under the influence of cannabis; the physician commented on this, saying it was unlikely to help with bowel problems

Emotional responses
- Physical and emotional pain
- Intense fear and anxiety
- Shock and despair
- Trauma
- Shame and embarrassment
- Disgust

Disruption in cognitive processes
- Finds it "difficult to get his head around" multiple triggering events
- Can't think properly or reflect, especially when emotionally overwhelmed, which, he notices, is happening a lot at this stage
- Thinking seems to be becoming "unbalanced"
- Has become increasingly "self-focused" and/or "other focused"
- Worries others might somehow smell or hear (stomach gurgling) or otherwise detect his ongoing bowel problems and disapprove of him
- Notices he's becoming a lot more wary of others
- Has started thinking the somehow "should have known" something horrible was going to happen to him
- Heightened perception and sense of impending doom and wondering "What's coming next?"
- Racing thoughts, especially about other people's intentions toward him

Anomalous conscious experiences
- Feels personally significant (i.e., senses that whatever's going to happen, it's going to happen to him)
- Becoming harder to tell whether his inner critical voice is his own voice, and notices it seems to be changing somehow, as though it is similar to language used by his physician

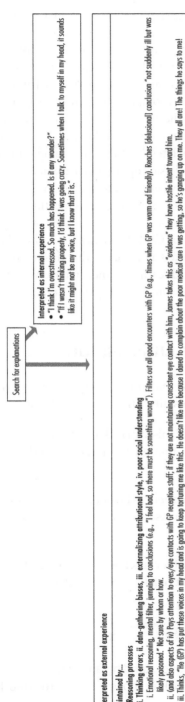

FIGURE 17–3. James's formulation.

2000)—it can nonetheless be applied in a systematic and helpful way to support forensic patients' recovery from the distress and other difficulties associated with their delusional thinking. Furthermore, it seems apparent that the application of CBT for delusions with this specific population can help reduce the risk of future violence. It therefore seems somewhat ironic that, arguably, the very area in which this complex intervention may be expected to have the most impact is also the area in which it is also most underresearched (Cawthorne 2019) and potentially underused. In contrast, low-intensity treatment programs (which tend to focus, for example, on delivering psychoeducation and building basic coping skills) are noted to be frequently delivered within forensic services (McIntosh et al. 2018); however, these are unlikely to have an impact on the big delusions that appear to drive serious violent behavior (Cawthorne 2019). It is therefore hoped that future increased implementation of CBT for delusions within these services will be encouraged and supported and, ideally, that this treatment will be offered to forensic patients much earlier in their recovery journey in order to maximize treatment outcomes and guard against a rapid decline in their future prognosis.

Questions for Discussion

1. Consider the possibility of forensic patients having earlier access to CBT for delusions. How might this affect the nature of this work?

2. What about the complex nature of this work? How can this be simplified and operationalized such that all the patient's underlying needs are addressed in therapy?

3. What, if anything, might the consequences be of failing to work with delusional ideation that has given rise to serious violent behavior (medication notwithstanding)?

4. How do therapists *really* know whether risk has been reduced following a modification or abandonment of a former delusional belief?

KEY POINTS

- Delusions often are significantly long-standing and entrenched and are often implicated in violence risk in those who are referred for CBTp within forensic services.

- Forensic patients often experience lack of trust or suspiciousness; have a high degree of co-occurring problems; and may tend to minimize the extent of their illness symptoms, trauma, or culpability for having committed acts of violence (particularly when this is driven by delusional ideation).

- Demonstrating flexibility, starting by working from the patient's own perspective, and shortening sessions if they become too arousing or disturbing can help at the early stage in the development of a therapeutic alliance.

- The therapist works to clarify the context for the onset of the delusion and makes a detailed analysis of its impact. The delusion can then be formulated using a bespoke forensic CBTp intervention. Highest priority is given to identifying and targeting associated behaviors that increase risk to self or others.

- Patients are supported to use a variety of CBT change strategies to help tackle their delusional thinking. Where applicable, a reevaluation of the impact of holding a significantly modified or entirely new (nondelusional) belief is then undertaken and used to inform and update the patient's risk assessment.

References

Allan K, Gumley A, Cawthorne P: Cognitive Behavioural Therapy for Psychosis: Assessment and Treatment Protocol. Unpublished treatment manual, Lanark, UK, The State Hospital, 2002

Benn A: Cognitive behaviour therapy for psychosis in conditions of high security, in The Case Study Guide to Cognitive Behaviour Therapy of Psychosis. Edited by Kingdon D, Turkington D. Chichester, UK, Wiley, 2002, pp 159–179

Bentall R, Haddock G: Cognitive-behavioural therapy for auditory hallucinations, in Forensic Mental Health Care: A Case Study Approach. Edited by Mercer D, Mason T, McKeown T, McCann G. London, Churchill Livingstone, 2000, pp 67–75

Birchwood M, Todd P, Jackson C: Early intervention in psychosis: the critical period hypothesis. Br J Psychiatry Suppl 172(33):53–59, 1998 9764127

Bjørkly S: Psychotic symptoms and violence toward others: a literature review of some preliminary findings, part 1: Delusions. Aggress Violent Behav 7(6):617–631, 2002

Cawthorne P: A process evaluation to determine the barriers and facilitators to implementation of a cognitive behavioural therapy for psychosis treatment programme in a high secure setting. Unpublished doctoral thesis, University of Stirling, Stirling, UK, 2019

Davidson KM: Cognitive Therapy for Personality Disorders: A Guide for Clinicians. Hove, UK, Routledge, 2000

Garety PA, Kuipers E, Fowler D, et al: A cognitive model of the positive symptoms of psychosis. Psychol Med 31(2):189–195, 2001 11232907

Garrett M, Lerman M: CBT for psychosis for long-term inpatients with a forensic history. Psychiatr Serv 58(5):712–713, 2007 17463357

Haddock G, Barrowclough C, Shaw JJ, et al: Cognitive-behavioural therapy v. social activity therapy for people with psychosis and a history of violence: randomised controlled trial. Br J Psychiatry 194(2):152–157, 2009 19182178

Link BG, Stueve A: Psychotic symptoms and the violent/illegal behavior of mental patients compared to community controls, in Violence and Mental Disorder: Developments in Risk Assessment. Edited by Monahan J, Steadman HJ. Chicago, IL, University of Chicago Press, 1994, pp 137–158

McIntosh LG, Slesser M, O'Rourke S, Thomson LDG: On the Road to Recovery psychological therapy versus treatment as usual for forensic mental health patients: study protocol for a randomized controlled feasibility trial. Pilot Feasibility Stud 4:124, 2018 30009040

National Institute for Health and Care Excellence: Psychosis and schizophrenia in adults: prevention and management (Clinical Guideline CG178). National Institute for Health and Care Excellence, March 1, 2014. Available at: https://www.nice.org.uk/guidance/cg178. Accessed June 12, 2017.

National Institute for Health and Care Excellence: Rehabilitation for adults with complex psychosis (Clinical Guideline CG181). National Institute for Health and Care Excellence, August 19, 2020. Available at: www.nice.org.uk/guidance/ng181. Accessed January 21, 2021.

Schwartz RC, Petersen S: The relationship between insight and suicidality among patients with schizophrenia. J Nerv Ment Dis 187(6):376–378, 1999 10379725

Scottish Intercollegiate Guidelines Network: Management of Schizophrenia (SIGN Publ No 131). Edinburgh, Scottish Intercollegiate Guidelines Network, 2013

Zaytseva Y: Critical period and duration of untreated psychosis. Cutting Edge Psychiatry in Practice 1:41–45, 2011

18

Using Digital Health Technology to Facilitate Measurement-Based Care in the Treatment of Delusions

Laura M. Tully, Ph.D.
Karina Muro, Ph.D.
Christopher Komei Hakusui, B.A.
Leigh Katharine Smith, Ph.D.

In the early twenty-first century, the phrase "There's an app for that" became common parlance—an acknowledgment of the exponential increase in smartphone applications available to users looking to address a wide variety of life challenges, such as building social connections, finding romantic partners, monitoring finances, and managing physical and mental health. As smartphones and associated wearable devices have become increasingly ubiquitous, public health scientists have looked to digital and mobile technologies for a variety of health solutions. This has sparked a rapidly growing field of digital health technology research and development; academic researchers and industry actors alike are racing to see who can produce the best viable and scalable solutions for global mental health needs. One such global mental health need is improving outcomes for individuals experiencing psychosis, and we argue that digital health technology has the potential to address long-standing challenges of access to, engagement in, and effectiveness of treatment for psychosis.

Although adaptations may be necessary, the idea that common psychotic symptoms such as paranoia make individuals with psychosis unwilling to use or uninterested in using technology as part of their care has been thoroughly debunked. A large body of research clearly demonstrates that people with psychosis use smartphones and apps as part of their daily lives and are interested in using digital health tools as part of their care (Torous et al. 2019). However, although the number of tools available continues to increase and the data indicate these tools hold a lot of promise, there is a lack of practical guidelines on how to choose the right tool and how providers can effectively incorporate digital health technology into clinical practice. Given the fast pace of development of digital health technology, often driven by for-profit companies that do not necessarily submit their tools to the rigorous evaluation of randomized controlled trials, it is important that as providers we have a framework for evaluating the available tools and determining when and how to use them as part of care.

In this chapter, we briefly review the status quo on digital health technology available for use in the treatment of psychosis, with a specific focus on the treatment of delusions, and provide guidelines for readers interested in keeping up with the latest research findings. We illustrate how digital health technology can help facilitate and enhance measurement-based care (MBC) and discuss key considerations when choosing a tool as part of a treatment approach, such as data protections and privacy, cost, ease of use, and cultural considerations. We finish with a detailed case example of integrating technology as part of cognitive-behavioral therapy (CBT) with a young adult Latinx individual experiencing suspiciousness and paranoia.

We cannot provide an exhaustive list of the ways in which technology can be used to support the treatment of individuals experiencing delusions and other symptoms of psychosis, nor can we expect this chapter to remain up-to-date given the rapidly evolving field of digital health technology. Instead, we aim to give you a framework for understanding how technology can be used in treatment and how to choose a tool that best fits your treatment goals. We provide practical examples of how clinical techniques and practices that you are currently using can be enhanced with technology as part of your standard clinical approach. All recommendations are provided in the context of a cognitive-behavioral framework—the recommended evidence-based practice for the treatment of delusions and associated symptoms of psychosis.

Status Quo of Digital Health Technology for Psychosis

At the time of publication, the status of digital health technology developed for psychosis and related symptoms can be divided into three categories:

1. Smartphone applications or web-based social media–style platforms designed to promote wellness, prevent relapse, and reduce hospitalizations via monitoring symptoms, providing educational content, and/or prompting coping skills use. These platforms range from those designed to be used independent of current treatment to those meant to be used in tandem with an individual's treatment team.
2. Brain game–style cognitive training software (either application or web based) designed to address common cognitive impairments characteristic of psychotic disorders (e.g., impairments in attention, working memory, executive functioning, face and emotion recognition).
3. Immersive video game–style and/or virtual reality (VR) technology designed to be used therapeutically to target specific symptoms (e.g., VR environments for threat belief testing).

To date, research has focused primarily on the first two categories. Overall, studies indicate that digital health technology tools can facilitate treatment engagement, symptom monitoring, reduction in paranoia and suspiciousness, reduction in negative symptoms, and improvement in social and occupational outcomes (for a recent trial using digital CBT to address paranoia, see Garety et al. 2021; for a brief and accessible review, see Torous et al. 2019). Similarly, cognitive training leads to improvements in global cognition that appear to last after training is finished and are associated with changes in brain structure and function. However, *how* cognitive training is delivered matters when it comes to generalizing gains to the real world: the largest gains are achieved when cognitive training is done as part of other treatment approaches (supported education and employment services, skills training, cognitive therapy); simply doing brain games on an app in the absence of other supportive treatments does not appear to lead to meaningful real-world benefits (Green et al. 2019).

The third area of research examines the potential of immersive video game and VR technology for alleviating specific symptoms of psychosis. For example, AVATAR therapy targets auditory hallucinations using a computer-generated character meant to personify a particularly distressing auditory hallucination. This character is voiced and controlled by the therapist, which enables the individual and provider to test various scenarios and ways of responding to and coping with hallucinations. Compared with a control group that received supportive counseling, individuals who received AVATAR therapy reported lower levels of auditory hallucinations and associated distress (for a review, see Rus-Calafell and Schneider 2020). Studies directly addressing the impact of VR interventions on delusions are limited, but findings are promising, in particular for addressing suspiciousness and paranoia. Overall, studies indicate that conducting behavioral experiments, such as threat belief testing sessions, in the VR environment (vs. in vivo) leads to a greater reduction in paranoia compared with treatment as usual (Geraets et al. 2020; Pot-Kolder et al. 2018) and compared with those who are exposed to the VR platform without belief testing sessions (Freeman et al. 2019). This supports VR as a promising intervention platform, in particular in cognitive-behavioral approaches, because the virtual environment offers a real-world analogue for repeatedly testing beliefs and conducting behavioral experiments. However, video game–style and VR technologies currently have significant and cost-prohibitive barriers to implementation, including the need for complex head-mounted displays and high-powered computing resources. Until these barriers are removed, AVATAR therapy and VR are unlikely to be widely available and accessible treatments for psychosis.

However, the use of technology in the treatment of delusions and other psychotic symptoms does not need to be as technologically complex as VR or require specially designed applications or wearable devices. Simple text message reminders have been shown to increase treatment engagement (D'Arcey et al. 2020), and integrating existing digital tools into care to facilitate MBC is accessible and can range from relatively simple approaches (e.g., supporting individuals in using the notes app on their smartphone to track their symptoms) to complex approaches (e.g., using an application specifically designed to prompt people to practice daily coping skills). Indeed, we argue that the potential for digital health technology to help individuals with psychosis reach their recovery goals is less about the specific tool and more about how providers can use digital health technology to support and enhance existing evidence-based approaches within an MBC framework.

Measurement-Based Care

What Is Measurement-Based Care?

MBC is the methodical collection of information on an individual's symptoms, day-to-day experiences, and activities that is then used to drive recovery-oriented clinical decision-making. MBC at the individual level is known to improve outcomes, and MBC at the aggregate level guides system-level changes in treatment delivery (Fortney et al. 2017). When working with individuals with psychotic symptoms, you likely will encounter multiple streams of information that must be integrated into a single conceptualization of their strengths and challenges to guide treatment. Integrating multiple streams of information is challenging; indeed, clinicians report that one of the primary barriers to feeling more empowered in their jobs is being asked to juggle too much information at once and not having the time to focus on the pieces that matter most. At its core, MBC involves identifying *which* information you think is the most important to attend to and then finding a way to assess it systematically. This is typically done through administering validated scales that have already been designed and calibrated to obtain specific information, including details that change over time (e.g., symptoms), details that tend to stay the same (e.g., personality), their positive experiences (e.g., life satisfaction), their negative experiences (e.g., depression), their experiences with you (e.g., the therapeutic alliance), and their response to treatments (e.g., the effectiveness of interventions). The information you gather is data, and collecting data is like creating a collective memory that reflects the lives and stories of the individuals you work with. The more data you collect and the more people you collect them from, the richer and more inclusive that collective memory becomes. Integrating technology into your treatment approach can help transform the information you gather into insights that matter.

How Can Technology Facilitate Measurement-Based Care?

First, technology can help you gather information more efficiently through things such as digital note-taking applications or private online journals in which people can record their thoughts and feelings. You can also streamline your data collection by administering surveys and questionnaires through online software (e.g., Qualtrics, SurveyMonkey) instead of with a pen and paper; this may seem like a trivial shift, but using technology to collect data allows you to consolidate all your information in a central location and then easily download your results so they can be quickly prepared for review.

Second, technology now facilitates the collection of information in ways that are actively engaging rather than passive and impersonal: from using beautiful applications and websites that summarize information in visually appealing and easy-to-understand formats, to providing automated feedback in real time, to using VR headsets that lead people through treatment exercises. Using interfaces that inspire individuals to share their stories with you rather than dragging them through the process reluctantly can increase both the quality and the quantity of the information you obtain.

Third, technology can help you communicate key takeaways faster through features such as graphs and data visualizations. Humans process images approximately 60,000 times faster than they process text, so using software to visualize the most important information can make communicating (and understanding) key takeaways much easier.

Fourth, despite some criticism that technology is pushing humans apart, when it is used thoughtfully it is unparalleled in its ability to bring people together. For example, practitioners can now connect individuals to broader communities of support in which they can interact with other people who are having similar experiences. Most recently this has been done via social networking platforms developed specifically for individuals experiencing psychosis, including platforms that promote peer-to-peer interactions, such as Horyzons and Prevention through Risk Identification Management and Education (PRIME) (both for individuals with recent-onset schizophrenia), Creating Live Interactions to Mitigate Barriers (CLIMB) (for individuals with chronic psychotic disorders), and Momentum (for individuals at clinical high risk for developing psychosis). For a review of peer-to-peer social networking interventions, see Biagianti et al. (2018).

Last, massive advances in computing technology have automated many complex processes that historically had to be done manually. For example, machine-learning algorithms can be used to make predictions about what a person will need, want, hate, and enjoy—and although this is most effectively done in conjunction with the guidance and opinions of humans, it can drastically lighten the load of designing treatments that are more uniquely tailored to an individual's particular needs.

How Might We Integrate Measurement-Based Care and Technology Into CBT?

As an example, let us consider how a cognitive-behavioral therapist might integrate technology into a treatment plan. CBT is information heavy by nature: we are encouraged to critically examine our thoughts, feelings, and behaviors; develop a logical narrative for how they are linked; and complete exercises and activities to strengthen self-awareness, evaluate maladaptive thinking patterns, and develop adaptive coping skills. MBC is a core principle of CBT, and providers traditionally use worksheets and associated paper-and-pen tools for facilitating symptom tracking and skill development.

Imagine that instead of using static, unresponsive worksheets, people could complete their exercises on their smartphones and receive immediate feedback that branches them to certain follow-up exercises depending on their responses. Imagine that they could receive alerts to complete their exercises at the times of day that work best for them based on real-life input such as their sleep schedule or when they are most active on social media. Imagine that they could view a graph of how their thoughts, feelings, and behaviors have changed over time and be given data-rich predictions about what to expect moving forward. Digital health technology can be designed to support individuals in telling a richer, more complete version of their own story and help them fill in areas that might otherwise be blank.

We propose six treatment areas in which digital health technology can enhance CBT: increasing engagement during assessment and information collection, providing innovative options for individuals to monitor delusional thoughts and engage in self-reflection, creating more immersive practice options for cognitive restructuring and building coping skills, facilitating more accurate predictions of symptoms and behaviors (i.e., relapse prevention), visualizing important takeaways, and building broader social networks. Table 18–1 summarizes current practices in these six treatment areas, provides tips on how technology could enhance or facilitate these activities, and provides different options for technology based on comfort level with technology (beginning, intermediate, advanced).

Considerations When Choosing a Digital Health Tool

We recommend considering the following factors to help you choose the most appropriate digital health tools as part of your practice: cost and access, ease of use and user experience, data protections and privacy, and cultural and linguistic considerations. We provide some guidelines for each of these considerations in this section. We also recommend checking One Mind PsyberGuide (www.psyberguide.org) for the latest developments in digital health technology. One Mind PsyberGuide is a nonprofit project that provides best practice guidelines for the development of mental health technology and publishes rigorous evaluations of new tools, including scores for many of the considerations listed here.

Cost and Access

Cost is a very practical barrier worth considering when choosing a digital health tool. If there is a cost, it is important to determine who is responsible for paying it. Is this a service your clinic needs to budget for (e.g., an annual licensing fee for a certain number of users), or is it a tool that individuals can buy themselves (e.g., an application on their smartphones)? Beware of free tools; many free applications make their money through advertisements that can disrupt the user experience, by selling user data to third parties, or by asking users for permission to mine data on their social media profiles. This is not to say that a free tool should never be used, but we recommend first investigating what "free" really means by reading the terms and conditions and making an informed choice (see "Ethical Considerations").

TABLE 18–1. Ways to integrate technology into cognitive-behavioral therapy practice

Technology benefit and options	Clinical practice or intervention	What we do now	What technology could help us do	Technology options
1. Increase engagement during data collection	Building a case formulation Intervention selection Psychoeducation tailored to the experiences and symptom profile	Complete clinician-directed assessments in session Administer questionnaires or homework exercises that can be long and hard to track with paper forms and/or workbooks	Create user-friendly questionnaires using software in which the layout (colors, fonts, display) can be customized Use survey-building software that allows clinicians to show or hide questions on the basis of previous answers, which saves time and energy Use smartphone applications that send surveys automatically at selected intervals for information collection Provide feedback on responses in real time with automated scoring (e.g., display an activity score with a short explanation, generate a battery score with a description of what it means) so questionnaires feel more interactive and personalized	**Beginner** Interactive PDF forms ($) **Intermediate** Survey design software ($$) Smartphone application for survey delivery ($–$$) **Advanced** Develop your own application ($$$; not recommended)

TABLE 18–1. Ways to integrate technology into cognitive-behavioral therapy practice *(continued)*

Technology benefit and options	Clinical practice or intervention	What we do now	What technology could help us do	Technology options
2. Provide innovative options for self-reflection	Symptom monitoring Building a case formulation Intervention selection Intervention design (e.g., designing behavioral experiments)	Assess any symptoms experienced since the previous session as part of session check-in Promote self-reflection by posing introspective questions in sessions using Socratic methods Assign homework to track symptoms using paper forms between sessions; encourage individuals to keep a paper journal or track symptoms between sessions on paper in some way	Ask individuals to write things down in an electronic platform as simple as Microsoft Word or the notes application on their smartphone, which can be quicker and easier for them than using a paper and pen Allow individuals to search multiple entries for keywords or ideas if they want to find a thought or return to an idea they have previously recorded Make sharing reflections with others nearly effortless Use apps to ping individuals at preset times to remind them to take a moment to self-reflect Use apps with preset questions designed to prompt deeper thinking	**Beginner** Digital note-taking software ($) Note-taking apps that set alarms for reflection reminders ($) **Intermediate** Online reflection journals that can be private or shared ($) Habit-tracking apps that help individuals reflect on behaviors over time ($) **Advanced** Audio transcription apps that convert spoken words into text ($$)

TABLE 18–1. Ways to integrate technology into cognitive-behavioral therapy practice *(continued)*

Technology benefit and options	Clinical practice or intervention	What we do now	What technology could help us do	Technology options
3. Create more immersive practice options for building coping skills	Relaxation skills Mindfulness skills Emotion identification skills Emotion regulation skills Distress tolerance skills	Use worksheets that describe the skill Practice skills live in session Use publicly available relaxation or mindfulness guidance videos (e.g., on YouTube); few options for engaging individuals in somatic work currently exist	Provide structured guidance for simple breathing exercises at appropriate points in a session with apps that offer preset options for different breathing intervals accompanied by soothing sounds or images to keep individuals on track Provide biofeedback to individuals in session through the use of simple devices for cardiovascular monitoring (HR, pulse oximeter) so they develop a stronger connection between their mental and physiological states Use VR headsets to submerge individuals in calming or stimulating spaces or transport them to different environments and worlds when they feel anxious, stuck, or shut down	**Beginner** Meditation or guided breathing apps ($) **Intermediate** HR monitors, pulse detectors ($$) **Advanced** VR or augmented reality headset experiences ($$$)

TABLE 18–1. Ways to integrate technology into cognitive-behavioral therapy practice *(continued)*

Technology benefit and options	Clinical practice or intervention	What we do now	What technology could help us do	Technology options
4. Predict behavior more accurately	Wellness planning/ relapse prevention Creating cope-ahead plans Selecting appropriate interventions	Provide psychoeducation on the vulnerability–stress model Identify symptom patterns on the basis of in-session assessments and homework assignments (typically completed on paper) Use paper worksheets to create a personalized wellness plan; we use key pieces of information when making assessments and plans, but what we attend to and remember can be subject to information overload, cognitive bias, selective attention, and memory loss	Explore how different variables are and are not related to each other Use data analysis software to describe individual experiences and predict outcomes Develop machine-learning algorithms that can anticipate individuals' behaviors and needs (e.g., how likely they are to respond to a particular type of treatment, what types of exercises they are most likely to enjoy)	**Beginner** Data spreadsheets such as Excel that allow for formula entry and analysis ($) **Intermediate** Statistical software programs ($–$$$) **Advanced** Analytic software that allows for complex model-building ($–$$$)

TABLE 18–1. Ways to integrate technology into cognitive-behavioral therapy practice (*continued*)

Technology benefit and options	Clinical practice or intervention	What we do now	What technology could help us do	Technology options
5. Visualize important takeaways	Building a case formulation Evaluating the outcome of interventions (e.g., reviewing results of homework assignments) Planning new interventions	Use a case formulation worksheet in session to visualize relationships among triggers, symptoms, maintenance factors Use a whiteboard in session to visualize key concepts discussed in session Engage in verbal discussions around treatment progress and change	Present graphs and other visualizations of quantitative data that represent important takeaways, such as how an individual's experiences are changing over time or how their experiences compare with other relevant groups Use text analysis software to analyze qualitative data to identify what words an individual uses most when writing in a self-reflection journal or responding to open-ended questions in a survey (e.g., word clouds) Use more sophisticated technology to create diagrams that represent social networks, the relationships between ideas, and customized decision trees	**Beginner** Data spreadsheet software (e.g., Excel) ($) Free word cloud generators ($) **Intermediate** Statistical software programs ($–$$$) **Advanced** Analytic software that allows for complex model building ($–$$$)

TABLE 18–1. Ways to integrate technology into cognitive-behavioral therapy practice *(continued)*

Technology benefit and options	Clinical practice or intervention	What we do now	What technology could help us do	Technology options
6. Build broader social networks	Increasing social support Normalization and stigma reduction Behavioral activation Social skills training	Assign socialization homework in session Provide psychoeducation about symptoms to normalize and destigmatize Engage the individual in peer support groups Engage the individual in cognitive-behavioral social skills training and facilitate family engagement in treatment	Organize group messaging chains to share resources, advice, or important information Connect individuals to broader social networks via discussion boards, social media pages, or community workspaces Build customized or private websites with discussion boards that are professionally moderated	**Beginner** Group messaging platforms such as text or email ($) Peer-led communities on social media platforms (typically free) **Intermediate** Apps and software that allow for group interaction and collective workspaces ($) **Advanced** Professional website software ($$)

Note. CV=cardiovascular; HR=heart rate; VR=virtual reality.

Related to the cost of the tool is access. Is special equipment needed to use the tool, such as a particular model of smartphone or access to a laptop or personal computer? Do you and the individual you are working with need to create profiles and log-ins? Does the tool work via cellular data or include the sending and receiving of text messages, and what are the implications for cell phone costs? The answers to these questions can help you estimate the level of technical support that might be needed to get started with the tool. With this information you can make an informed decision about which tool has the lowest access barriers for the individuals you are working with.

Ease of Use and User Experience

Onerous sign-up and log-in processes, glitchy software, or complex features that lack intuitive design will reduce motivation to use the selected tool (Kumar et al. 2018). Simple, intuitive designs that require little up-front learning and have streamlined log-in access are likely to work best. You do not have to select the most complex, feature-rich tool; simple surveys about mood, symptoms, and daily experiences that are summarized in the application or on a web-based dashboard can provide rich data sets for identifying early warning signs of symptom exacerbations and help guide treatment progress (Torous et al. 2019). We recommend testing out the tool before introducing it to your practice so that you can get hands-on experience with it and evaluate whether it is relevant for your treatment approach. If the tool you wish to test is behind a paywall, we recommend contacting the developers, because many companies can provide a free trial or demonstration.

Ethical Considerations: Data Protections and Privacy

When deciding to use digital health technology as part of treatment, it is important to consider how the technology in question handles user data, both in terms of security and privacy (i.e., where and how the data are stored, what protections and protocols are in place in case of a data breach) and in terms of data ownership and control (i.e., does the user own the data, and can the user request the deletion of their data from the database?). This is particularly important when working with vulnerable populations. For example, many smartphone applications targeting physical and/or mental health are offered for "free" in that there is no price the user must pay to install the app on a device. However, the hidden cost is often in what data are being collected about the individual and how those data are handled. Companies offer the product for free; in return, the user agrees—typically via a long and obtuse terms-of-agreement document (the end user license agreement [EULA])—to give the company access to their data. Depending on the tool, this access may be very broad and include multiple types of data from the user's device, such as GPS location data, movement data, device use data (e.g., screen time, time spent in certain applications), and communications data (e.g., number of phone calls or text messages sent and received). The upside to this approach is that companies can leverage the power of big data to develop important insights about their users, which could lead to individualized health recommendations and improved outcomes. This has been termed *digital phenotyping*, that is, the describing of a person's health and behavior using multiple types of digital data, often mined from devices without active user input (Onnela and Rauch 2016). Digital phenotyping is the holy grail of mental health technology research because it has the potential to solve big questions about mental health with minimal burden on the user. The darker side to this approach is that users may be unaware of the extent of data sharing that they have agreed to, and companies often support their products financially by selling user data to third-party companies. High-profile cases of data misuse (e.g., Facebook's highly criticized nonconsensual collection of user data with Cambridge Analytica in the 2010s) have brought this aspect of digital technology into stark reality, eroding trust and highlighting the importance of user informed consent, guidelines for ethical data use, and privacy practices.

Despite the inherent risks, concerns about data privacy should not deter you from using technology as part of your treatment approach. With new regulations that have come into effect (e.g., the implementation of the General Data Protection Regulation in the European Union in 2018 and the analogous California Consumer Privacy Act, which became enforceable in July 2020) and a growing field of stakeholder-driven mental health tools with clear and ethical data use practices detailed in their EULAs, safe and ethical options are becoming more available. The point here is to learn how to be an informed consumer in this field. How do you evaluate what the technology in question is doing with user data, and what are some key considerations when choosing a tool? We provide five key questions to ask of a potential tool. Most of the answers will be found in the EULA, specifically the section on data privacy, which can typically be found on the company's website or in the application itself. We estimate it will take approximately 10–15 minutes to determine the answers to these questions.

1. What data will the application or technology gather from users?

    a. Will it gather active input data, such as survey responses, ratings, diary entries, and/or pictures?

    b. Will it gather passive data, such as GPS and movement data, IP addresses, or screen time?

2. Will those data be identifiable or deidentified?
3. How will the company or software developer use the data?

   a. Will data be used for quality improvement efforts, such as bug fixing and product improvement (which is common for many applications and typically means the data remain internal to the company and are deidentified)?

   b. Will data be used for advertising efforts, such as capitalizing user data to identify other products users may be interested in?

   c. Will the data be sold to third parties for revenue?

4. What control do users have over the data?

   a. Can users request to see their own data? If so, how do they do this, and in what format do the data come?

   b. Can users request to delete their data? If so, how is this done?

   c. Can users specify which data are being used (i.e., if the application has the capacity to collect passive data from multiple sources on a device, do users have the option to turn off some of this data sharing)?

5. Does the company detail any limitations to privacy and confidentiality of data? Companies often have clauses in their EULAs around the disclosure or transfer of user data, including in instances of suspected illegal activity; in cases of breaches of terms and conditions; or when using outside third-party services to manage business operations such as email lists, website development and maintenance, and marketing.

Once you have the answers to these questions, you can make an informed decision about whether and how to use the technology. People will vary in their level of comfort—some may be unfazed by wide data sharing, and others may feel strongly about data control. Being prepared for this discussion and knowing how to find out the answers to these questions will help you choose the right tools for your work and help you and the individuals you work with to become informed digital consumers.

Cultural and Linguistic Considerations

Most digital health tools available in the United States are developed by English-speaking groups for use in English-speaking populations; for those whose primary language is a language other than English, this presents a significant barrier. Similarly, access to technology and the digital world varies markedly by race, ethnicity, and socioeconomic status: 2015 census data demonstrated that 36.4% of Black and 30% of Hispanic individuals did not have access to a computer or a broadband internet connection, compared with 21% of whites (U.S. Census Bureau 2017). This pattern persisted through 2019: 82% of white individuals reported having access to a computer compared with 58% of Black and 57% of Hispanic individuals (Atske and Perrin 2021). Non-white ethnic/racial minorities consistently have limited access to digital tools, which creates numerous barriers to them taking part in the digital world. The barriers have become even more visible now during the global COVID-19 pandemic, with significant ethnic and racial disparities in education, employment, and health care.

In addition to access, it is important to consider cultural factors, beliefs, and attitudes around digital health technology when thinking about using digital health tools as part of clinical care. In marginalized communities, historical abuses by the medical system, such as the 40-year-long Tuskegee syphilis study that exploited Black men and the nonconsensual use of Henrietta Lacks's cells for the advancement of in vitro fertilization technology, have led to an understandable mistrust of digital health technology and the institutions promoting it. Among Latinx individuals, undocumented status and evolving immigration policies contribute to a fear of seeking medical care, including a fear of providers using digital health technology tools that elicit concerns around government monitoring. This historical perspective, combined with current sociopolitical contexts in the United States, is an important consideration when proposing digital health technology as part of a treatment approach with individuals from marginalized communities.

Cultural and linguistic considerations should be at the forefront of our practice as providers: the United States continues to diversify rapidly, with 4 in 10 Americans identifying as non-white in 2020 (U.S. Census Bureau 2020). In California, approximately 60% of the population, many new immigrants to the United States, identifies as non-white, and 44% of Californians speak a language other than English (Bhushan et al. 2020). As we as providers work to integrate digital health tools into mental health services, it is imperative that we consider cultural and linguistic factors. In the following subsections, we focus on specific considerations regarding digital health technology when working with Latinx individuals, one of the fastest growing ethnic groups in the United States.

Specific Considerations for Working With Latinx Individuals and Families

Latinx individuals are the second-fastest-growing ethnic group in the United States, making up about 18% of the total U.S. population. They are a culturally heterogeneous group and are from various geographic backgrounds in Latin America, including Mexico, South and Central America, and the Caribbean (Fortuna 2021).

For many Latinx individuals, having a mental health diagnosis is stigmatizing, and access to and utilization of mental health services are challenging. In combination with a thorough understanding of relevant cultural values and factors (i.e., a cultural formulation), digital health technology has the potential to improve access to, utilization of, and quality of mental health services for this underserved population.

Many Latinx households are characterized by a mixed status (i.e., undocumented parents and U.S.-born children) and often are multigenerational, comprising both immediate and extended family members. In a clinical setting, it is common to work with adolescents and young adults who are bilingual, speaking both Spanish and English, while their parents are monolingual, speaking only Spanish. Thus, there may be varying degrees of English language proficiency and literacy between the individual and their family, and these differences should be considered when using digital health technology.

Even though Latinx families are heterogeneous, important shared cultural beliefs, values, and attitudes shape and impact mental health care and in turn the use of technology in MBC. A few of the core Latinx cultural values that influence treatment and the utilization of mental health services include *familismo* (the value placed on family and loyalty), *personalismo* (the importance of interacting with others in a warm and caring manner), and *respeto* (respect for others and especially authority figures). The cultural value of *familismo* is especially crucial because immediate and/or extended family members may need to help with the use of technology during sessions (e.g., logging on to a telehealth session, connecting to the internet, setting up reminders on a smartphone app, communicating via text messaging). Furthermore, having a clear understanding of who is part of the family system is important because certain family members may need additional technology-based education presented in their preferred language or in a manner that is tailored to their level of English proficiency. These cultural values need to be both thoroughly assessed and considered with each Latinx individual because they will affect each person differently.

Acculturation level also needs to be assessed because it can shed light on the best and most practical ways to provide education and support when using digital health technology tools. For example, is the Latinx individual a first- or second-generation American who may need more time to understand the importance of mental health services and, in turn, additional time to learn and practice using digital health tools? Other Latinx individuals may already be savvy about the use of technology and need a completely different level of guidance when using digital health technology as part of their treatment. Likewise, assessing access to technology (internet availability, laptop vs. smartphone access) as well as their level of comfort and familiarity with digital technology is key. Keep in mind that the cultural value of *respeto* (respect for authority figures) might inhibit Latinx individuals from initiating a conversation about their needs. As clinicians, we must create a space for them to share their concerns about technology. Larger social and political contexts, such as mental health stigma and immigration policies and enforcement, should also be considered. These contexts contribute to the fear and mistrust that Latinx families often have about disclosing and sharing their information.

Practical Considerations for Telehealth With Latinx Individuals and Families

During the global coronavirus pandemic that began in 2020, there was a rapid move toward the provision of mental health services predominantly via telehealth (e.g., video-conferencing software). In our experience, Latinx families benefit from additional opportunities to learn and practice how to set up telehealth sessions. The following are some practical considerations:

- Take some time to learn whether the individual and their caregiver have a working email address, and help them create an email address if needed.
- Have a written, step-by-step guide to the telehealth platform in Spanish and English.
- Smartphones are widely used among the Latinx population, and text messaging can be the most efficient and practical way to share telehealth information.
- Change the language settings on the telehealth platform to help reduce the language barrier.
- To prepare for technological challenges with a primary device, explore whether there are family members who may allow the individual to borrow another device.
- Schedule additional time during your first telehealth session for a debrief to learn about the successes and challenges of using technology.
- Latinx families encounter ongoing barriers to engagement in mental health treatment. Frequently revisit the additional resources and supports they may need related to changes in housing stability or living situation, financial resources, and access to digital health technology.

Personal Reflection

Consider the ways in which you might already use digital health technology in your own life. Perhaps you use a fitness-tracking app to monitor your running progress, a menstrual cycle tracker to track ovulation, or a meditation app to remind yourself to practice mindfulness at the beginning of your workday. How have these applications helped you reach your goals or stay on track with habits you are trying to form? What value do they add to your day-to-day routine? For many people, the appeal of an application that both collects useful data about a behavior they are engaging in (e.g., running) and summarizes progress in visually appealing dashboards (e.g., increases in distance or endurance over time) reinforces the behavior and results in progress being made over time. Alternatively, perhaps you have tried to use an application to support a new habit (e.g., meditation practice) but keep forgetting to use it. What factors influence how likely you are to use the app in your daily life? Does not using the application lead to any negative automatic thoughts about your ability to take care of yourself? What actions have you taken to try to promote use of the application as planned (e.g., setting reminders or alarms)? Reflecting on your own use of digital health technology and how it has positively impacted your life can help in supporting people to whom you provide services in benefiting from technology as well. If someone expresses concern about using technology as part of their care, asking them about the ways in which they might already use digital technology in their life could alleviate their concerns and help them understand how it could be helpful for mental health recovery.

Now consider the restrictions you have placed on the technology in your life. What is your comfort level with sharing your activity on social media? Have you changed your privacy settings or requested that your data be deleted from a particular tool? Do you try to manage your screen time by limiting time spent on certain applications? Are there aspects of your life you keep entirely analog? What about your approach to the terms and agreements for software tools and websites that you use? Do you read them closely or happily accept without investigation? Finally, how do your answers to these questions differ from those of other people in your life? It is important to recognize that each of us has different comfort levels and limits when it comes to digital health technology in our lives, and this is true for the people we worth with clinically as well. Exploring their comfort level will help you identify the best way to integrate technology into care while also respecting personal limits.

Case Example

Fernanda was a 15-year-old bilingual (Spanish and English) Latinx, female-identifying individual who was experiencing psychotic symptoms, including suspiciousness and paranoia. Fernanda's goal for treatment was to reduce suspicious thoughts of feeling watched and feeling that someone was trying to hurt her when nobody was around. In therapy sessions she spoke English; at home she spoke Spanish. Fernanda attended sessions with her mother, who spoke Spanish only. Fernanda had sought treatment at a specialty early psychosis clinic that used the coordinated specialty care treatment model, including CBT for psychosis with a bilingual (Spanish and English) clinician.

Supporting the Individual and Family in Using Telehealth

To help reduce transportation barriers, Fernanda and her mother agreed to telehealth sessions. Although Fernanda and her mother had their own smartphones, Fernanda's mother struggled to remember her email password to set up a telehealth platform account. After an assessment of access to digital technology tools, primary language, and preference, as well as comfort and familiarity with technology, Fernanda's mother was open to setting up a new email address with the clinician during the session. A plan was made to ensure that if Fernanda's mother's email address did not work, then the telehealth platform information would be sent via text. Education about the telehealth platform was reviewed in Spanish with Fernanda's mother and in English with Fernanda. Informational handouts about the telehealth platform were also sent via text and email. After a few practice sessions with the support of the clinician and Fernanda's guidance at home, both Fernanda and her mother learned how to navigate the telehealth platform. A debrief checkout was incorporated into the end of each practice session to ensure that concerns about technology use and access were discussed. This additional time also allowed Fernanda's siblings to greet the clinician (*personalismo*) and to share successes about using telehealth. During some of the practice sessions, it was common for Fernanda's older sister to help their mother log in to their telehealth account for collateral sessions. Now Fernanda's mother could join telehealth sessions when she was at work. Both Fernanda and her mother expressed that this digital method allowed Fernanda to attend sessions consistently and decreased Fernanda's guilt about her mother missing work for in-person appointments.

Using Technology to Facilitate Therapy Homework

During therapy, Fernanda identified that it would be helpful to track the frequency of her suspicious thoughts using a notebook. However, she often did not complete her therapy homework because she either had forgotten to carry her notebook with her or could not find it in the moment. Fernanda agreed to use the notes app on her smartphone for tracking. Fernanda's mother also agreed to track symptom frequency in her smartphone to support Fernanda. Both Fernanda and her mother shared that using their smartphones was helpful because Fernanda did not like talking about symptoms in Spanish; sharing her experiences in English was less anxiety provoking. Using her smartphone allowed Fernanda to write about her symptoms in English while the clinician mediated between Fernanda and her mother when reviewing the homework together. This method facilitated Fernanda's and her mother's communication about symptoms in their preferred languages. With the switch to the smartphone, Fernanda completed her homework assignment consistently because she had her phone with her all the time. An additional and unanticipated benefit was that Fernanda felt more comfortable knowing that her information was private and protected by the passcode for accessing her phone.

Tracking her suspicious thoughts helped Fernanda and her clinician to develop a case formulation in Spanish and English. Fernanda's mother also contributed by tracking the observed impact on behaviors at home (hypervigilance, difficulty leaving the house for social occasions, sleeping difficulties, anxiety and panic attacks, and limited communication with family members). With the integration of digital technology, new discoveries were made about Fernanda's triggers, emotions, and beliefs. Specifically, Fernanda identified that on the days that her suspiciousness increased, she had more school-related stress due to exams and difficult homework assignments. This information was discussed in session, which allowed Fernanda's mother to better understand where Fernanda's anxious emotions and behaviors were coming from. Fernanda's mother was then able to externalize Fernanda's behaviors instead of internalizing them (i.e., believing that Fernanda did not care about the family).

Using Digital Tools to Support Cognitive Restructuring

Using the audio-recording and notes apps on her smartphone, Fernanda practiced cognitive restructuring by recording the evidence for and against her suspicious thoughts in real time. Using her smartphone also helped her overcome memory difficulties when recalling past situations and cognitions related to suspiciousness. The audio recordings and notes app were reviewed in sessions and incorporated into thought records to further examine the suspiciousness. Fernanda identified the belief that "if someone starts a conversation with me during family gatherings, then this means they are trying to plot a way to share information with someone to harm me." Fernanda was able to discern that sometimes her suspicious thoughts were not accurate or helpful. This led to the development of alternative thoughts regarding why family members might start conversations with her (e.g., "They want to get to know me or spend quality time with me"; "They are also making conversations with others, and no one is getting hurt"). As a result, her social anxiety decreased. Ultimately, when Fernanda was struggling to identify alternative cognitions in social situations, she practiced evaluating the pros and cons of paying attention to her suspicious thoughts in social situations. Fernanda then used a phone alarm for a daily reminder to practice this cognitive skill regardless of whether or not she was in a social situation.

Supporting Individuals in Choosing the Right Digital Technology Tools

Over time, Fernanda and her clinician explored different smartphone apps that would remind her to track her symptoms and practice a variety of coping skills as part of her recovery. Fernanda's clinician supported her in exploring her level of comfort and knowledge around data sharing and privacy practices, and together they researched possible apps that could support Fernanda in consistently implementing her wellness plan.

In the end, it was evident that without access to and utilization of digital tools such as a smartphone device, Fernanda would have struggled tremendously in practicing cognitive and behavioral skills in her everyday life. Similarly, treatment progress would have been slower and problematic, which would have made the possibility of cognitive shifts in the treatment of her delusions challenging. Importantly, Fernanda was able to continue using digital health technology to independently manage her wellness after graduating from therapy.

Summary and Conclusions

Digital health technology has the potential to address long-standing challenges in access to, engagement in, and effectiveness of treatment for psychosis. Research evidence at the time of writing demonstrates that individuals with psychosis are interested in and willing to use digital technology as part of their treatment and that digital health technology can facilitate treatment engagement and symptom monitoring, improve negative and cognitive symptoms, and improve social and occupational outcomes. Integrating digital health technology into clinical practice does not have to involve complex software applications or expensive wearable equipment. Incorporating existing applications on smartphones, such as note-taking apps, reminders, and voice memo recordings, into the treatment approach can facilitate MBC and support individuals in remembering to complete therapy homework and practice coping skills. When you are choosing a digital health technology tool to use, we recommend considering such aspects as cost, access, ease of use, data security and privacy, and any relevant cultural and linguistic factors that could have an impact on willingness to use the selected tool. Using digital health technology tools to enhance and support standard treatment approaches can lead to more effective and meaningful interventions tailored to individuals' daily experiences and recovery goals.

Questions for Discussion

1. Think about an individual whom you are currently treating. How might you use digital health technology to support their treatment progress?

2. What are some of your own preconceived notions and cultural biases about technology that might impact the way you use digital health technology tools in your treatment approaches?

3. When working with Latinx individuals, who come from a heterogeneous group, it is essential to complete a comprehensive assessment of cultural values and beliefs, acculturation, language preference, and access to technology (smartphone, laptop, or tablet). What are some of your anticipated concerns in completing an assessment of cultural and language needs around the use of technology in clinical care?

KEY POINTS

- Research indicates that digital health technology tools can address long-standing challenges in access to, engagement in, and effectiveness of treatment for psychosis.

- MBC is the methodical collection of information on an individual's symptoms, day-to-day experiences, and activities that is then used to drive recovery-oriented clinical decision-making.

- Digital health technology is uniquely poised to facilitate MBC, in particular in the context of CBT, in which providers traditionally use worksheets and associated paper-and-pen tools to facilitate symptom tracking and skill development.

- We propose six treatment areas in which digital health technology can enhance CBT: increasing engagement during assessment, providing innovative options for the individual to monitor delusional thoughts, creating more immersive practice options for cognitive restructuring and coping skills, facilitating more accurate relapse prediction and prevention, visualizing important takeaways, and building broader social networks.

- Consideration of data security and data ownership is imperative when choosing a digital health tool. New regulations coupled with stakeholder-driven product designs have prompted more consumer-centered ethical data use policies in the digital health technology industry.

- Given that most digital health technology has been developed by primarily English-speaking teams and that access to the digital world in the United States varies markedly by race, ethnicity, and socioeconomic status, cultural and linguistic considerations are imperative when integrating digital health technology tools with treatment plans.

References

Atske S, Perrin A: Home broadband adoption, computer ownership vary by race, ethnicity in the U.S. Pew Research Center, July 16, 2021. Available at: www.pewresearch.org/fact-tank/2021/07/16/home-broadband-adoption-computer-ownership-vary-by-race-ethnicity-in-the-u-s. Accessed September 28, 2021.

Bhushan D, Kotz K, McCall J, et al: Roadmap for Resilience: the California Surgeon General's Report on Adverse Childhood Experiences, Toxic Stress, and Health. Office of the California Surgeon General, December 9, 2020. Available at: https://osg.ca.gov/wp-content/uploads/sites/266/2020/12/Roadmap-For-Resilience_CA-Surgeon-Generals-Report-on-ACEs-Toxic-Stress-and-Health_12092020.pdf. Accessed September 28, 2021.

Biagianti B, Quraishi SH, Schlosser DA: Potential benefits of incorporating peer-to-peer interactions into digital interventions for psychotic disorders: a systematic review. Psychiatr Serv 69(4):377–388, 2018 29241435

D'Arcey J, Collaton J, Kozloff N, et al: The use of text messaging to improve clinical engagement for individuals with psychosis: systematic review. JMIR Ment Health 7(4):e16993, 2020 32238334

Fortney JC, Unützer J, Wrenn G, et al: A tipping point for measurement-based care. Psychiatr Serv 68(2):179–188, 2017 27582237

Fortuna L: Working with Latino/a and Hispanic patients. American Psychiatric Association, 2021. Available at: www.psychiatry.org/psychiatrists/cultural-competency/education/best-practice-highlights/working-with-latino-patients. Accessed September 28, 2021.

Freeman D, Lister R, Waite F, et al: Automated psychological therapy using virtual reality (VR) for patients with persecutory delusions: study protocol for a single-blind parallel-group randomised controlled trial (THRIVE). Trials 20(1):87, 2019 30696471

Garety P, Ward T, Emsley R, et al: Effects of SlowMo, a blended digital therapy targeting reasoning, on paranoia among people with psychosis: a randomized clinical trial. JAMA Psychiatry 78(7):714–725, 2021 33825827

Geraets CNW, Snippe E, van Beilen M, et al: Virtual reality based cognitive behavioral therapy for paranoia: effects on mental states and the dynamics among them. Schizophr Res 222:227–234, 2020 32527676

Green MF, Horan WP, Lee J: Nonsocial and social cognition in schizophrenia: current evidence and future directions. World Psychiatry 18(2):146–161, 2019 31059632

Kumar D, Tully LM, Iosif A-M, et al: A mobile health platform for clinical monitoring in early psychosis: implementation in community-based outpatient early psychosis care. JMIR Ment Health 5(1):e15, 2018 29487044

Onnela J-P, Rauch SL: Harnessing smartphone-based digital phenotyping to enhance behavioral and mental health. Neuropsychopharmacology 41(7):1691–1696, 2016 26818126

Pot-Kolder RMCA, Geraets CNW, Veling W, et al: Virtual-reality-based cognitive behavioural therapy versus waiting list control for paranoid ideation and social avoidance in patients with psychotic disorders: a single-blind randomised controlled trial. Lancet Psychiatry 5(3):217–226, 2018 29429948

Rus-Calafell M, Schneider S: Are we there yet?! A literature review of recent digital technology advances for the treatment of early psychosis. mHealth 6:3, 2020 32190614

Torous J, Woodyatt J, Keshavan M, Tully LM: A new hope for early psychosis care: the evolving landscape of digital care tools. Br J Psychiatry 214(5):269–272, 2019 30739613

U.S. Census Bureau: The digital divide: percentage of households by broadband internet subscription, computer type, race and Hispanic origin. Suitland, MD, U.S. Census Bureau, September 11, 2017. Available at: www.census.gov/library/visualizations/2017/comm/internet.html. Accessed September 28, 2021R.

U.S. Census Bureau: Quick Facts. Suitland, MD, U.S. Census Bureau, 2020. Available at: www.census.gov/quickfacts/fact/table/US/PST045222#qf-headnote-b. Accessed February 28, 2023.

19

Cognitive-Behavioral Therapy–Informed Skills Training for Families Caring for a Loved One With Delusions

Sarah Kopelovich, Ph.D.
Maria Monroe-DeVita, Ph.D.
H. Teresa Buckland, Ph.D., M.Ed.

Delusions are profoundly isolating. By their nature, delusions serve to alienate their holders from those around them. The holders' convictions about what is truth and what is falsehood are unshared at best; are commonly challenged by even the most well-intentioned; and at worst expose them to risk of loss of civil liberty, relationships, and self-determination. Active involvement of family or other natural supports is critical to the process of recovery and is now widely recommended as a standard of care (Keepers et al. 2020).

The terms *family* and *natural supports* are often used interchangeably. Both include unpaid, nonprofessional relationships identified as important sources of love and support by the individual. Although it is the case that family can include nonadopted and nonbiological relationships (e.g., family by choice), the term *natural support* is intended to refer more broadly to individuals in the person's broader communities. In this chapter, we use the term *natural supports* to encompass both family and social support systems and the term *family interventions* to refer to interventions intended for those natural supports whom the individual receiving care has identified as their primary support system.

Unfortunately, mental health researchers and clinicians have historically perpetuated theories that familial dynamics cause schizophrenia. The consequent blaming and shaming of family members often led to therapeutic misalliance between treatment providers and service users. We now have decades of cross-cultural research that indicates that high *expressed emotion* can increase the likelihood of relapse and rehospitalization but that psychosis is not caused by family dynamics and that the etiologies of psychoses are complex and multifaceted (Canavan 2000). Comprehensive care that includes family psychoeducation, skill-building to improve the emotional tone in the home, and the involvement of natural supports in both therapeutic interventions and—when possible—therapeutic decision-making should be implemented as early as possible in the pathogenesis of a psychotic disorder. When families remain involved, individuals with psychosis have better physical health outcomes, social and occupational outcomes, and engagement in mental health treatment and reduced rates of relapse and rehospitalization. In some cases, effect sizes for family interventions for psychosis are comparable to those in psychopharmacological trials for schizophrenia (McDonagh et al. 2017). For the 50%–60% of adults with a serious mental illness and co-occurring disorder, family contact and/or familial financial support is correlated with a reduction in or discontinuation of substance use (Clark 2001).

Family psychoeducation as a stand-alone treatment for schizophrenia and other psychoses was developed in the 1970s and is now included in national treatment guidelines in a number of countries. Although these treatment guidelines have established psychoeducation with identified natural supports as the minimum standard when working with an individual with delusions, ideally, members of the core support network of the patient should be enlisted as *active partners* to both the care team and the patient. Such a partnership is mutually beneficial to all parties. From the care team's perspective, the ability to understand and conceptualize strengths, resources, challenges, and barriers to recovery is facilitated by the perspectives of the natural supports and a better understanding of the biopsychosociocultural factors at play. Moreover, the clinical team can share clinical tasks with natural supports to enhance uptake of illness self-management and core therapeutic interventions. We discuss this function later in the chapter during the discussion of coaching families in skills informed by cognitive-behavioral therapy (CBT). Inclusion allows natural supports who are in the role of caregiver to share additional helpful perspectives the patient may not be able to share, to reinforce clinical interventions, to model or co-rehearse new skills, and to help their loved one with symptom monitoring and wellness planning. The opportunity for inclusion in discussions of care provided to a loved one can enhance the caregiver's sense of self-efficacy and ability to support their loved one. When executed skillfully, selective involvement of the family can preserve the bonds between family members by changing the dynamic.

Although the literature provides ample evidence that family engagement in clinical care is beneficial to the individual receiving services in terms of symptom and functional outcomes, clinicians should ensure that natural supports are engaged in a manner consistent with recovery-oriented care to enhance the perceived benefits and the relationships between and among the three parties. Strategies for maintaining a focus on the individual and their preferences for treatment are discussed later in this chapter.

Case Example of Co-rehearsal of Skills

Jenny, a 32-year-old woman residing with her 65-year-old mother, Martha, was becoming increasingly paranoid toward her. Jenny complained frequently to her care team that she was at her wits' end with her mother because "she's always on my case about taking my meds. It's all she cares about." Jenny's psychiatrist requested that Martha attend the next appointment. During the appointment, the psychiatrist shared how common it is for adults in the general population to miss medication doses. These figures surprised Martha, and she acknowledged that she sometimes forgets to take her blood pressure medication. Together Martha and Jenny worked with the psychiatrist on practical approaches to help them both remember to take their medications as prescribed. Because they adopted the same system (moving the medications to the opposite shelf on a spice rack in the kitchen after each dose), they were both more successful at remembering to take their medications without prompts. More important, Jenny felt respected as an autonomous adult, and she and her mother were able to talk about more enjoyable topics now that the focus was off Jenny's medication use.

What Gets in the Way of Engaging Natural Supports?

Despite the fact that the majority of adults with a serious mental illness live with a family member and many report a preference for familial involvement in their treatment, natural supports are not routinely engaged in their loved one's care. In fact, so pernicious are the impediments to clinical engagement of natural supports that estimates suggest that less than 2% of families are even receiving diagnostic psychoeducation (Interdepartmental Serious Mental Illness Coordinating Committee 2017). Impediments to family interventions include systems-, provider-, patient-, and family-level barriers. At the systems level, family engagement may not be a reimbursable service depending on the payer, staff may be unwilling or unable to provide interventions at times that accommodate working family members, or decision-makers may not be attuned to the benefits of family intervention. Because coordinated multidisciplinary specialty care is often exclusive to either assertive community treatment or early intervention for psychosis programs, family programming is rarely found in traditional outpatient behavioral health services. Moreover, supervisors rarely set the expectation that natural supports are involved in the care of adult loved ones, and in their supervision of frontline clinicians, they rarely discuss the benefits of including them. At the provider level, clinicians are seldom trained in family interventions, may lack the time or motivation to administer them, or may hold pejorative views of family engagement (e.g., deeming family members overinvolved). At the patient level, although many service users report a desire for family education and skills training, they also express concerns that greater family involvement will lead to diminished privacy and agency in their treatment. They are not informed of the benefits or the proposed terms of family involvement and may therefore view family engagement in all-or-nothing terms. Finally, at the family level, high rates of refusal, withdrawal, and nonadherence further complicate efforts to involve family supports (Smith and Birchwood 1990).

Addressing Barriers to Including Family in Treatment

Although systematic implementation of family interventions is needed to help redress the issues noted previously, individual clinicians can and should enhance their support of families in the clinic. Clinicians can supplement clinic-delivered family interventions with bibliotherapy; advocacy organizations; support groups; web-based or in-person caregiver training programs; and an emerging cadre of mobile health interventions that provide education, connection, and skills coaching. Finally, for both natural supports and the individual receiving services, making the time for occasional joint sessions that facilitate the processes of sharing information, being heard, and having values and preferences taken into account is affirming. This affirmation promotes hope and helps reduce stress related to feelings of disenfranchisement, exclusion, or fear of doing or saying the wrong thing. Stress reduction is an important part of the recovery process for the entire support system.

Personal Reflection Based on a Lived Experience With Care Inclusion

My adult son lives with my husband and me (H.T.B.). We often share meals, and we see one another and talk with one another every day. As part of my son's treatment, his psychiatrist welcomes our participation in his medication management appointments. This provides hope and stress reduction for many reasons:

- My husband, son, and I know the psychiatrist is getting a complete picture of our son's symptoms.
- We all feel good about being treated respectfully as part of a collaborative team; our ideas are worth considering, and the psychiatrist is willing to allow the three of us to come up with a plan for treatment that reflects our needs and desires.
- We have the opportunity to ask questions about medications so we feel more confident managing disconcerting and uncomfortable side effects.
- We feel empowered to use the therapeutic communication strategies we have been taught when strongly held distressing beliefs arise or get worse. We are not afraid of saying or doing the wrong thing because we have the provider's input and can call for help if needed.

Key Techniques for Family Engagement

The research literature is clear: clinical neglect of the natural support systems of patients who present for the treatment of psychotic symptoms is a critical missed opportunity with deleterious effects on service users, their primary support systems, and clinical teams. In the remainder of this chapter we focus on key strategies for involving natural supports as active agents in the care and recovery of their loved one with delusions.

Given the empirically supported clinical, relational, and functional benefits of family interventions for psychosis, clinicians should consider incorporating key techniques into standard clinical practice with this patient population. We outline several techniques for engaging natural supports in the recovery process of their loved ones with strongly held beliefs, but fundamentally, family engagement extends beyond a set of techniques. It is a way of working with patients that views the patient as part of their family system, communities, and cultural groups. To not activate and engage these systems in their recovery is to swim against a strong and seductive current whereby individual find greater value and safety in their strongly held beliefs than in their interactions with others. When the clinician operates from a service model in which family engagement is normative, the clinician is then naturally inclined to identify existing support systems and integrate them into treatment and to generate ways to overcome obstacles such as refusal to authorize the release of information. Techniques for normalizing family engagement, listed in a more or less sequential manner, include the following: 1) engaging patients in a discussion of the risks and benefits of engaging natural supports, 2) developing a mini-formulation related to patients' reactions to engaging natural supports, 3) promoting a family-involved shared decision-making model of care, 4) using motivational enhancement techniques to resolve ambivalence among all stakeholders, 5) providing recovery-oriented psychoeducation and normalization to reduce stigma and promote hope, 6) addressing caregiver stress and expressed emotion, and 7) coaching natural supports in CBT-informed skills.

Informed Consent for Family Engagement

Provide patients with information about the risks and benefits of including family in treatment. The risks and benefits demonstrated in the empirical literature, some of which were described in the preceding sections of this chapter, should be shared by the clinician, and perceived risks and benefits should also be elicited from the patient. Ensure that patients understand that they can dictate the terms of who, when, how, and for what purpose family are involved in their care. As with other applications of informed consent, patients can be assured that consent is dynamic and that they can reevaluate the extent of familial involvement at any point. Such an approach enhances trust and mutual respect between the clinician and patient and promotes agency and empowerment, which are central to a recovery-oriented system of care. Clinicians can invite their patients to consider who they would like to include in their treatment plan. Once the patient has identified the individuals they would like to be included, the patient and the clinician can jointly extend that invitation to the natural support(s).

Assessment of Automatic Thoughts, Feelings, and Behaviors Pertaining to Engaging Natural Supports

Assessing automatic thoughts, feelings, and behaviors related to engaging natural supports can help you to develop a mini-formulation that can be addressed collaboratively (Figure 19–1). Clinicians should be particularly attuned to themes of shame and self-stigma, which are common among individuals who experience strongly held beliefs that are not shared by others. When such themes are observed, it is important that they be labeled and that clinicians work with the patient to identify the ways in which

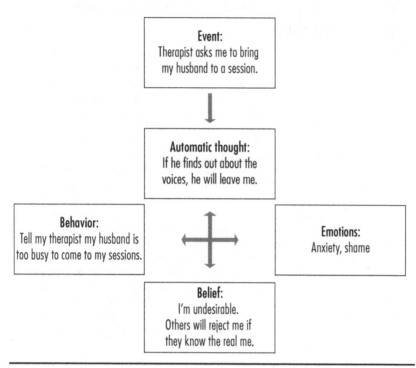

FIGURE 19–1. Mini-formulation of a patient's reluctance to involve her husband in her clinical care.

shame and self-stigma are being reinforced by their behavior of excluding family from their recovery process. According to prominent shame researcher Dr. Brené Brown, shame thrives on secrecy, silence, and judgment. Exposing shame and testing the underlying beliefs that fuel it by providing natural supports with psychoeducation, normalization, and communication coaching can promote relief from shame.

Family-Involved Shared Decision-Making

Clinicians must be mindful of delineating and communicating boundaries to individuals and the natural supports they choose to include. This is particularly important for adult patients who elect to involve parents. Patients should retain the locus of control in shared decision-making regarding their treatment. In this family-involved shared decision-making mode, the patient is seen as the expert in their experience, and the clinician is viewed as an expert by virtue of their education. Like all experts, the patient-clinician team considers information from credible sources, which in this case should include natural supports.

Case Example: Family-Involved Shared Decision-Making

Serena is 48 years old and was diagnosed with schizoaffective disorder when she was 28. She had always been a star performer in school and at work, but severe bouts of depression, mania, and psychosis have caused multiple interruptions to her career and her personal life since their onset. She has taken numerous medications over the past 20 years to control her symptoms, has been hospitalized on 12 occasions, and has received a course of electroconvulsive therapy. Although Serena can recall some helpful clinical providers, she primarily recounts a traumatic and stressful treatment history. Serena communicated to her primary provider that one of her chief concerns is that she will be hospitalized involuntarily, put in restraints, and administered antipsychotic medication against her will. She recalls that this occurred during one of her early hospitalizations, and she has remained so fearful that this will occur again that she has refrained from disclosing to her family when her mood or psychosis is getting worse.

On the basis of this disclosure, Serena's primary provider helped her create a mental health advance directive as well as a crisis plan. After Serena and her provider collaborated on this document, they invited her family to participate in sharing their observations of Serena's triggers, early warning signs, and treatment options. For Serena's self-identified family (two siblings and a close friend from childhood), the opportunity to engage with Serena and her providers was a lifeline. The team all agreed on the shared goal of preventing rehospitalization and forced treatment. Once these documents were established and talked through, with input from all stakeholders, Serena felt more comfortable having open and honest conversations with her treatment team and natural supports.

Motivational Interviewing

Motivational interviewing techniques are flexible strategies that can be used to resolve ambivalence among clinicians and patients who are contemplating family engagement. They can also be integrated into sessions that include family members to help them explore their own ambivalence related to changing their behaviors toward or around the patient (Belmontes 2018). Motivational interviewing can be particularly helpful in enhancing personal choice, clarifying values, and establishing personal goals among patients and their families. Interventions can then be framed in terms of shared values and goals, which enhances the likelihood that the family system will align in their pursuit of these goals.

Recovery-Oriented Psychoeducation

Psychosis is arguably one of the most misunderstood and stigmatized sets of mental health symptoms. Myths and misconceptions about psychosis and strongly held beliefs abound. One of the most common misconceptions is that psychotic and nonpsychotic beliefs are categorically different from each other. As was articulated in Chapter 1 ("Delusional Beliefs and the Madness of Crowds"), delusions lie along a continuum from "normal" to eccentric beliefs. Although many people think of delusions as fixed false beliefs, delusions are not considered to be categorically false (indeed, as illustrated elsewhere in this text, many beliefs that are classified as delusions contain a grain of truth) and do fluctuate over time. Psychoeducation on delusions is critical to addressing the stigma, avoidance, and maladaptive communication patterns that can emerge between well-intentioned natural supports and their loved ones who assert unusual or odd beliefs. Family members may alternate between confrontation (e.g., trying to convince the person that their belief is untrue), collusion (e.g., trying to align with the person by agreeing with the belief), and patronizing mollification (e.g., trying to distract the person every time they raise the concern or urging them to "think happy thoughts").

In addition, because delusions can be preoccupying for the individual and highly distressing to the family, interactions may revolve around the discussion of the delusions or their treatment (e.g., frequent checks on medication use). Recovery-oriented psychoeducation is critical to addressing these misconceptions and to reducing the overattention they are paid. Although it may seem counterintuitive to some clinicians, in particular those who have learned to see delusions and non-delusions as binary classifications, clinicians should engage in non-collusive normalizing of unusual beliefs. Normalization of unshared or bizarre beliefs is a key CBT technique that serves two main purposes: 1) it is the antidote to stigma, in that we as clinicians can begin to understand that these beliefs, although unusual, are not all that uncommon and are capable of being understood, and 2) it aids in the management of worry thoughts (e.g., "My son will wind up in the back ward of a mental hospital if he goes around saying these things"), which in turn can reduce anxiety and promote a more helpful dynamic between individuals and their natural supports. Clinicians can prepare family materials that include links to videos and reading materials that expose families to individuals with psychosis who can promote hope for meaningful recovery.

Assessment and Addressing of Natural Support Stress and Expressed Emotion

As noted earlier in this chapter, there is robust evidence that reducing caregiver stress and levels of expressed emotion—which includes expression of hostility, criticism, and emotional overinvolvement—can reduce the risk of relapse and hospitalization among individuals who have been hospitalized previously for a serious mental illness. Lebert (2018) proposed five pillars of caring for others who need support: self-care (defined as self-compassion and self-nurturing), communication and befriending, work-life balance, emotional neutrality, and hope. Clinicians can support the efforts of natural supports to engage in self-care by connecting families with family peer supports (individuals or organizations), providing referrals for their own individual or family therapy, and conveying the importance of caregiver self-nurturing and self-compassion in terms of modeling effective wellness strategies and engaging more effectively with their loved one. Research has demonstrated that family members who use a variety of strategies—including guided self-help—to manage their own well-being are able to reduce expressed emotion (Kopelovich et al. 2021). Engaging in discussion of pleasant or emotionally neutral topics can improve the relationship and decrease stress levels in the home. This point can be modeled in session, and clinicians can help teach family members how to engage in befriending sessions and how to substitute assumptions with benevolent, open-ended, nonjudgmental curious questions.

Cognitive-Behavioral Skills Coaching

Because families spend more time with their loved ones than the clinical team does, they are in the best position to support skill development and mastery. It can be helpful to teach a range of skills to the family and friends of those with strongly held beliefs. We focus on a set of skills that target communication, problem-solving, and coping strategies and were specifically designed for the natural supports of individuals with delusions and other psychotic and psychotic-like experiences. These skills were derived from the training Psychosis Recovery by Enabling Adult Carers at Home (Psychosis REACH; Kopelovich et al. 2021; Turkington et al. 2018). The skills are organized by the acronym FIRST: falling back on the relationship, inquiring curiously, reviewing the information and putting it together, skill development, and trying out the skill and getting feedback (Eisen et al. 2021).

FIRST Skills

Aptly named, the FIRST skills can be used *first* by families to help support their loved one experiencing delusions and other psychotic symptoms. Although the skills clearly build on one another (e.g., starting with shared goals typically helps with targeting skills teaching and practice), they can be applied nonlinearly as families become more adept at using them. Clinicians should emphasize that the FIRST skills cover core therapeutic techniques that are used by clinicians (e.g., fostering a strong therapeutic alliance, befriending, normalizing, adopting a Socratic style). However, in using these skills, family members are not serving as substitutes for clinical service delivery but rather are adopting and adapting these clinical skills to ensure that the home environment is conducive to recovery, to restore peace in the home, and to facilitate the translation of cognitive and behavioral skills to the individual's home environment.

F: Falling Back on the Relationship

The F skill focuses on helping families and natural supports take a step back to build from and/or improve their existing relationship with their loved one experiencing psychosis to enhance engagement and motivation. Clinicians can encourage families to start by *identifying their loved one's strengths* (e.g., families might ask "What do/did they enjoy doing? What are/were they good at? What do they value?") to look beyond current challenges.

Similarly, families should be encouraged to engage in *self-exploration of their own strengths* to see whether there is alignment with their loved one (e.g., "Is there something we both do well or enjoy doing together?") or to simply help them to leverage their own strengths as they begin applying the FIRST skills (e.g., "I'm actually a really good listener. That will help me when it comes to curious questioning").

Encouraging families to *identify shared goals* with their loved one can then help them to get beyond what are often hot button issues (e.g., medication nonadherence, substance use, unemployment) to work collaboratively with their loved one toward a shared vision. For example, the shared goal of greater independence can set the stage for identifying the steps toward independence, which may eventually include addressing hot button concerns such as medication nonadherence that have gotten in the way.

Last, clinicians should encourage families to apply many of the effective relationship-building practices described earlier, including *befriending* (e.g., "Tell me about your day"; "Remember that time...."), *normalizing* (e.g., "Actually, a lot of people tend to have the sense that others are out to get them. Research shows this is more common than we previously thought"; "It makes a lot of sense that you would feel that way about the police, given what happened the first time you were hospitalized"), and *expressing empathy* (e.g., "That sounds like an understandable response to feeling like someone is watching you"). Natural supports should also be coached in the liberal use of strategies such as *validation* and *praise* (e.g., "That sounds really scary. It sounds like you handled it as well as you could in the moment"), which set the stage for the other skills.

I: Inquiring Curiously

Many clinicians know the I skill as Socratic questioning, but using the term *curious questioning* can help families to better understand the importance of being genuinely curious about their loved one's experience, including the loved one's symptoms and challenges. Often families feel unsure about whether they should ask questions about their loved one's symptoms. It is helpful for clinicians to educate families that curious questioning not only is OK but is essential to both building the relationship and better understanding what is at the heart of the delusions. Clinicians should encourage families not to overthink their questions but to reflect on and *be genuine with their curiosity* (e.g., "You know, I didn't know how to ask before, but I've been thinking about your worry about the cars that keep driving by our house. Can you tell me a little bit more about who you think they are and what you're worried about?").

Curious questioning can help families to *drop assumptions* and strike a balance between challenging symptoms (e.g., "This is not true. This is not really happening") and colluding with their loved one about the symptoms (e.g., "You're right. Someone *is* out to get you") by *offering a midpoint of collaboration* (e.g., "So you are concerned that they're out to get you. Tell me more about what you're worried they'll do. Have you noticed whether there is something that makes you feel less distressed about the concern or makes it go away?"). If family members notice they are making assumptions about their loved one's experience, encourage them to back up and ask more about it (e.g., "I've always assumed you thought the cars driving by our house were just random people wanting to harm you, but the other day you mentioned something about a past coworker you also thought had it in for you. Can you tell me more about whether you see these two as linked?").

People who experience delusions often jump to conclusions and form strong beliefs without considering the evidence. Clinicians can encourage families to explore those conclusions sensitively with a series of questions that examine a broader range of evidence and clearer perspective on the situation (e.g., "What do you notice? What is your interpretation? What is this based on? Do you always think this or only in certain situations? How do you make sense of this experience? Can you remember the first time you came to this conclusion? What do you do to feel safe in the moment? Can you help me understand step by step what happens? Are there other possible explanations, no matter how unlikely they may seem?").

R: Reviewing the Information and Putting It Together

By working from a place of shared goals and understanding of their loved one's experiences, families can be in a better position to work collaboratively toward making sense of the experiences and addressing the loved one's needs through fostering targeted skills. To help them do this, clinicians can educate families on how to identify and link thoughts, feelings, and behaviors with their loved one. Firmly grounded in CBT, this step is called *developing a maintenance formulation* (see Figure 19–1). Encouraging families to examine these patterns together with their loved one sets the stage for collaborative planning for the next step of skill development. For example, when an individual with strongly held beliefs notices someone staring at them while at the bus stop (event) and interprets this as "They want to hurt me" (automatic thought) and "I'm not safe" (belief), the individual may feel worried or even frightened (feelings/emotions) and decide to miss the bus because of it (behavior). This formulation can help to examine bidirectional linkages, such as how avoidance of the bus and increased isolation at home (behaviors) result in increased anxiety and depression (emotions). Making these linkages can then help to identify the specific skills that can be used to reduce distress and support shared goals.

S: Skill Development

The S skill focuses on developing strategies and tools to support goal attainment and is based on a shared understanding of the problem, guided by the preceding step. In determining these strategies and tools, families should first assess their loved one's level of distress. If the loved one is in a heightened state of arousal, it is essential to focus first on regulating the distress, which will then facilitate the processing of new information and learning of new skills. Families should collaboratively *identify and implement effective coping strategies* to reduce the intensity of emotions (e.g., doing grounding exercises; practicing paced breathing; doing something enjoyable such as exercising, going for a walk, listening to music). Clinicians can coach families in the use of some or each of the skills listed here. These can be taught individually, in a live group (in person or virtual), or by posting online brief recorded skills coaching demonstrations that are made available to patients and their families.

- **Skills to enhance mental flexibility:** Families can now work with their loved one to generate multiple explanations for common events. In the earlier example of the bus stop, asking about other possible explanations for why someone was staring at them at the bus stop can help to expand the person's perspective on the situation. The goal is not to come to a firm conclusion about the "right" explanation. Rather, the idea is to generate as many alternative explanations as possible without concern for which ones are right or wrong. It may be helpful to start with a nonactivating event to help the loved one stay focused on learning rather than having to deal with the emotion it creates. The family can later shift to more personally relevant examples. Along the way, the clinician should encourage the family to reinforce the cognitive model within the formulation by posing hypothetical changes to the scenario and walking through how different reactions to the event affect the interplay among thoughts, feelings, and/or behaviors.

- **Collaborative empiricism:** One of the hallmarks of a CBT approach is to engage in collaborative empiricism with the patient. Clinicians will want to teach this approach to families as they move forward with skills teaching and development. A key step is *gathering the evidence* about the delusional belief. Families can ask their loved one, "How might we gather new evidence about what's going on? What should we consider credible sources? How do others handle these kinds of decisions?" For example, courts hear evidence and ask experts, and scientists form a hypothesis, design an experiment, and test the hypothesis. Next families can assess whether and to what extent their loved one is interested in exploring the belief. If the loved one is interested in exploring their interpretation of the situation, the family can collaboratively examine whether other explanations may be at play. They should then take in all available information, asking which data support the conclusion and which data do not, as well as considering any cognitive biases that might be influencing their interpretation. If their loved one is unwilling to explore the interpretation (e.g., "You never believe me. This is true"), the family can explore the underlying belief (e.g., "I am unsafe"), then collaboratively examine whether that belief is true in all situations, whether there are exceptions to the rule, and how they can create more experiences in which those exceptions stand true. Next they can *engage in a behavioral experiment and test it out*. The family can ask their loved one questions such as "How can we check this out? What would indicate if it was or was not occurring? What do you predict will happen? What did you observe? What did I observe? What might this mean?"

- **Activity scheduling:** The more active we are, the less time we have to focus on a persistent concern and the more we are engaged in a life worth living. Thus, families can help to ensure that daily routines are maintained. Within those routines, the loved one should be encouraged to engage in at least one activity each day that brings them joy and one activity that brings a sense of accomplishment, as well as activities that meet the function of the underlying belief (e.g., worth, connection, safety). Families should be encouraged to reinforce even the smallest of activities, which can also shape the loved one's behavior toward more complex or longer activities (e.g., "Wow, when you did the dishes today, it let me know you really care about our home"; "It was so nice spending time with you this weekend. I really value our time together"). This also serves to continue to build and strengthen the relationship and sense of shared goals.

- **Problem-solving skills:** Both natural supports and their loved ones who are struggling with preoccupying and distressing beliefs are confronted with a number of challenges that arise on a daily basis. As stress levels increase, the ability to identify the most pressing and actionable problems and the ability to take appropriate action are impaired. Co-learning and co-rehearsal of a stepwise approach to problem-solving are beneficial to both individuals with delusions and their support systems. The steps of problem-solving should be reviewed and rehearsed using personal examples from the natural supports. These steps include 1) learning how to define the problem, 2) identifying and evaluating potential solutions, 3) making an informed decision about the best possible response to the problem, 4) implementing the preferred solution, and 5) evaluating the results.

- **Coping strategies:** The following tools can be used with families to help their loved one cope with distressing beliefs. *Distraction techniques* may be the first place to start, given that they are likely the most accessible techniques and most typically used. These can include listening to music, practicing a hobby, exercising, or engaging in other activities that keep the loved one from perseverating on the distressing belief. *Metacognitive techniques* include mindfulness (observing and describing the thought without reacting to it), diffusion (gaining some distance from the thoughts, such as "I am having the thought that my phone is being tapped" rather than "My phone is being tapped"), and acceptance (recognizing that delusions are viewed as a part of everyday life and that people choose what power to give them). *Focusing* techniques include creating a rational response to the distressing belief (e.g., "I am safe in this moment") and using positive imagery to focus on affirming or relaxing thoughts (e.g., imagining oneself on a beach). The last coping strategy focuses on *addressing worry*. Clinicians should encourage families first to work with their loved one on jointly identifying that they are worried (rather than getting stuck in the validity of the worry thought), then to identify how much they are worrying as well as when and where the worry occurs. Families can then shift into discussing strategies such as worry postponement, which involves deliberately setting aside time each day for worry (e.g., 30 minutes at lunchtime), leaving the other 23.5 hours in the day to let go of the worry until it is "worry time."

T: Trying Out the Skill and Getting Feedback

Like the practice of any skill, it is critical to encourage families to work with their loved one to try out different skills and see how they are working. It is critical to reinforce with the loved one that not all skills will work equally well; the only way to figure out which skills are most effective for the person is to try them out. Assessing together what worked well, what did not work, and why or why not is a key part of the puzzle. For example, further collab-

orative assessment may reveal that the reason a skill did not work was because it was not fully implemented. The next steps here would be very
different from those in the case where the skill was fully implemented but
just did not help the situation. Initially practicing the skill outside the activating event can help build mastery so that it is easier to apply during times
of crisis. Typically, skills training includes 1) modeling and demonstrating
the skill, 2) practicing the skill, and 3) providing feedback. Although these
steps are typically conducted in this order, provision of feedback can also
be interspersed throughout the practicing of the skill, when conducted together. Clinicians can practice skills training with families, who can then
use that same model to help their loved ones with practicing skills.

Case Example: Inclusion of Family Caregivers— Core Therapeutic Interventions

Manuel was a 24-year-old second-generation Mexican American man who
resided with his parents and two younger sisters. Over the past 3 months, he
had become increasingly concerned that gas stations in his city were ripping
off people with disabilities by overcharging them for gas paid by credit card.
He repeatedly went to the police department to express his concerns and
complained to employees at several gas stations around town. Recently, these
encounters had escalated to the point where police were called to the scene,
culminating in an arrest and subsequent involuntary hospitalization. Manuel's concerns persisted after he was discharged to his parents' home 72 hours
later. In fact, he had now developed the concern that the gas stations were
part of a larger conspiracy involving all branches of the government. However, he was agreeable to following up on his outpatient appointment because he recognized that his tactics were not having the desired effect, and
he was open to receiving advice from a psychologist about "how to use mind
tricks on others to get them to do what I want."

Manuel's mother accompanied him to his initial appointment, during
which the therapist, Dr. Alvi, modeled the skills of building the relationship,
engaging in curious questioning, developing a shared understanding of the
problem ("I'm vulnerable; others are trying to take advantage of me"), and
rehearsing a concrete skill to help Manuel manage his own distress to more
effectively engage with others. With Manuel's permission, Dr. Alvi set aside
time to meet via telehealth with both parents and Manuel's sisters to provide
psychoeducation, counsel them on self-care, and coach them in the FIRST
skills. Dr. Alvi inquired about government mistrust among other members
of the family in an effort to normalize concerns about financial exploitation.
Manuel's parents reported that institutional mistrust was quite common in
their hometown, and they had often made comments to that effect. They
found it comforting to learn from Dr. Alvi that such concerns were quite
common and that there were strategies to help "check out the facts" that
they could implement alongside Manuel.

Over the course of the next 4 months, Manuel's parents made a consistent effort to engage in befriending sessions (sharing mutual concerns about

being taken advantage of financially), engage in curious questioning (asking about other possible reasons this discrepancy in gasoline prices might be occurring), and finally test out some solutions (going to the gas pumps to actually measure how much gas was purchased by a credit card vs. cash). Once they tested the solution it became apparent that the amounts of gas were equal. Manuel's sisters started spending more time with Manuel cooking together and going through old family photo albums. Although Manuel's concerns resurfaced from time to time, he experienced far less preoccupation and sense of urgency. He decided that he wanted to focus on further developing his cooking skills by attending a culinary program.

Discussion

The inclusion of natural supports in the care of individuals with psychosis is a worthy topic because families have been poorly integrated into routine care practices for individuals with serious mental illness despite the inclusion of family interventions for psychosis in national practice guidelines. Natural supports are key to counteracting the profound isolation that is common when individuals hold beliefs that are misaligned with those of their social groups. The research affirms that family interventions for psychosis can enhance the health of the individual with delusions and the family system. Clinicians must work collaboratively with their administrators, patients, and patients' families to identify the barriers to these interventions. At a minimum, clinicians should provide digestible, factual information about psychosis to defuseconfusion, stigma, and self-blame. Clinicians can address common myths and misconceptions about psychosis and share statistics and first-person accounts that normalize unusual and strongly held beliefs. When normalizing psychoeducation and information about self-care strategies are provided in universally accessible modalities (e.g., on the clinic's web page or in print brochures), then access to this information is not dependent on patient authorization. Clinicians can engage in motivational enhancement strategies and discuss what is meant by *family-involved shared decision-making* with patients who are reticent about permitting the clinical team to engage their natural supports. Finally, the FIRST skills provide a helpful framework for guiding natural supports in concrete, evidence-based strategies to restore the relationship, improve the dynamic in the home, and address distress or impairment related to a host of stressors.

Questions for Discussion

1. Consider the barriers to administering family interventions that were reviewed in this chapter. What barriers have you experienced in your role? What do you need to overcome these obstacles?

2. Create a SMART (specific, measurable, actionable, realistic, and timely) goal for incorporating family into treatment services.

3. After familiarizing yourself with the FIRST skills, make a plan to rehearse teaching these skills to families. Solicit feedback from a colleague, a supervisor, or the families with whom you work.

KEY POINTS

- Family involvement in care is correlated with better mental and physical health and quality of life for those experiencing delusions and other symptoms of psychosis. Outcomes for those with family support include higher rates of treatment engagement, reduced rates of relapse and rehospitalization, and higher rates of employment.

- Despite the fact that the majority of adults with chronic delusions and other symptoms of psychosis live with a family member and familial involvement is requested, family members are not routinely engaged in care.

- Family psychoeducation with a normalizing approach to understanding a loved one's delusions should always be provided.

- An emphasis on training family members in self-care and skill-building in the domains of communication, problem-solving, and coping strategies can further enhance the recovery trajectory.

References

Belmontes KC: When family gets in the way of recovery: motivational interviewing with families. Fam J 26(1):99–104, 2018

Canavan J: The role of the family in schizophrenia. Trinity Student Medical Journal 1(1):31–39, 2000

Clark RE: Family support and substance use outcomes for persons with mental illness and substance use disorders. Schizophr Bull 27(1):93–101, 2001 11215552

Eisen K, Kharrazi N, Simonson A, et al: Training inpatient psychiatric nurses and staff to utilize CBTp informed skills in an acute inpatient psychiatric setting. Psychosis 14(1):70–80, 2021

Interdepartmental Serious Mental Illness Coordinating Committee: The Way Forward: Federal Action for a System That Works for All People Living with SMI and SED and their Families and Caregivers (Publ No PEP17-ISMICC-RTC). Rockville, MD, Substance Abuse and Mental Health Services Administration, 2017

Keepers GA, Fochtmann LJ, Anzia JM, et al: The American Psychiatric Association Practice Guideline for the Treatment of Patients With Schizophrenia. Am J Psychiatry 177(9):868–872, 2020 32867516

Kopelovich S, Stiles B, Monroe-DeVita M, et al: Psychosis REACH: effects of a brief CBT-informed training for family and caregivers of individuals with psychosis. Psychiatr Serv 72(11):1254–1260 2021 34015942

Lebert L: The five pillars of caring for psychosis, in Back to Life, Back to Normality, Vol 2: CBT Informed Recovery for Families With Relatives with Schizophrenia and Other Psychoses. Edited by Turkington D, Spencer HM. Cambridge, UK, Cambridge University Press, 2018, pp 41–50

McDonagh MS, Dana T, Selph S, et al: Treatments for Schizophrenia in Adults: A Systematic Review (AHRQ Publ No 17[18]-EHC031-EF). Rockville, MD, Agency for Healthcare Research and Quality, 2017

Smith J, Birchwood M: Relatives and patients as partners in the management of schizophrenia: the development of a service model. Br J Psychiatry 156(5):654–660, 1990 2095942

Turkington D, Gega L, Lebert L, et al: A training model for relatives and friends in cognitive behaviour therapy (CBT) informed care for psychosis. Cogent Psychol 5(1):1497749, 2018

20

Decoding Delusions

Demonstration of Key Skills for Working With Unusual Beliefs

Douglas Turkington, M.D.
Kate V. Hardy, Clin.Psych.D.
Latoyah Lebert, M.Phil.
Sarah Robinson, B.Sc.

In this book, chapter authors have highlighted a number of key skills that are helpful for working with patients with delusions and other strongly held beliefs. The chapter authors provide clinical case examples to emphasize how to implement these skills in a clinical setting. In this chapter we provide descriptions of and links to filmed video vignettes that demonstrate key skills in action across the four main areas of intervention: 1) befriending, 2) developing a formulation, 3) delivering change strategies, and 4) maintaining change. Although all roles in the filmed vignettes are played by actors (typically therapists and research assistants), they emulate real-life clinical scenarios while preserving the confidentiality of clinical encounters. We recognize that although

The authors of this chapter would like to thank Dr. Alison Brabban, Dr. Rob Dudley, Ms. Helen Spencer, and Dr. Thomas Christodoulides.

clinical role-plays are an important element in clinician training, there is an artificiality inherent in acted-out interactions. In order to ensure that the skills are demonstrated in short and accessible clips, the encounters are brief and very focused. It is likely that the skills demonstrated in the clips might take longer to employ in a live clinical encounter. We have endeavored to ensure that each patient is represented in a manner that demonstrates key areas of focus in therapy, but we recognize that an acted role does not fully capture the individual lived experience of psychosis.

The video demonstrations can be accessed at www.appi.org/Hardy.

Befriending, Normalizing, and Questioning

Befriending

As described in Chapter 7 ("Collaboration, Not Collusion"), befriending is fundamentally an approach that can reduce distress linked to delusions by fostering the development of a respectful and unchallenging interpersonal relationship. When befriending the patient, the clinician does not attempt to question or test the content of the delusion but instead falls back on areas of personal strength, humor, pleasant memories, and positive emotions. Exploring and addressing strongly held beliefs in cognitive-behavioral therapy (CBT) can only be done when the patient perceives evidence of a trusting therapeutic relationship. Although befriending is a core component of CBT for psychosis, it is also an approach used across different therapies and may also be offered as a stand-alone treatment. Video 1 demonstrates a brief befriending example between a nurse and an individual on an acute inpatient unit. Rather than trying to convince the patient to go to a group session, the nurse identifies a shared interest with them and uses this to start to form a relationship. This results in increased engagement and interest from the individual, allowing for exploration of the barriers to group attendance and buy-in to spending some time exploring some options to help them meet their goal of being discharged from the unit.

 Video 1: Befriending

Normalizing

Normalizing is discussed in Chapter 7 and is presented as a core element in supporting patients toward a better understanding of their experiences. Termed "an antidote to catastrophization" by Kingdon and Turkington

(2005, p. 94), this approach allows exploration of the prevalence of experiences consistent with psychosis as well as enables the clinician to emphasize these experiences in the context of an understandable reaction to extreme situations. In Video 2, Toyah opens by discussing her belief that she is being bullied at work by her line manager. She is saddened, anxious, and angry and is having trouble sleeping because the bullying is always on her mind. Dr. T empathizes with this experience and normalizes Toyah's distress as understandable in the context of the difficulties she is experiencing. He shows her that it is normal to begin to take things personally, such as the wearing of a red dress or a curt email ending, when under stress in the workplace. This is a useful strategy to support joining with Toyah and provides a nice entry to beginning to engage in peripheral questioning with Toyah around her experience with her line manager.

 Video 2: Normalizing

Demonstration of Collusion as an Approach to Avoid

Establishing a strong therapeutic relationship allows the clinician to begin to explore and show curiosity regarding the strongly held beliefs of the patient. A frequent concern of novice therapists working with psychosis is the challenge of sitting on the collaborative fence and neither colluding with nor confronting the patient. As Video 3 shows, collusion can be highly problematic. Although the clinician may engage in collusion with the hope of strengthening (or repairing) a relationship, it is rarely beneficial in the long term. Video 3 highlights this. Dr. T (a psychiatrist) is interviewing Pamela, who has been newly admitted to the ward under the U.K. Mental Health Act, which allows involuntary hospitalization if a person is deemed to be at risk of harm to themselves or to others. Pamela believes that numerous different species of aliens have been chasing her with a view to abducting her and stealing her organs. Pamela is not willing to talk about any other subject, and to settle her down and reduce her anxiety, Dr. T discloses his own beliefs that there have probably been gray aliens visiting the Earth since the 1947 Roswell incident and that numerous different species probably do exist but assures her that the ward is totally safe from aliens. Dr. T states that the nurses are trained to deal with any hostile aliens, including any aliens that might get past security, so Pamela is totally safe and can relax. Initially, this collusive approach does seem to reduce Pamela's anxiety, but she becomes increasingly agitated about what she has heard from Dr. T and asks how the aliens will be controlled because they use telepathy that will immobilize the nurses. Pamela tells Dr. T that he knows nothing about these hostile aliens who have hands that come out of their eyes. Pamela's speech becomes increasingly bizarre and hard to follow, and both her conviction in her delusion and her level of distress seem to increase.

Video 3: Collusion as an Approach to Avoid

Demonstration of Confrontation as an Approach to Avoid

At the other end of the spectrum from collusion is confrontation, and it should go without saying that confrontation rarely results in strengthened therapeutic rapport. In fact, it is not uncommon for collusion and confrontation to go hand in hand if the clinician has not committed to working on the relationship and is struggling to demonstrate genuine curiosity about the individual's experience. Video 4 shows an example of the therapist being pulled into a confrontation with a patient who holds strong beliefs that he is John the Baptist. The patient has a grandiose delusion that he is acting on by burning pornography and attempting to preach in churches. He has no interest in therapy and invites the therapist to join his anti-pornography team. Although the therapist is highly skilled and attempts to engage the patient and make genuine progress in therapy, the patient appears to take almost everything the therapist says as a confrontation. Ultimately, the only course of action for the therapist is to terminate the session because there is no further opportunity for collaborative exploration of the belief.

Video 4: Confrontation as an Approach to Avoid

Collaborative Exploration

Video 5 provides a beautiful insight into the collaborative exploration of a belief. Here the therapist is demonstrating genuine curiosity about the experience of the individual. She is nonjudgmental in her questioning, checks with the patient that she has permission to engage in further questioning, provides summaries of what she has heard the patient say, and gives opportunities for the patient to correct these summaries, yet there is no sense that the therapist is colluding in the belief. Ultimately, this collaborative exploration sets the scene for the patient and therapist to create a jointly developed plan to further understand the patient's experience. The collaborative fence serves as a place from which curious questioning can occur, which is demonstrated in Video 5. Other questioning techniques can be used to enhance exploration of the belief using guided and shared discovery.

Video 5: Sitting on the Collaborative Fence

Downward Arrow

In Video 6, Dr. B uses the downward arrow technique with Cheryl, who is presenting with a belief that she is being held back in life by forces unknown to her. Dr. B prefaces this exercise with an explanation of the downward arrow technique so that Cheryl understands why she is continuing to pursue a specific line of inquiry. This technique results in the discovery that Cheryl holds a core belief of "I am a failure." Using an inference-chaining questioning style, it is often possible for the clinician to find the seed at the heart of the delusion, and often affect is expressed when this happens. In this case the affect is sadness.

Video 6: Downward Arrow

Socratic Questioning

Another frequently used questioning technique is Socratic questioning. In Video 7, peripheral questions are intermingled with more probing questions that begin to introduce doubt and allow alternative explanations to be considered. As can be seen, Socratic questions can lead to the identification of holes in the belief, and in this case Cheryl responds with some confusion and an indication that she is trying to understand this further. Clinicians should be careful to ensure they are eliciting feedback frequently from the patient to determine how the questioning is being received.

Video 7: Socratic Questioning

Developing a Formulation
Construction of a Morrison Formulation

Each of the clinical chapters highlights the core role that formulation plays in cocreating meaning and understanding the role of strongly held beliefs. Formulation is the means by which therapist and patient create meaning out of experiences and identify specific areas for intervention. In Video 8, the therapist and patient are working together to support a shared understanding of the patient's delusion and its impact on his day-to-day life. In this clip, the patient is too paranoid to travel on the bus and activates numerous safety behaviors. The therapist and patient construct a Morrison formulation together, and as a result of the use of guided discovery, it becomes apparent how to proceed in a homework exercise.

 Video 8: Formulation

Timeline Review

Another approach to developing a formulation is to examine past experiences and better understand how they connect with current symptoms. The timeline review is essential when working with trauma (as described in Chapter 16, "Trauma and Delusions") and can be particularly helpful when working with systematized delusions (as shown in Chapter 12, "A Bizarre and Grandiose Delusion"). In Video 9, we return to the scenario of the therapist working with the patient who believes he is John the Baptist. Exploration of the timeline highlights that at the time the patient developed beliefs about being John the Baptist, he was experiencing several significant stressors, including the breakdown of his relationship and the failure of his business. Inductive questioning supports further understanding that the patient made links between seeing an advertisement for pornography and an illuminated cross, which was connected with a strong energized feeling. It is likely that further exploration over time would reveal the relevance of the religious elements of these beliefs, although it is apparent in the video that the patient is not ready to engage in that level of exploration. See Turkington et al. (2015) for a detailed case presentation.

 Video 9: Timeline Review

Developing Change Strategies

Behavioral Experiment

As mentioned in the previous section, the formulation serves a dual purpose. It allows for enhanced understanding of the patient's experience, and it also highlights where interventions should be targeted to support the patient in moving toward their goals. Several chapters provide examples of behavioral experiments to explore the accuracy and helpfulness of a belief. In Video 10, we return to the patient who believes that people can hear his thoughts. Following careful exploration of this belief, the therapist asks the patient how they could test it. Through the use of Socratic questioning, the therapist supports the patient in coming up with a behavioral experiment to test whether people can hear his thoughts. Importantly, in this process we see the therapist explore possible outcomes, including preparing for the possibility that they may find evidence that people can indeed hear the patient's thoughts. This is an important element of the development of a behavioral experiment because it demonstrates that the therapist has bought in to the experiment and is prepared to accept all potential outcomes as possibilities. This is in contrast to an experiment designed to prove the patient wrong. Experiments set up in that manner are likely to be less successful and may potentially harm the therapeutic relationship. The patient is helped to begin to drop unhelpful safety behaviors to allow the experiment to proceed.

 Video 10: Behavioral Experiment

Coping Skills

In Video 11, Dr. L demonstrates a brief CBT session with Miguel, who believes that a hitman is hiding somewhere in his neighborhood and is going to attempt to shoot him. Miguel states that a red sighter dot from a sniper's rifle went along the top of his bedroom wall. He was terrified and refused to go near the windows or doors. He hid away in safe areas of his apartment. He coped by repeatedly saying three prayers for protection every time he moved to a different room and by shouting out three times every hour telling the hitman to go away. A discussion about the helpfulness of his strategies ensues, and Miguel seems interested in thinking about some other strategies. Dr. L gives Miguel a list of 60 coping strategies and explains them to him. Miguel suggests his own strategy: salsa dancing (he says that he was a very good dancer in the past), which he can do in a safe area of the house.

Video 11: Coping

Schema Intervention

Another intervention that can be used is addressing underlying core schemata. Using inference chaining or when exploring the timeline, it is sometimes possible for the clinician to discover an Achilles' heel—a belief linked to the delusion. The Brief Core Schema Scales (Fowler et al. 2006) can also be used to detect a linked schema. It is then possible to work at the schema level, and this often will help reduce the distress linked to the delusion. In Video 12, Dr. B returns to the belief "I am a failure" with Cheryl. She explores the accuracy of this belief using the continuum approach to work at the schema level that underlies the systematized delusion that a sinister organization is always preventing Cheryl from succeeding.

 Video 12: Schema Intervention

Role-Play

Chapter 13 ("Who Are You?") includes discussion of a Capgras delusion and formulation and a related intervention. Video 13 demonstrates an intervention approach to this presentation. In this video, Robert lives in the same house as his mother and has the delusion that she has been replaced by someone who looks similar. He refers to his mother as "her upstairs." Progress in therapy comes while Robert and the therapist are creating a timeline; he remembers the time when he saw a *Crimewatch* program in which the clothing of a murdered woman was shown, and in a state of delusional mood he recognized it as his mother's nightdress. From this timeline further information is elicited, and the therapist suggests a role-play of an important memory to see whether there might be any other explanations that can be considered. Robert's conviction in the Capgras delusion decreases to some degree, and he becomes less distressed by it.

 Video 13: Capgras Delusion

Metacognitive Techniques

Video 14 demonstrates the use of metacognitive techniques to reduce worry linked to a persecutory delusion. Worry and rumination are frequently found to be ineffective and exhausting safety behaviors linked to delusions. In this video, the worry and rumination, rather than the delusion itself, are targeted, with a discussion of the pros and cons of worry and the identification of an alternative activity (listening to music) to engage in rather than worrying.

Video 14: Metacognitive Techniques

Maintaining Change

The final stage in working with strongly held beliefs should focus on functioning and wellness planning. This allows the patient and therapist to review gains and create a plan for maintaining them while also being prepared for future challenges. As demonstrated in Video 2, Toyah had a delusional belief of being persecuted by her line manager, Janet. She had delusions of reference and marked anxiety. She was struggling to keep up the quality of her work and had insomnia and severe rumination about the persecution. Early sessions were difficult, with Toyah maintaining a high level of conviction in the belief. The final session, shown in Video 15, focuses on the progress Toyah has made and reviews effective coping skills she has learned. In addition, a wellness plan is developed, and it is agreed that rising anxiety and insomnia are signs that Toyah should initiate the regular use of coping strategies and further exploration of any tension at work with Janet. Verbal information is written up on an action card, which Toyah keeps in her purse.

Video 15: Maintaining Change

Conclusion

The techniques and skills described in this book are just a few of the myriad strategies clinicians can use to support an individual with delusions or strongly held beliefs. A handful of these are presented as live examples, with an emphasis on working from a collaborative and recovery-oriented stance.

References

Fowler D, Freeman D, Smith B, et al: The Brief Core Schema Scales (BCSS): psychometric properties and associations with paranoia and grandiosity in non-clinical and
psychosis samples. Psychol Med 36(6):749–759, 2006 16563204

Kingdon D, Turkington D: Cognitive Therapy of Schizophrenia. New York, Guilford, 2005

Turkington D, Spencer H, Jassal I, Cummings A: Cognitive behavioural therapy for
the treatment of delusional systems. Psychosis 7(1):48–59, 2015

Index

Page numbers printed in **boldface** type refer to figures and tables.